OUR
VETERANS

OUR VETERANS

Winners, Losers, Friends, and Enemies on the New Terrain of Veterans Affairs

SUZANNE GORDON, STEVE EARLY,

AND JASPER CRAVEN

DUKE UNIVERSITY PRESS *Durham and London*   2022

© 2022 DUKE UNIVERSITY PRESS
All rights reserved
Printed in the United States of America on acid-free paper ∞
Typeset in Minion Pro and Trade Gothic
by Westchester Publishing Services

Library of Congress Cataloging-in-Publication Data
Names: Gordon, Suzanne, [date] author. | Early, Steve, author. |
Craven, Jasper, [date] author.
Title: Our veterans : winners, losers, friends, and enemies on the new
terrain of veterans affairs / Suzanne Gordon, Steve Early, and Jasper Craven
Description: Durham : Duke University Press, 2022.
Includes bibliographical references and index.
Identifiers: LCCN 2021047747 (print)
LCCN 2021047748 (ebook)
ISBN 9781478015901 (hardcover)
ISBN 9781478018544 (paperback)
ISBN 9781478023142 (ebook)
Subjects: LCSH: Veterans—United States. | Veteran reintegration—United
States. | Veterans—Services for—United States. | Veterans—United States—
Social conditions. | Veterans—Medical care—United States. | Veterans—
Mental health—United States. | BISAC: MEDICAL / Health Policy |
SOCIAL SCIENCE / Disease & Health Issues
Classification: LLC UB357 .G673 2022 (print) | LLC UB357 (ebook)
DDC 362.860973—dc23/eng/20211220
LC record available at https://lccn.loc.gov/2021047747
LC ebook record available at https://lccn.loc.gov/2021047748

Cover art: Veterans Day parade held on New York's 5th Avenue.
Spencer Platt / Getty Images.

This book is dedicated to the unsung heroes and heroines of the veterans' healthcare system.

CONTENTS

ABBREVIATIONS

ACA	Affordable Care Act
ADA	Americans with Disabilities Act
AFGE	American Federation of Government Employees
AIR	Asset and Infrastructure Review
AMVETS	American Veterans organization
APWU	American Postal Workers Union
AVC	American Veterans Committee
BLM	Black Lives Matter
CARES Act	Coronavirus Aid, Relief, and Economic Security Act
CCN	Community Care Network
CDC	Centers for Disease Control and Prevention
CFPB	Consumer Financial Protection Bureau
CIA	Central Intelligence Agency
CNAS	Center for a New American Security
COVID	Coronavirus Disease
CVA	Concerned Veterans for America
CVN	Cohen Veterans Network
CWA	Communications Workers of America
DAV	Disabled American Veterans

DCCC	Democratic Congressional Campaign Committee
DCO	direct commission officer
DEA	Drug Enforcement Administration
DNC	Democratic National Committee
DOD	Department of Defense
DOJ	Department of Justice
DSCC	Democratic Senatorial Campaign Committee
EMN	Eisenhower Media Network
EPA	Environmental Protection Agency
FBI	Federal Bureau of Investigation
FDA	Food and Drug Administration
FEC	Federal Election Commission
FEMA	Federal Emergency Management Administration
FY	fiscal year
GAO	Government Accountability Office
GOTV	Get Out the Vote
GWOT	Global War on Terror
IAVA	Iraq and Afghanistan Veterans of America
IED	improvised explosive device
IG	Inspector General
IPV	intimate partner violence
IVAW	Iraq Veterans Against the War
MFSO	Military Families Speak Out
MHS	Military Health System
MST	military sexual trauma
NATO	North Atlantic Treaty Organization
NDAA	National Defense Authorization Act
NIH	National Institutes of Health
NLRB	National Labor Relations Board
NNU	National Nurses United
NVLSP	National Veterans Legal Services Program

OSHA	Occupational Safety and Health Administration
P.L.	public law
PAC	political action committee
PDAT	Post Deployment Assessment Treatment
POGO	Project on Government Oversight
PPE	personal protective equipment
PTSD	posttraumatic stress disorder
PVA	Paralyzed Veterans of America
ROTC	Reserve Officers' Training Corps
SNAP	Supplemental Nutrition Assistance Program
SWAN	Service Women's Action Network
TBI	traumatic brain injury
TIF	The Independence Fund
USA	United Spinal Association
VA	Department of Veterans Affairs
VBA	Veterans Benefits Administration
VFP	Veterans for Peace
VFW	Veterans of Foreign Wars
VHA	Veterans Health Administration
VOI	Veterans Organizing Institute
VOW	Veterans Opportunity to Work
VSO	veterans' service organization
VVA	Vietnam Veterans of America
VVAW	Vietnam Veterans Against the War
WIC	Special Supplemental Nutrition Program for Women, Infants, and Children
WWP	Wounded Warrior Project

PREFACE

The coauthors of this book believe that readers are owed some explanation for how and why we came to write a book about veterans, without ever having served in the military ourselves. In a 2017 book about his first campaign for the presidency, a Sixties antiwar activist named Bernie Sanders described his engagement with veterans affairs in a way that reflects our own perspective:

> Some may see it as incongruous for a strong progressive to be a fierce advocate for veterans rights. I don't, and never have. I will continue to do everything I can to make sure that the United States does not get entangled in wars that we should not be fighting. But I will never blame the men and women who do the fighting for getting us into those wars. If you don't like the wars we get involved in, hold the president and Congress responsible. Don't blame the veterans.[1]

Like Sanders, Suzanne Gordon was very involved, as a college student, in protests against the Vietnam War. After becoming a journalist, she covered the GI Coffeehouse movement and related expressions of antiwar sentiment by active-duty military personnel in the early 1970s. Over the years, her free-lance work has appeared in the *New York Times*, the *Boston Globe*, the *Los Angeles Times*, the *Washington Post*, *Washington Monthly*, the *Atlantic*, the *Nation*, the *Hill*, *Mother Jones*, *Jacobin*, *American Prospect*, the *Village Voice*, the *Toronto Globe and Mail*, and many other publications. She has also been a past commentator for CBS Radio and American Public Media's *Marketplace*.

In the 1980s, Suzanne helped trade unionists in the United States and Europe—some of whom were veterans—promote "economic conversion." Working with them, she organized an international conference on this subject and coedited *Economic Conversion: Revitalizing America's Economy* (1984). This book critiqued the cost and wastefulness of global military spending. Its cross-border contributors showed how factories engaged in arms manufacturing could be converted to the production of socially useful goods and services.

Over the last thirty years, Suzanne has been an advocate for a publicly funded national healthcare system in the United States. As coeditor of a Cornell University Press book series on the culture and politics of healthcare work, she has published studies of her own and by other authors that deal with patient safety, hospital funding and administration, home care and long-term care, nursing and medical education, and health systems in other industrialized countries.

In books like *Life Support, Nursing against the Odds*, and *Safety in Numbers*, Suzanne has written extensively about the invisible work of nurses—members of our largest healthcare profession. In her research, writing, and public speaking before tens of thousands of RNs and allied professionals, she has long stressed the importance of caregivers speaking up on behalf of patients and their families. And she has described how private hospital administrators and managers, including some "nurse leaders," have used their organizational influence to thwart much-needed workplace improvements and systemic change.

Suzanne's exploration of our veterans' healthcare system began with a series of "team-building" workshops that she conducted for staff at the Department of Veterans Affairs (VA) Medical Center in Palo Alto, California. Since then, she has published two books about the VA—*The Battle for Veterans' Healthcare: Dispatches from the Frontlines of Policy Making and Patient Care* (2017) and *Wounds of War: How the VA Delivers Health, Healing, and Hope to the Nation's Veterans* (2018). In 2017, Suzanne also coauthored a report for the American Legion titled "VA Healthcare: A System Worth Saving," and helped found the Veterans Healthcare Policy Institute (VHPI) to provide ongoing analyses of VA-related developments. In 2019, she wrote a nationally distributed guide for Rotary Clubs about how they can better partner with the VA on local programs to support veterans. Suzanne is a frequent speaker before audiences of veterans and VA staff members, healthcare union members, and healthcare reformers around the country.

Jasper Craven first started writing about veterans' issues while working as a stringer for two Vermont newspapers. He was assigned to cover the Senate

Veterans Affairs Committee, then chaired by Senator Bernie Sanders, and Sanders's subsequent campaign for the presidency in 2016. Over the past six years, Jasper has published investigative reports on the problems of military personnel and veterans in a wide range of publications, including the *New York Times*, the *Nation*, *Politico*, *Washington Monthly*, *American Prospect*, the *Intercept*, *Task and Purpose*, *Vice*, *Reveal*, and many others. In 2020, he launched *Battle Borne*, a weekly online newsletter, which provides investigative reporting and commentary on veterans' issues and the military.

In his freelance work, Jasper has chronicled leadership misconduct and workplace harassment within the National Guard, local controversy over the deployment of F-35 fighter bombers, Capitol Hill lobbying involving the VA, White House attacks on VA employees (and misconduct by some VA police officers), the declining political clout of veterans' service organizations, and the courting of military voters by both major political parties. As a fellow at the Veterans Healthcare Policy Institute, Jasper collaborated with Suzanne on a widely distributed *Congressional and Reporters' Guide to Veterans' Healthcare*, plus other VHPI reports on VA staffing issues, mental health care, and mainstream media coverage of the VA.

Steve Early is the author of four previous books about labor or politics. Although the beneficiary of a draft deferment at the time, he enrolled in the Reserve Officers' Training Corps (ROTC) at Middlebury College in 1967. His one-semester experience as an ROTC cadet made him a staunch advocate of removing ROTC from campus, abolishing the draft, and ending the Vietnam War, in whatever order any of those goals could be achieved, locally or nationally. In May 1970, he was a local organizer of the national student antiwar strike that involved more than 4 million college and high school students. This formative experience demonstrated the power and potential of collective action for political or workplace change and, in his case, helped inspire fifty years of labor-related activism.

While attending law school in the 1970s, Steve worked with union members—some of them recently returned Vietnam veterans—in a high-risk industry (coal mining). In that and other labor organization roles, he assisted campaigns for workers' rights, safer and healthier workplaces, and affordable healthcare. Because of his long experience in difficult contract negotiations and strikes over job-based medical benefits, he is a strong supporter of Medicare for All.

As someone with a union background, Steve was drawn to the subject matter of this book because of the overlap between labor and veterans' issues in three areas. They include military service as a form of work (albeit nonunion), the occupational health and safety hazards faced by military personnel, and how their later need for medical care and disability benefits is addressed through a national system of "workers' compensation" (aka the VA) which is, in many ways, superior to state programs for injured private-sector workers.

Steve has also been struck by the parallel erosion of veteran organization influence and infrastructure, nationally and locally, and labor union decline in the United States. As documented in this book, both trends have had adverse consequences for an overlapping working-class constituency. One upside has been the emergence of newer groups advocating for younger veterans or nonunion workers. While some of these new formations are more promisingly "progressive" in their politics, they also tend to be less membership based, self-financed, or democratically run.

We have collaborated on *Our Veterans* not just because of our shared interest in the issues explored herein but also to amplify the voices of veterans we've met whose commitment to helping each other *and* their fellow citizens is a true public service. As readers will discover, the heroes and heroines of this book tend to be independent thinkers, critics of the status quo, and catalysts for new forms of advocacy. But among them, readers will also meet men and women, equally committed and courageous. They've tried to work within the structures of existing public institutions or nongovernmental organizations to achieve many of the same goals—whether better healthcare for veterans, a smoother transition from their military service to civilian life, or reduced use of military force, because of its profound and lasting impact on millions of people in the United States and abroad.

AUTHORS' NOTE AND ACKNOWLEDGMENTS

To write this book, we personally conducted many interviews with veterans and others involved in the field of veterans affairs. When quotes appear around interview material and are not followed by a citation, these are from original interviews. We also drew on the interviewing work of other authors, journalists, videographers, and hosts of podcasts, cable TV, and radio shows, particularly in cases where our own requests for interviews with public figures quoted in this book were denied.[2] In some cases, at the request of a particular interview subject, we have concealed his or her identity via the use of a fictitious name, which is identified as such by an asterisk next to it.

This book would not have been possible without the help of many friends, colleagues, and valuable sources acknowledged below—and a few who wish to remain anonymous. Some will be thanked more than once, in their different capacities. All three of us would like to recognize everyone connected with the Veterans Healthcare Policy Institute (VHPI). We thank Russell Lemle for his consistent support and insight into veteran suicide and many other mental health issues. Paul Cox and Lou Kern have shared their varied experiences as Vietnam veterans and advocates for veterans' causes. Paul Sullivan, national vice-chair of Veterans for Common Sense, has generously shared his expertise about VA benefits, burn pit exposure, and many other issues.

We also want to recognize VHPI's first executive director, Brett Copeland, and Justin Straughn, who joined the staff later. Since VHPI was founded, its steering committee has included—in addition to Lemle, Cox, Kern, and Sullivan—Ian Hoffmann, Bridget Lattanzi, Essam Attia, and Joan Zweben. On the VHPI advisory board, we are indebted to Andrew Pomerantz, Joe Ruzek, Dorothy Salmon, Kenneth Watterson, Jay Youngdahl, H. Westley Clark, Larry Cohen, Charlene Harrington, Mark Jwayad, Charlynn Johns, Phil Longman, and Eddie Machtinger. For more information on VHPI's work, see https://www.veteranspolicy.org.

At the Department of Veterans Affairs, a long and distinguished list of current and former employees has assisted our research and writing. Among those who've served in VA headquarters in Washington, DC, are Ken Kizer, Robert McDonald, David Shulkin, Rajiv Jain, Maureen McCarthy, Kayla Williams, Stephen Trynosky, and Terrence Hayes. We also want to thank the following past or present staff members at VA medical centers and clinics around the country: Rebecca Shunk, Russell Lemle, Andy Pomerantz, Jason Kelley, Jeff Kixmiller, Dirk Woods, Tom Kirchberg, Harold Kudler, Bonnie Graham, Judi Cheary, Linda Ward Smith, Ralph Ibsen, Lana Zera, Donald Kollisch, Joe Ruzek, Will Martin, Tom Horvath, and Jessica Early. There are too many other VA caregivers to thank by name, but this book is dedicated to you.

In veterans' advocacy organizations, we are indebted to dozens of people who took time out from their busy schedules to answer questions, clarify issues, and put us in touch with other helpful contacts. Foremost among them are stalwart advocates for their fellow female veterans—Tammy Barlet, Veterans of Foreign Wars; Maureen Elias, Paralyzed Veterans of America; Joy Ilem, Peter Dickinson, and Adrian Atizado, Disabled American Veterans; and Katie Purswell, American Legion. Rick Weidman, now retired from Vietnam Veterans of America (VVA), and Kris Goldsmith, founder of High Ground Veterans Advocacy and former VVA staffer, both displayed endless patience with our queries. Steve Robertson, former national legislative director for the American Legion, helped us better understand the Legion's past work in Congress and the handling of veterans affairs on Capitol Hill.

At the San Francisco–based Swords to Plowshares, many thanks to Michael Blecker, Bradford Adams, Maureen Sieder, and Kate Richardson. At Veterans for Peace, the "Save Our VA" (SOVA) campaign has relied on an exemplary network of volunteers. Special thanks, for those efforts and for book-related help in many forms, go to Paul Cox, Susan Schnall, Jeff Roy, Dave Cooley, Bruce Carruthers, Essam Attia, Arlys Herem, Bob Anderson, Bob Suberi, Jim Brown, Dan Shea, Mark Foreman, Bill Peterson, Pat Scanlon, Maurice Martin, Mick Cole, Dan Luker, John Ketwig, Buzz Davis, Denny Riley, Joshua Shirley, Peter Branson, Skip Delano, Liz Weisen, and Tarak Kauff. Among VFP national leaders and staff members, Adrienne Kinne, Garrett Reppenhagen, and Colleen Kelly were most helpful, along with VFP Advisory Board member Anne Wright.

At Common Defense and its Veterans Organizing Institute, we are very grateful for all the assistance we received from Alex McCoy, Jose Vazquez, Kyle Bibby, Naveed Shah, and Janice Jamison. Britany DeBarros at About Face and Nancy Lessin, cofounder of Military Families Speak Out, were both very informative about the politics of post-9/11 antiwar organizing among veterans, active-duty military personnel, and their families. Lory Manning at Service Women's Action Network, Derek Coy, veterans' health officer at the NY State Health Foundation, and Dana Montalto, at the Veterans Legal Clinic at Harvard Law School, were valued sources of information as well.

We owe a big debt of gratitude to all of the following authors, researchers, and writers on military or veterans affairs: Carl Castro, Andrew Bacevich, Danny Sjursen, Eric Edstrom, W. J. Astore, Matthew Hoh, Rory Fanning, Larry Wilkerson, Kayla Williams, Ellen Moore, Stacey Bannerman, John Ketwig, Jerry Lembcke, David Kieran, Jamie Rowan, Michael Messner, Nan Levinson, C. J. Chivers, Aaron Glantz, Tom Englehardt, Andrea Mazzarino, Kenneth MacLeish, David Swanson, Nick Turse, Medea Benjamin, Jennifer Mittelstadt, Joseph Hickman, Vince Emanuele, Joe Allen, Spencer Ackerman, Isaac Arnsdorf, David Philipps, Jennifer Steinhauer, and Quil Lawrence.

Stephen Trynosky, already mentioned above, deserves special thanks for the insights provided by his monograph, *Beyond the Iron Triangle: Implications for the Veterans Health Administration in an Uncertain Policy Environment.* Stephen has spent years in the Army Reserves while working in various federal agencies including the VA and has always been on call for authorial queries of all kinds. Retired Delta Airlines captain Patrick Mendenhall, a former Navy pilot, provided much insight into career transitions from military to civilian aviation when he collaborated with Suzanne on *Beyond the Checklist,* a 2013 book about aviation safety.

Writers for specialized publications directed at members of the military have been a particular source of insight and inspiration. Among them we would like to recognize: Leo Shane at *Military Times*; Nikki Wentling at *Stars and Stripes*; the contributors to *Task and Purpose* and *Military.com*, including Steve Beynon, Haley Britzky, and Jeff Schogol; Kelly Kennedy and her colleagues at *The War Horse*. We urge all readers of this book to check out the always hilarious *Duffel Blog*. Edited by former Marine Paul Szoldra, it was created to help "military members and civilians advance critical thinking in national security through satire and smart humor." In the world of veteran-run podcasts, there are none better than *Fortress on a Hill*, a collaboration between Danny Sjursen, Chris Henrikson, and Keagan Miller, and *Hell of a Way to Die*, hosted by Francis Horton and Nate Bethea.

In the labor movement, we have had many helpers and supporters. Special thanks to Marilyn Park, now retired from the American Federation of Government Employees (AFGE), and our dear friend and ally, former AFGE rep Ian Hoffmann. AFGE is very lucky to have past or present activists like Linda Ward Smith, Alma Lee, Eric Gerkin, Betsy Zucker, Adam Pelletier, Elliot Friedman, Matt Sowards, Matt Muchowski, Jim Martin, Bob Fetzer, Barb Galle, Nick Keogh, Jackie Simon, and Julie Tippens. At National Nurses United, it has been a privilege to work with Bonnie Castillo, Corey Lanham, Ann Marie Lunetta, and other advocates for VA nurses. At the Communications Workers of America, we would like to thank Chris Shelton, Sara Steffens, Brooks Sunkett, Biruk Assefa, and their union's Veterans for Social Change Network. At the AFL-CIO's Veterans Affairs Council, Will Attig provides a key link between labor and veterans' organizations. We would also like to thank Dennis O'Neil and Keith Combs, from the American Postal Workers Union, and former APWU staffer Katherine Isaac for connecting us with retired member Roger Bleau. In the UK, a longtime union friend (and former "squaddie"), Tim Webb, shared his views on veterans' healthcare issues in his country.

We would like to recognize the following past or present members of Congress for their critical role in veterans affairs: former Michigan congressman and House Whip David Bonior, Senator Bernie Sanders, and current House members Nancy Pelosi, Raúl Grijalva, Alexandria Ocasio-Cortez, and Mark Takano. Very special thanks to Kathryn Becker Van Haste and Essam Attia in Senator Sanders's office. Elizabeth MacKenzie and Matt Reel, from Congressman Takano's, both added much to our understanding of the legislative process as it affects veterans' healthcare. Thanks also to Sophie Friedl who worked for the Senate Veterans Affairs Committee. Iraq War veterans Tyson Manker and Dennis White shared their perspectives on veterans in politics and helped with other book-related topics. Griffin Mahon, from the Veterans Working Group of Democratic Socialists of America, was similarly informative. In California, Mike Matlock was an invaluable guide to veterans' organizations and politics in the Golden State.

Last but not least, there were many valued editors who published material in various media outlets that now appears in different form in this book. Special thanks go to Robert Kuttner, David Dayen, Gabrielle Gurley, and Harold Myerson at the *American Prospect*; Phil Longman and Paul Glastris at *Washington Monthly*; Katrina vanden Heuvel, Emily Douglas, and Emily Hiatt at the *Nation*; Bhaskar Sunkara, Micah Uetricht, Shawn Gude, Meagan Day, and Emma Fejgenbaum at *Jacobin*; Aaron Glantz, formerly at *Reveal*; Honor Jones, Siddhartha Mahanta, and Lauren Katzenberg at the *New York Times*; Paul Szoldra at *Task and Purpose*; Jonathon Sturgeon and Jess Bergman at *The Baffler*; Pat Caldwell and Adam Weinstein at the *New Republic*; Nick Baumann at *The Atlantic*; Dick Price and Sharon Kyle at *LA Progressive*; Randy Shaw at *Beyond Chron*; Jeffrey St. Clair and Josh Frank at *CounterPunch*; Wade Rathke at *Social Policy*; Alexandra Bradbury, Dan DiMaggio, and Saurav Sarkar at *Labor Notes*; Michael Albert at *Znet*; and the moderators at *Portside*.

At Duke University Press, we want to thank Director Dean Smith and Editorial Director Gisela Fosado for their encouragement and support, along with their editorial and marketing staff colleagues Alejandra Mejia, Jessica Ryan, Chad Royal, Laura Sell, Christopher Robinson, and Aimee Harrison. (Three cheers also for the DUP Workers Union!) Our East Bay neighbor Denise Logsdon and Christi Stanforth were our copyeditors; Elliot Linzer was our indispensable indexer. At the Borchardt Agency in New York, Anne, Georges, and Valerie Borchardt were trusted allies, as always. Last but not least, we'd like to thank one of our favorite New York editors, Carl Bromley, now at Melville House in Brooklyn, who provided much valuable feedback on this project in its early stages.

INTRODUCTION

FRIENDLY FIRE

Wow, wouldn't this be something. I fight in Iraq and Afghanistan
just to be killed in the House of Representatives.
—TONY GONZALES, a newly elected House member, after
a pro-Trump mob including fellow veterans stormed
Capitol Hill on January 6, 2021

Anybody who's ever served in the military—or even just read a book or seen a movie about waging war—knows that one of its occupational hazards is coming under fire from your own side. Being shot at, shelled, or strafed mistakenly by fellow soldiers during training exercises or combat can be a fatal problem for even the most formidable of generals (Stonewall Jackson, for instance).[1] Active duty has also been the source of service-related injuries and illnesses, postwar personal woes, and political betrayals not caused by any hostile nation. Millions of US military veterans have experienced such "friendly fire," first in uniform and later as veterans. Our mission in this book is to assess the resulting loss and damage many suffer in their work and personal lives and the political harm caused by some institutions and individuals who advocate for veterans or purport to be on their side.

The disconnect between patriotic celebration of veterans and how re-turning soldiers are actually treated has a long history in the United States. In the 1780s stalwart survivors of George Washington's Continental Army were paid in paper currency that was nearly worthless and not accepted by banks, merchants, or local governments demanding overdue property tax payments. Many citizens who had volunteered to liberate the colonies from British rule ended up impoverished as a result. Some suffered humiliating eviction from their small farms or postwar incarceration in debtors' prisons. High-ranking officers fared better, as they always do. They received pen-sions, some of which were transferable to their widows and orphans.[2]

After the Civil War, hundreds of thousands of demobilized Union soldiers had great difficulty supporting themselves and their families. Only the severely disabled were eligible for care in a few newly created soldiers' homes. The *Army and Navy Journal*, a military publication, offered the helpful advice that vet-erans should avoid becoming "dirty loafer[s]" if they wanted to succeed in civilian life. Those who developed "new muscular habits," rather than suc-cumbing to personal despair and reliance on charity, would eventually find jobs and housing; those who sought any special help would end up fatally dependent on it.[3] When, in 1890, members of the Grand Army of the Re-public were finally awarded pensions not tied to death or disability while on active duty, the *Nation* proclaimed, "The ex-Union soldier is . . . a helpless and greedy sort of person, who says that he is not able to support himself and whines that other people ought to do it for him."[4]

After the First World War, 3.6 million veterans were promised bonus payments—but not until twenty-seven years after their service. When the Great Depression began, that was too long for many to wait. So in 1932, twenty thousand impoverished former soldiers descended on Washington, DC, to petition Congress and the White House for immediate payment. Conservative national groups representing veterans, like the American Legion, criticized their multiracial encampment and refused to support it. President Herbert Hoover, a Republican, denounced the protest organizers as communists and criminals. Under his orders, the so-called Bonus Marchers were brutally at-tacked and dispersed by Army units led by three midcareer officers destined to become our most famous World War II generals.[5]

The losers of that one-sided domestic battle helped others who served abroad after them. Not only did Congress authorize payment of $2 billion in bonus money to World War I veterans four years later, but the Servicemen's Readjustment Act of 1944—better known as the GI Bill—was enacted, in part, to avoid similar or worse postwar unrest among the next generation of returning veterans. As one historian explains, "If the twelve million veterans of World War II had been dumped off the boats like the nearly four million from the previous world war and given only $60 and a train ticket home, with neither educational nor economic opportunity awaiting them when they got back, violent revolution might have easily been sparked."[6]

Yet one generation after a broad swath of former "citizen soldiers" gained greater access to housing, healthcare, and higher education via the GI Bill, veterans of the most unpopular conflict in US history felt less well treated when they returned home. Their alienation from the war that hundreds of thousands were drafted or enlisted to fight began on active duty in Vietnam and military bases located in what are now called "red" states. As US intervention in Southeast Asia turned into a bloody quagmire, dissent within the military took the form of desertions and equipment sabotage, rioting in military stockades, and deadly assaults on officers known as "fragging"—a grenade-assisted form of friendly fire that was not unintentional.[7]

On the home front, uniformed foes of the Vietnam War created a nationwide network of off-base coffeehouses where they could listen to music, read GI-written leaflets and newsletters, and socialize with each other and their civilian allies. This helped break down the military/civil society divide, which is far wider today—largely because of the postwar creation of an "all-volunteer force" to replace the dissident draftees of fifty years ago. While histories of the period highlight campus unrest, soldiers on active duty and reservists opposed the war with growing fervor and, ultimately, greater impact. By 1970, according to Vietnam-era veteran and University of Notre Dame historian David Cortright, this rank-and-file rebellion "played a decisive role in limiting the ability of the U.S. to continue the war."[8]

A year later, Vietnam Veterans Against the War (VVAW) created a Bonus March–style encampment in Washington, DC. Ridiculed and red-baited by older veterans' groups, they demanded peace in Vietnam and recognition of their own postwar needs. Their brave stand signaled the beginning of a long struggle for expanded GI Bill coverage, veterans' healthcare reform, and compensation for exposure to Agent Orange—the chemical herbicide widely used in Vietnam with toxic aftereffects for combatants and civilians alike. Survivors of the hazards of World War II and Korea now represent less than 10 percent of all veterans. About half served during the Vietnam era or periods of peacetime before or after it. And the fastest-growing veteran cohort, which includes 2 million women, was part of the professional military deployed during the first and second Gulf Wars, the occupation of Afghanistan, and other conflicts around the globe.[9] By 2021, about 11 percent of all US veterans were female.[10]

Prior to 1973, military service was a burden more widely shared by the entire adult male population, even with draft deferments that unfairly privileged college students. For better or worse, abolition of conscription, while maintaining selective service registration by men, ended a two-century-old tradition of citizen soldiering. It helped the Department of Defense (DOD) reduce the risk of political dissent within its ranks—and society at large—by putting "distance between the army and the American people."[11] This post-Vietnam reorganization of the military has been the single greatest influence on where and how modern-day soldiers are recruited and what kinds of problems they experience when transitioning back to civilian life.

Architects of the all-volunteer force, like Army Secretary Stanley Resor, were initially concerned that "a political draft would be replaced by an economic draft of the poorest Americans," leaving the military attractive only to those "on the economic margin."[12] To encourage wider enlistment, particularly during periods when patriotic fervor would be an insufficient incentive, the Pentagon built what historian Jennifer Mittelstadt calls "a military welfare state." Pay, pensions, and housing allowances for career soldiers were much improved, and veterans' benefits, as a "reward for faithful service or compensation for loss," were emphasized far more than in the past. Via the Department of Veterans Affairs (VA), millions of former service members gain access to free higher education, job training and counseling, home mortgage assistance, and medical care in the nation's largest public healthcare system. When seeking employment in both the public and the private sector, veterans enjoy hiring preferences that give them an edge over other workers in the civilian job market. According to Mittelstadt, such arrangements have the effect of "differentiating the veteran from the civilian and elevating him as worthy of entitlement."[13]

The veteran community jealously guards these entitlements, sometimes to the detriment of its own 19 million members, who now constitute just 7 percent of the adult population, down from 18 percent in 1980. Passage of the original GI bill, which benefited all who served during World War II, was initially opposed by several groups fearful that assistance to disabled combat veterans would be underfunded as a result. As noted later in this book, fewer than half of all veterans today receive healthcare coverage through the VA. Yet past attempts to extend the VA's system of socialized medicine to more veterans or their families have been thwarted by some of their own organizations. As one Washington, DC, advocate for veterans told us, he even gets angry when proponents of Medicare for All cite the VA as a good functioning model of single-payer healthcare. VA benefits belong to us, he exclaimed, because we earned them. If other Americans want free higher education or VA-style medical coverage, they should enlist, he argued. Any universalization of these benefits would, in his view, be tantamount to breaking the sacred promise, made by Abraham Lincoln and now carried out by the VA, to care first "for him who shall have borne the battle, and for his widow, and his orphan."

When political homage is paid to veterans, no speech is more often invoked than Lincoln's Second Inaugural Address, which contained those few words but a larger message as well. Like more than half of all US presidents, Lincoln was himself a veteran—of brief home-front service in the Illinois Militia. Speaking on March 4, 1865, on the eve of Confederate surrender to a vast citizen army, Lincoln asked Union supporters to approach their next challenge "with malice toward none" and "do all which may achieve and cherish a just and lasting peace, among ourselves, and with all nations."[14]

According to Civil War historian and Princeton University professor Allen Guelzo, Lincoln had no intention of carving out a special space, in postwar society, for veterans or their survivors. His overriding concern was implementing a process of national reconciliation. Former service members were part of this process, for sure, but not its sole focus. Lincoln's call to "bind up the nation's wounds" was not limited to those soldiers injured on the battlefield, but addressed the need for broader healing. Despite his deep personal connection to those who served under him, the nation's greatest nineteenth-century commander in chief did not favor putting veterans on a pedestal or turning them into a privileged caste.[15]

THE ALL-VOLUNTEER FORCE

As revealed in the chapters that follow, this is not the attitude of many veterans' organizations today, modern politicians pursuing the "veteran vote," or corporations and philanthropies branding themselves as "veteran friendly." In the past fifty years, many former soldiers have gone from seeing themselves as representative of the civilian society they served to feeling quite estranged from it. That larger society, in turn, has less connection with the experience of military service than ever before. During the First and Second World Wars, the US military, made up of citizen soldiers, largely reflected the US population. During the Vietnam War, although draft deferments favored those who could go to college or graduate school, the burden of service was nonetheless still shared by more than 1 percent of the US population. All of that changed in 1973 when the United States ended conscription and shifted to an all-volunteer military. As military historian Andrew Bacevich explains this shift, "The viability of the all-volunteer force depended . . . on the army's ability to create credible paths to career success for those who were not white and not male."[16]

The US military has thus developed far greater gender, racial, and ethnic diversity. After much struggle, it was also forced to accept more women as well as openly gay and transgendered recruits. According to DOD statistics, nearly a third of the 1,304,418 men and women on active duty in 2018 identified themselves "as a racial minority (Black or African American, Asian, American Indian, or Alaska Native, Native Hawaiian, or Other Pacific Islander, Multi-racial, or Other/Unknown)."[17] Other estimates put the percentage of people of color in uniform even higher—at 43 percent.[18] The Armed Forces now employ more women than ever before, including in combat roles since that ban was lifted in 2013. About 280,000 women have served in Iraq and Afghanistan since those post-9/11 deployments began. About 16 percent of all enlisted personnel and 18 percent of all officers are female.

Reflecting gender discrimination, the legacy of their exclusion from combat, or both, far fewer women serve as higher-ranking officers; only six have ever attained four-star rank. Black officers face their own obstacles to career advancement, particularly in the Marines. In the past they have "typically specialized in logistics and transportation, like moving supplies or driving trucks, and not in combat arms specialties like infantry or artillery," where their white counterparts are able to win faster and higher promotions. As of 2020, only two of the forty-one most senior commanders in all branches were Black. Yet, reflecting the overall demographic shift in the enlisted ranks, a quarter of all veterans are now nonwhite.[19]

Meanwhile, military service remains as much motivated by the economic draft as appeals to patriotism and public service. According to the Council on Foreign Relations, only 17 percent of recruits come from families that have a household income of $87,000 or more. Most come from families with a household income between $41,000 and $87,000, and 19 percent from households with an income lower than $41,000 a year.[20] Military recruiters sign up poor and working-class Americans in disproportionate numbers from particular states and regions where a tradition of military service remains strong and local economies are weak. As Matt Kennard revealed in his 2015 book, *Irregular Army*, the manpower needs of the simultaneous US military occupations of Iraq and Afghanistan required a lowering of physical and mental fitness standards and a dangerous "loosening of enlistment regulations on criminals, racist extremists, and gang members" (some of whom later wreaked havoc at home and abroad, with unauthorized acts of violence).[21] As we report later in this book, recruiters today meet their quotas by playing up the future job market advantages of having military training and access to GI Bill coverage, as opposed to crushing student debt. Plus, there is the immediate lure of medical insurance and other benefits better than any offered in the private sector to minimum-wage workers with a high school diploma or less.

When seventeen-year-old Cruz Gonzalez,* the daughter of undocumented Mexican immigrants, checked out the Army Reserves, she was told that enlisting would help her parents become citizens. (An asterisk will be used throughout the text to indicate that a person requested a pseudonym.) Her recruiter stressed that military service would "open up a lot of doors education-wise, give me free healthcare and job security. . . . I would be at the top of every single pile when employers are looking for new employees because everyone wants workers who are self-motivated, which is what you become in the military." West Virginia native Dennis White was a high school dropout working at Wendy's for $5.15 an hour before he joined the Army and its infantry surge in Iraq in 2007. "When you come from nothing, the military doesn't seem so bad," he says. "You get fed three times a day and you get paid pretty well, so it wasn't a bad move for me because I got to escape a crazy economy at the time of the recession."[22]

In the left-behind precincts of rural and urban America, military service has become a family business. In 2019 nearly 80 percent of all new Army recruits reported that they had a family member in the military, and 30 percent disclosed that it was a parent. In Dennis White's case, both his father and grandfather served before him and then became blue-collar workers. As two military family members explain in a book called *AWOL* about the "unexcused absence of America's upper class from military service," a major influence on enlistment decisions is recruits' past personal contact with veterans or active-duty service members they personally admired.[23]

Only about one-third of all Americans under thirty today have any such familial or community connection to the military, which is not surprising: the percentage of veterans in the adult population has shrunk by half since 1990, to 7 percent or less.[24] Four out of ten young people say they have never personally considered joining the military. In 1974 about half of all Americans who did so came from the South or Southwest. Today that figure is closer to 70 percent. Not surprisingly, the states with residents overrepresented in the military are also those with a disproportionate number of DOD facilities and military families living around them—Texas, Nevada, Arizona, Virginia, Alabama, Georgia, and North and South Carolina.[25]

The burden of military service is not just shared by a much narrower slice of the total population. The 1 percent who serve have been fashioned into what Army Major Daniel Sjursen (now retired) calls "a homegrown foreign legion." One architect of that transformation was the infamous Donald Rumsfeld, secretary of defense under President George W. Bush, who argued on the eve of the US invasion of Iraq that a "smart and nimble force" could "do more with less."[26] The simultaneous US occupation of Afghanistan, which continued over two decades, poured many of the same troops into both countries, often more than once. As former assistant secretary of defense Lawrence J. Korb points out, multiple deployments without adequate "dwell time" or relief periods between each combat tour increased the risk of veterans suffering from posttraumatic stress disorder (PTSD) by 50 percent.

The active-duty component of the all-volunteer force was insufficient to meet the personnel demands of the Global War on Terror, as waged in open-ended fashion by Presidents George Bush, Barack Obama, and Donald Trump. National Guard and Reserve units, which carry about 800,000 Americans on their rolls, were repeatedly tapped for combat-zone service. As Korb notes, "When these men and women complete their deployments, they are normally deactivated and lose their U.S. Department of Defense (DOD) military health care benefits and are thrown back into the civilian health care system."[27] As a result, they often lacked support structures and services available to active-duty families living on or near military bases.

Pentagon planners succeeded in keeping overall death tolls down among troops deployed to Middle Eastern combat zones by privatizing military functions. What researcher Heidi Peltier calls the "camo economy" enables US war planners to announce troop withdrawals while simultaneously maintaining or expanding our military presence abroad by "relying more heavily on contractors." According to Peltier, during the final year of Trump's presidency, contract employees actually outnumbered active-duty troops in the Central Command region that includes Iraq and Afghanistan by 53,000 to 35,000.[28] By mid-2020, the total number of combat-zone deaths among private contractors since September 2001 numbered about eight thousand, versus seven thousand soldiers killed while wearing a uniform. Fortunately, advances in medical care ensured that "the ratio of severely wounded service members surviving potentially fatal injuries" was "more than five times higher in the wars in Iraq and Afghanistan than in any previous war."[29]

ADJUSTMENT PROBLEMS

Hundreds of thousands of post-9/11 veterans returned home after repeated deployments, but some were no longer "nimble." Doing "more with less" for them as veterans did not work out any better than Donald Rumsfeld's Iraq invasion plan. Between 2006 and 2015, the number of veterans requiring VA-provided mental health care rose from 900,000 annually to 1.6 million, a reflection of the ongoing collateral damage from "forever wars." Other VA patients had gunshot wounds, lost limbs, traumatic brain injuries, PTSD, or respiratory problems from burn pit exposure. Women who served and were subjected to sexual harassment, physical assault, and rape bore the scars of military sexual trauma. Veterans of all types experience higher-than-average rates of joblessness, homelessness, chronic pain, mental illness, and substance abuse. These problems were particularly acute among formerly enlisted men and women who returned to poor and working-class communities slow to recover from the Great Recession of 2007 and 2008. Their experience of military service added new wounds of war to the not-so-hidden injuries and preexisting conditions of class.

Not surprisingly, 44 percent of post-9/11 veterans reported reintegration problems after leaving the military, as compared to only 25 percent of earlier veterans.[30] Some retained a strong sense of civic responsibility and a continuing desire to serve a higher purpose. For others, service-related injuries or emotional problems were personally crippling. Novelist Elliot Ackerman, a Marine officer who completed five combat tours in the Middle East, describes the soldier who, as a civilian, "must reintegrate into society, find happiness and a new purpose . . . in a job at Home Depot, going to college, working in real estate. Nothing compares to what he has just done. . . . A certain depression sets in: the knowledge that the rest of his days will be spent sitting on his front porch, sipping Coors Light, watching life pass by."[31]

Instead of feeling comfortable in civilian society, some veterans—regardless of their political leanings—experience feelings of alienation, anger, and resentment toward fellow citizens. In their view, the 99 percent who do not serve too often display little understanding or concern for those who did, beyond obligatory displays of what Daniel Sjursen calls "performative patriotism."[32] In his memoir, *Touching the Dragon*, former Navy SEAL James Hatch recalls being "forced to reintegrate into a society that I had spent two decades defending, but in which I didn't feel I had a place." Hatch enlisted in the Navy at age eighteen and was so disdainful of fellow sailors who just wanted to "gain skills they could use later on as civilians" that he became a real "warfighter," always "close to the enemy."[33] Before devastating injuries ended his career, Hatch survived 150 direct-action missions in Bosnia, Africa, Iraq, and Afghanistan. According to Hatch, in addition to experiencing a "serious volume of fighting," his generational cohort of special operators face "a serious volume of aftermath. Marriages falling apart. Alcoholism. Guys getting kicked out of their houses. Guys drowning in opioids. The real recoil hasn't even hit yet."[34]

Kayla Williams was a "rare open progressive" when serving as an Arab-speaking linguist in the Army's 101st Airborne Division. Yet after returning from Iraq, she found "the shallow pettiness of so many Americans" to be "incredibly off-putting." She had, after all, "watched a man bleed to death, been shot at, heard mortars fall nearby, endured the fear and privation of a year at war, put up with the sexual harassment and the isolation of being the only woman around for months on end. What did these selfish civilians with their insignificant concerns understand about that? I had nothing in common with them. . . . I only felt normal when I was with others who had been in combat."[35]

Jason Kander, a liberal Democrat and lawyer from Missouri who served in Afghanistan for just four months, returned home without physical injuries to pursue a career in state politics. Nevertheless, he felt saddled with survivor's guilt. He remembers "going out to dinner and seeing people having a good time with friends and thinking, 'Don't these people know what's going on over there? How can everyone act like everything's fine? . . . How can everyone act so normal?'"[36] When Erik Edstrom got home, the West Point graduate turned Afghan War critic received "thudding back slaps and free beers from well-meaning civilians" in bars and restaurants. But over time, he felt that "when it comes to our military, the mantra of the public is: thank, don't think. To most of them, war—the war my friends died for—was elevator music."[37]

POLITICAL ALIENATION

As sociologist and Vietnam vet Jerry Lembcke told us, "This generation of veterans went off to Iraq and Afghanistan with more hoopla than any generation since World War II. But a lot of them, particularly the men, came back deflated and disappointed with the experience they had. It did not live up to the mythology of what war is supposed to be, because there is no glory in these inglorious wars." According to Lembcke, the resulting feelings of depression, alienation, or betrayal experienced by some veterans have been turned into generic "anger against the government" because "they've got to blame somebody" for putting them in harm's way.

During his first presidential campaign, Donald Trump unexpectedly tapped into this vein of veteran discontent, despite his own lack of military service and what appeared to be a series of fatal political gaffes. While running for the White House in 2016, Trump famously dissed a Gold Star family who lost a son in Iraq. He called Senator John McCain, America's most famous prisoner of war, a "loser" for being captured in Vietnam. When asked about widespread sexual assault in the modern-day military, he said it wasn't a serious problem. After a Trump campaign event held for the ostensible purpose of aiding veterans' charities, the candidate had to be publicly shamed into making his own promised donation. By contrast, while serving as New York's junior senator Hillary Clinton helped members of the National Guard and the Reserves gain greater access to health benefits. During her 2016 campaign for the presidency, she released a comprehensive, twelve-page policy paper for veterans. Trump's was less than one page long. Clinton won endorsements from 110 former military leaders, far more than favored Trump. But, in multiple ways, the Clinton campaign did not regard veterans—who vote in disproportionate numbers and represent about 13 percent of the nation's active electorate—as a constituency worth cultivating. Her phone bankers failed to collect information about past military service that could be used to make targeted follow-up calls; instead of veteran-focused messaging, her campaign employed generic "get out the vote" (GOTV) scripts. And Clinton, unlike Trump, was not a campaign critic of the forever wars in Iraq and Afghanistan, which she, as a leading US senator, had strongly supported.

The Republican ground campaign behind Trump easily out-organized the Democrats among veterans and military families. With a multi-million-dollar budget, the party-backed group known as GOPVets was tasked with boosting vet voter turnout, which ended up being 2.8 million greater in 2016 than four years earlier. GOPVets deployed fifty former members of the military to work as full-time organizers and set up task forces in swing states with large veteran populations, including North Carolina, Florida, New Hampshire, Ohio, and Pennsylvania. Hundreds of volunteers were trained on veterans' issues and then knocked on more than a million doors. An allied organization called Concerned Veterans for America (CVA) used its ample funding from the Koch brothers to knock on 250,000 more doors. Pro-Trump mailers were not just mailed out; they were handed out, one-on-one, by volunteers to fellow veterans at American Legion posts, NASCAR races, and Blue Angel air shows.

On Election Day in 2016, Trump lost the popular vote by more than 3 million, but veterans played a key role in his electoral college win over Clinton. Nationwide, 60 percent of all veterans cast their ballots for a wealthy recipient of five draft deferments, based on Republican promises that he would boost military pay, make America great again, and address concerns about veterans' healthcare. An analysis of 2016 voting data conducted by Francis Shen and Cornell University's Douglas Kriner found exceptionally high support for Trump in blue-collar communities that had suffered some of the highest post-9/11 combat casualty rates. Their findings suggested that this voter turnout was crucial to Trump's narrow defeat of Clinton in three decisive swing states: Pennsylvania, Michigan, and Wisconsin. Among former military personnel, Trump beat Clinton by a twenty-six-point margin nationwide, a bigger percentage of the vet vote than John McCain's share when he ran against Barack Obama in 2008. Trump also performed well in areas with large active-duty voting populations. For example, Montgomery County, Ohio—home to the city of Dayton and a significant portion of Wright-Patterson Air Force Base in nearby Greene County—went to Trump after favoring Barack Obama in 2008 and 2012. Trump also outperformed past Republican presidential nominees in North Carolina's Onslow County, home to the Marine Corps's Camp Lejeune.[38]

Once in office, Trump continued to make anti-interventionist head feints. Meanwhile, he packed his administration with former generals who earned their extra stars in the nation's failed forever wars. He proposed ever-larger Pentagon budgets and new weapons programs. At the VA, under the guise of giving veterans greater healthcare "choice," Trump empowered would-be privatizers of the agency. Trump's initial legislative achievements included passage of more than a dozen bills involving veterans. As his second VA secretary, Robert Wilkie, proclaimed, "No president in the post–World War II era has ever put veterans at the center of both his campaign and his administration until President Trump did."[39] A Pew Research poll conducted in mid-2019 showed that Trump remained popular among veterans even while US military intervention in Iraq and Afghanistan was viewed unfavorably by a majority of those surveyed.[40]

Fortunately, before the votes of 19 million veterans, plus an additional 2 million active-duty military personnel and their family members, were in play again, Trump became a self-proclaimed "wartime president." His poor performance in the domestic battle against COVID-19, its disastrous economic impact, and the White House response to nationwide protests against police brutality put wind in the sails of a 2020 presidential candidate with broader appeal than Hillary Clinton. Like Clinton, Joe Biden had been a senatorial supporter of US intervention in Iraq during the Bush administration; unlike Clinton, he later questioned the wisdom of a military escalation in Afghanistan while serving as Obama's vice president. Among other advantages, Biden benefited from being part of a military family. His oldest son, Beau, served as a Delaware National Guard major in Iraq; Beau's premature death at age forty-six after suffering a stroke and then brain cancer led his father to wonder whether burn pit exposure might have been a contributing cause.

As we recount later in the book, veterans in Congress—even when elected as proponents of greater bipartisanship—were sharply divided along party lines on issues related to Donald Trump. In the veteran population at large and among active-duty soldiers, growing anti-Trump sentiment found expression not just via support for other presidential candidates but in myriad forms of public disapproval.[41] By the fall of 2020, even retired generals and colonels, once part of his administration, had become critics of Trump's threatened use of the military—other than the National Guard—against Black Lives Matter protesters. Mindful of the all-volunteer force's growing racial diversity, these top officers and their successors at the Pentagon also broke with the White House over its resistance to rebranding military bases still named for Confederate traitors. And, for veterans who didn't think it was "fake news," Trump's private disparagement of dead soldiers as "suckers" and "losers" was a final pre-election insult.

Trump's even bigger defeat in the 2020 popular vote, plus his electoral college loss, didn't eliminate the continuing appeal and threat of Trumpism. One group that helped chip away at veteran support for Trump was Veterans for Responsible Leadership (VFRL), which recruited several thousand members during the presidential campaign.[42] Its cofounder, Naval Academy graduate and Vermont physician Dan Barkhuff, posted anti-Trump messages on YouTube that drew nearly 3 million views. As Barkhuff told the *New Yorker*, most of the group's initial supporters, who had served in the military, were "Republicans disgusted with Trump." VFRL asked all new recruits to abide by a Veteran Code of Conduct that commits signers to "stand for the equality and dignity of all" and to "hold all elected leaders, government servants, and law enforcement to the highest moral, ethical, and professional standards." After the 2020 election, but before its results were finalized, Barkhuff announced that VFRL was turning its attention to veterans who've "lost their way" and embraced the tribalism of right-wing paramilitary groups. Barkhuff expressed hope that VFRL could become a rival "tribe," capable of competing with "the white nationalism of Trump."[43]

Three weeks later, during the final stage of the presidential election process on January 6, 2021, Capitol Hill was stormed by a pro-Trump mob. Former military personnel were disproportionately represented in this crowd of thousands—and on later lists of those charged with criminal activity.[44] One participant was a retired Navy SEAL whose company taught SEAL-type tactics to local police departments; a month before the event, he posted a Facebook video proclaiming, "Once things start going violent, then I'm in my element."[45] Another who arrived early to case possible entrances was Keith Lee, an Air Force veteran, former private contractor in Afghanistan, later a police detective in Texas, and, by 2020, a sales manager laid off during the pandemic. Using a bullhorn, forty-one-year-old Lee helped direct right-wing militia members into the building, setting up a clash between veterans.[46] During this spasm of violence, Ashli Babbitt, a fourteen-year veteran of the Air Force, was fatally shot by a police officer when she tried to gain forcible entry to the House Speaker's Lobby. On the law enforcement side, an Iraq combat veteran, Eugene Goodman, became a Capitol Police hero by leading several senators to safety. Meanwhile, one of his colleagues, an Air National Guard member, was fatally assaulted. An Air Force Academy graduate and retired lieutenant colonel was among those later arrested and charged with invading the Senate chamber. A fifty-year-old former Marine from Ohio with a history of addiction, domestic violence, and racism pushed his way into the building wearing "a combat helmet, ballistic goggles, and a tactical vest with handheld radio."[47] His preferred tribes were the Ohio State Regular Militia, a local paramilitary group, and Oath Keepers, a national network of right-wing "patriots" created by a former Army paratrooper.

Tony Gonzales was one of the veterans in Congress risking friendly fire when they helped barricade House chamber doors and usher colleagues away from such assailants. A newly elected Republican from Texas, Gonzales was considered a "traitor" because he favored certification of Biden's victory. As Trump-incited rioters descended on his new place of employment, the former naval officer thought: "Wow, wouldn't this be something. I fight in Iraq and Afghanistan just to be killed in the House of Representatives."[48]

If there was any collective realization at that moment, bipartisan or otherwise, it was that the political allegiance of veterans and their families could not be ceded to right-wing extremists. To do so would mean electing more Donald Trumps and dooming future federal efforts to aid millions of poor and working-class Americans, whether they served in the military or not.

A SYSTEM WORTH SAVING—FOR ALL OF US

This pivotal confrontation on Capitol Hill—and the contest for the vet vote in 2020 that preceded it—should dispel any simplistic notion that US military veterans are monolithic in their political outlook. As we explain in this book, the field of veterans affairs is complicated terrain because of the latest fractures and failings of various institutions ostensibly devoted to veterans' well-being. The most influential players on this field include the Department of Defense (DOD), the former employer of all veterans; the Department of Veterans Affairs (VA), the federal agency officially charged with salving their postwar, service-related wounds and providing them with myriad benefits; the veterans' service organizations (VSOS), old and new; self-proclaimed veteran-friendly philanthropists and employers; investor-owned firms now positioning themselves to become caregivers for veterans at government expense; and both major political parties, their candidates, and wealthy donors, all wooing the vet vote during every election cycle, with varying results for themselves and veterans.

Within the federal government, the interplay between the DOD and the VA is critical. Think of America's wars, and related military service, as creating a huge funnel between its largest and second-largest federal agencies. Entering at the top of the funnel, via the DOD, are former draftees and enlisted men and women who've been discharged favorably. Hundreds of thousands carry mental or physical wounds of war associated with combat. Others—who served near or far from the front lines—sustained job-related injuries or illnesses similar to those experienced by millions of blue-collar workers in civilian life. Their common need for healthcare services or later disability benefits—what is called "workers' compensation" in the civilian world—is met at the other end of the funnel by the VA, which operates the Veterans Health Administration (VHA) and the Veterans Benefits Administration (VBA).

Many American workers who get hurt on the job or develop an occupational disease soon become familiar with the shortcomings of our state-based system of workers' compensation. In most states, benefit levels are too low. Private employers fight workers' claims. Rehabilitation services are fragmented and managed by private insurers. Workers who get approved treatment for specific work-related conditions may not be able to return to work. At some point this deprives them of job-based medical coverage for themselves and their families. So even successful workers' comp claimants can end up in personal bankruptcy due to unpaid bills for care. By contrast, veterans who become VHA patients, due to their low income, service-related health condition, or recent deployment in a war zone land on an island of socialized medicine within our larger system of private insurance and for-profit healthcare delivery.[49]

Like the National Health Service in the UK, the VHA is an integrated national network of public hospitals and clinics providing direct care. It's not a hospital chain competing with others for market share, nor is it a collection of physician practices or specialty services reimbursed by private insurers, Medicare, or Medicaid. All VHA doctors, nurses, therapists, and other professional and nonprofessional staff are salaried, not paid on a fee-for-service basis. VHA caregivers are trained to identify and treat the signature wounds of particular wars as well as other medical conditions resulting from military service at home or abroad. Its primary care providers and specialists know how to recognize conditions like Agent Orange–related diabetes or respiratory problems related to past toxic exposures. Every VHA employee receives some training on how to better recognize and assist patients who are suicidal. Thousands of VHA mental health providers are taught the latest evidence-based treatments for PTSD, while outside the VHA, only 30 percent of private-sector providers employ such treatments.[50]

About a third of the VHA's 300,000 staff members are veterans themselves, which helps create a unique culture of empathy and solidarity between patients and providers that has no counterpart in American medicine.[51] About 120,000 VHA employees are union members. Due to collective bargaining rights, VHA management must pay more attention to the kinds of occupational hazards that are widespread in healthcare work, particularly in private-sector hospitals without unions. The VHA was the first and remains one of the few US healthcare systems to install the kind of lift equipment that helps nursing staff avoid debilitating and often career-ending back, neck, and shoulder injuries.[52] Due to the troubled and occasionally violent behavior of some patients, the VHA takes exceptional measures to ensure safe conditions for its staff.[53]

Unfortunately, in Congress, the harm-inflicting DOD has a bigger fan club than the caregiving VHA. When the Pentagon seeks a bigger budget, the House and Senate, with few dissenting voices, conduct an annual contest to determine which body can allocate more funding faster. There's far less eagerness to acknowledge and address the full, long-term costs the nation has incurred as a result of its $5.8 trillion worth of post-9/11 military spending. In her 2021 study for the Costs of War Project, Harvard professor Linda Bilmes warns that the United States "risks defaulting on our financial obligation to this generation of veterans" because total expenditures on their healthcare and other benefits are now projected to reach $2.5 trillion by 2050.[54]

Instead of grappling with how to pay this growing tab, Republicans, who never find fault with the Pentagon, fixate on VHA failings, real or imagined. Democrats, who rarely challenge Big Pharma, for-profit hospital chains, or commercial insurers, often join their GOP colleagues in criticizing the VHA's handling of veterans' problems (while rarely crediting the DOD as the source of many of them). As we show later in the book, this political dynamic has helped shape media depictions of the VHA as an always "troubled," "dysfunctional," or "scandal ridden" federal agency, whereas the DOD is rarely described in these terms regardless of how many costly, wasteful, or failed wars it has waged.

The fact that most VHA patients strongly support public provision of their care creates a challenge for its would-be privatizers.[55] Legislation that has already diverted billions from the VHA's budget to the private healthcare industry had to be carefully framed as a way to empower veterans as patients by giving them more consumer "choice." Veterans have also been the target of a disinformation campaign designed to turn them against Medicare for All. Conservatives falsely claim that making existing single-payer coverage for seniors into a universal program would eliminate the veterans' healthcare system. In reality, as proposed by Senator Bernie Sanders and others, Medicare for All would maintain the VHA and help the majority of veterans who must now depend on private insurance, for themselves and their families, until they reach Medicare age because they are not VHA-eligible.

As Paul Sullivan, a Gulf War combat veteran and former deputy secretary of the California Department of Veterans Affairs, points out, "The forces against quality healthcare for all Americans know that a fully funded and staffed VHA would set a shining example for the national healthcare they bitterly oppose." By hindering the agency's ability to perform its basic mission, as the Trump administration did for four years, Republicans hope to discredit government-run healthcare in any form.

WHAT THE VA DOES WELL (AND STILL POORLY)

The modern-day VA has an overall budget of $243 billion (FY 2021), which funds not only VHA-provided medical care but higher education, job training and counseling, vocational rehabilitation, home loans, life insurance and burial services, pensions, and disability compensation. VA benefits are determined and administered by the Veterans Benefits Administration (VBA). The VA achieved cabinet status in 1989, not long after Ron Kovic's Vietnam War memoir, *Born on the Fourth of July*, was turned into a popular Hollywood movie starring Tom Cruise.[56] As that film vividly depicted, veterans' hospitals were not prepared for an influx of badly wounded soldiers, including Kovic, in the post-Vietnam era. Underfunding and understaffing left VHA facilities in shocking physical condition. Kovic's account of his experience as a VHA patient, shared by many others, helped propel the VA reform efforts, led by Michigan congressman David Bonior and others, that we describe in chapter 4. The resulting shake-up of the Department of Veterans Affairs bureaucracy, which took several decades, ultimately resulted in dramatic improvements in healthcare delivery, including making services more accessible via a network of community-based "Vet Centers."[57]

By the 1990s, under the leadership of Kenneth W. Kizer, a physician, public health expert, and veteran who was President Clinton's VA undersecretary for health, the VHA had expanded its hospital-based system to include primary care, mental health, and patient safety programs. Its IT staff created a pioneering system for electronic medical record–keeping. One group of healthcare experts studying these initiatives concluded that the VHA was "engaged in far-reaching and innovative changes in American health care."[58] By 2006 the VHA was even receiving accolades from the conservative business press. *Fortune* ran a story on veterans' healthcare with the banner headline "How the VA Healed Itself."[59] *Bloomberg Businessweek* declared that the VHA had "the best medical care in the U.S."[60] The *Harvard Business Review* described the VHA's "turnaround" as the largest and most successful institutional transformation of its kind in US history.[61]

Today the VHA delivers care to almost 9 million eligible veterans at over 1,255 sites, including 170 medical centers and 1,074 outpatient sites. Its facilities include primary care clinics, geriatric and palliative care services, surgery, rehabilitation facilities, nursing homes, inpatient residential programs, and campus- and community-based centers.[62] In spite of contemporary challenges like COVID-19, multiple studies confirm that the VA delivers care that is more integrated, more coordinated, and of higher quality and lower cost than almost any other healthcare system in America.[63] One source of cost-savings is the VA's singular ability to negotiate better drug prices for the 5 million veterans whose prescriptions it fills. As a 2020 study by the Government Accountability Office found, the VHA paid Big Pharma approximately 54 percent less than Medicare for hundreds of the same brand-name drugs.[64]

Unlike private-sector providers, the VA also addresses what are called the "social determinants of health" by helping its patients find job training, employment, housing, and other support services. The VHA's second major mission is research. Among the VA breakthroughs that have helped all patients are the development of the shingles vaccine, the nicotine patch, and the first implantable cardiac pacemaker. The VHA has launched the Million Veteran Program to explore the impact of genetics on health and is also on the front lines of COVID-19 research, involving long-term effects of the virus.

Since 1946 the VHA has been affiliated with major academic medical centers throughout the country. It now trains 70 percent of the nation's medical residents and 40 percent of all other healthcare professionals. The coronavirus pandemic showcased the VHA's additional and lesser-known mission as a backup for the private healthcare system during public health emergencies, natural disasters, and other crises. During the California wildfires of 2018, VHA facilities created command posts that did targeted outreach to thousands of veterans living in fire-endangered communities. In Puerto Rico the VHA medical center was one of the few fully functioning hospitals during and after Hurricane Maria in 2017. During the coronavirus crisis of 2020–21, the VHA set aside ICU and hospital beds for non-VHA patients in all its hospitals and dispatched more than a thousand of its own staff members to assist hospitalized civilians and patients in state-run veterans homes overwhelmed by COVID-19 cases.[65]

The VHA also continues to be the most transparent and accountable healthcare system in the country because it is closely monitored not only by its own Office of the Inspector General and the Government Accountability Office but also by the watchdog organizations we describe in chapters 4 and 5.[66] In addition, any veteran with a complaint about VHA care can take that concern to their own member of Congress, those serving on the House and Senate Committees on Veterans Affairs, and even a special White House hotline.

While many Americans assume that military service makes all veterans eligible for VA coverage, that is definitely not the case. Since 2008, veterans who served in any combat zone after 1998 have been granted five years of free VHA care if they received a discharge under other than dishonorable conditions. But getting longer-term treatment, related compensation, or noncombat veteran access to the VHA requires filing a successful claim with the Veterans Benefits Administration (VBA) based on a "service-connected disability."

The level of service connection can range from zero to 100 percent (in 10 percent increments).[67] A partial disability finding might result from back or knee injuries incurred while carrying 60- to 100-pound packs during basic training or combat—a problem few civilians connect to military service. Other, more serious, conditions warranting VHA coverage include amyotrophic lateral sclerosis (or Lou Gehrig's disease) or other diseases that were a side effect of Agent Orange exposure during the Vietnam War and the traumatic brain injuries (TBIS) and amputations suffered by targets of improvised explosive devices in Iraq or Afghanistan.

To be awarded a service-connected rating from the VBA, an eligible veteran must have a medical condition that was incurred or aggravated while on active duty. A veteran can, and often does, receive multiple service-connected disability ratings for each claimed medical condition identified. Every veteran has a right to appeal any VBA service-connected disability rating or denial through a claims process. Unfortunately, appeals can take months or years to be resolved, and many are ultimately denied.

Veterans are also eligible for VHA services if they have low incomes or are indigent. Over the objections of many veterans' organizations, Congress in 1986 mandated means testing for health benefits, a system which now employs "more than 3,000 different geographic based income eligibility thresholds across the nation."[68] Until 1996, the only people eligible to go to the VHA were economically indigent or had service connected conditions. In 1996 Congress enacted eligibility reform to allow more veterans to enroll in a system that was moving its primary focus from inpatient care toward outpatient and prevention care. At that time, all veterans were eligible for enrollment and were, according to specific criteria (military history, disability rating, income, among others), assigned to a specific Priority Group. Means testing today applies only to Priority Groups 5, 7, and 8. Because of underfunding, being in Priority Groups 7 and 8 effectively denies access to most veterans who have no service-connected disability or too high an income.[69] By 2019, all of these barriers to VHA access had left an estimated 1.53 million veterans without any health insurance and another 2 million reluctant to seek care because of out-of-pocket costs.[70]

To access the VHA and other benefits, former service members must first establish their official status as a "veteran." As Title 38 of the Code of Federal

Regulations explains, a veteran is "a person who served in the active military, naval, or air service and who was discharged or released under conditions other than dishonorable."[71] Someone who served in the National Guard or the Reserves is not considered a veteran by the VA unless they were called to active duty. Eligibility for various forms of VA assistance is much affected by military discharge status.

There are four administrative discharge categories: honorable, under honorable conditions (general), other than honorable, and uncharacterized. An administrative discharge is determined by a service member's commander and assigned without a court-martial. There are two punitive discharges: bad conduct and dishonorable. These cannot be assigned without a court-martial and cover very serious crimes like murder, treason, and rape.

The vast majority of service members receive honorable discharges, even if they were separated for medical reasons before their enlistment contract expired. Other-than-honorable and general discharges are given to people who were "chaptered out" by the military, meaning they left the service before their contract expired for other reasons. This form of discharge has increased fivefold since World War II. As we explain in chapter 1, this is because the military too often punishes soldiers for rules infractions that result from their mental health problems or other service-related conditions.

When the Servicemen's Readjustment Act—known as the GI Bill—was passed in 1944, Congress intended that any solider not discharged under dishonorable conditions should be given access to VA benefits. Veterans' advocates have argued that, with congressional acquiescence, the VA has instead ignored that original intent, as well as its own rules, and deprived hundreds of thousands of service members—more than 575,000 since 1980—of veteran status. These veterans are denied access to all VA programs, including healthcare and education benefits. Since 1980 over 600,000 have received general discharges, which give them only access to healthcare, but not GI Bill coverage or vocational rehabilitation, unless they have a proven service-connected disability.[72] All so-called "bad paper" discharges carry a permanent stigma for the men and women who get them. When veterans leave the military with a DD214 form containing an unfavorable "narrative of separation," they are not eligible for veterans' hiring preferences in public-sector jobs, and may have difficulty finding private-sector employment as well.

Even veterans who have honorable discharges and service-related health conditions must prove their VA eligibility in a system often backlogged with tens of thousands of claims. They have to provide documentation to VBA, often with the help of VSO representatives or lawyers specializing in the field.

They must fill out multiple forms and provide detailed medical evidence to claims processors and doctors who often work for outside contractors, not the VA itself. Too many veterans experience what one VA benefits expert, Paul Sullivan, calls "an adversarial, complex, and burdensome claims nightmare," which breeds anger and frustration among those forced to wait too long for needed healthcare, compensation, or other services. Nevertheless, by 2020, the VBA was dispensing disability payments to 5,905,865 veteran or family beneficiaries; total annual VBA spending on compensation and pensions was $110 billion.[73]

A WORD ABOUT THE P-WORD

On the battleground of veterans affairs, there is much obfuscation about the word *privatization*. As sociologist Paul Starr defined it in a 1988 essay, privatization is a spectrum of activities and goals. At the far end of that spectrum is the complete transfer of public functions or services to a private contractor. At the near end is an incremental shifting of "activities or functions from the state to the private sector" but falling short of any total dismantling of the agency involved.[74] Many Americans associate privatization with the more abrupt change of the first sort in local government service delivery. Their city council decides to contract out garbage collection and disposal. On a particular date, the local Department of Public Works stops picking up the trash. A private contractor like Waste Management takes over the job with its own workforce and equipment.[75]

In the process, as Starr notes, privatizers invariably seek to "break up public employee unions, blaming their members for broader institutional problems." They argue that private provision of public services will make them cheaper, more efficient, and of superior quality. Yet, as Starr points out, these claims belie or obscure well-documented downsides of privatization like lack of outside contractor accountability for inferior performance or the resulting downward pressure on wages and benefits that makes privatization a contributing factor to greater income inequality. Finally, and most perniciously, what Starr calls "privatization by attrition" can starve public education or healthcare programs of needed funds and personnel while further eroding public confidence in government's ability to meet basic citizen needs.[76]

"Privatization by attrition" is an apt description of the continuing threat to veterans' healthcare. Healthcare delivery by the federal government's second-largest agency can't be outsourced as simply or decisively as local solid waste collection. Nine million veterans can't become patients of Kaiser

Permanente or HCA Healthcare, instead of the VHA, overnight. The VHA's scale and complexity as a public institution—plus its popularity among veterans—is such that advocates of privatization must disclaim any intention of shutting down all veterans' hospitals, getting rid of their staff, buildings, and equipment, and shifting all taxpayer-funded treatment to the private sector.[77] Even Concerned Veterans for America, the Koch brothers' front group that helped elect Donald Trump in 2016, says it only favors "VA reforms and more health care options for veterans."[78] Like a smoke screen laid down on the battlefield, this disingenuous stance is designed to obscure, confuse, and mislead. If the damage already done to the VHA, under Presidents Trump and Obama, was better understood, partial outsourcing of its services would be no more welcome than total privatization.

A ROAD MAP FOR THE BOOK

In chapter 1 we describe lesser-known forms of "friendly fire" experienced by men and women on active duty, which create their later need for healthcare and other benefits. Many "wounds of war" like hearing loss, brain damage, or burn pit exposure were not inflicted by any foreign enemy. Instead, they result from the appalling malpractice of the military itself or its private contractors and equipment manufacturers. In this chapter we also explore why and how the workplace culture of the military has become particularly toxic and dangerous for many women. We reveal how conditions at Fort Hood and other such bases can spawn sexual harassment and assault, domestic violence, and self-harm. Rather than ameliorating such conditions or taking responsibility for those damaged by them, the military instead too often resorts to "bad papering"—sending soldiers home with other-than-honorable discharges that deprive them of VA benefits and hamper their later civilian job search.

In chapter 2 we look at life and work after the military, paying particular attention to how the experience of former officers differs from that of enlisted personnel. Military training and skills—and how they are viewed by employers—help shape the range of occupational choices for veterans, from executive positions in the private sector to civil service jobs in law enforcement or the postal service. We explore problematic aspects of the "vet-to-cop" pipeline and the related steering of military veterans into private security jobs. This chapter also describes psychological and physical problems that can hinder veterans' personal relationships, their continuing education, and employability in any field. We conclude by assessing the COVID-19 pandemic's impact on veterans' standard of living and prospects for the future.

In chapter 3, "Stolen Valor," we recount how soldiers deployed in post-9/11 conflicts have been simultaneously put on a pedestal, thanked for their service, and then ill served by a panoply of organizations and individuals purporting to be on their side. We show how self-styled helpers of veterans have at times actually jeopardized their access to better healthcare, a decent education via the GI Bill, and later employment with good working conditions and opportunities for advancement. We also profile a leading advocate for veterans in California who has repeatedly enlisted their organizations in corporate-funded campaigns against bills in Congress or ballot initiatives that would benefit veterans and their families.

In chapter 4 we introduce the American Legion and other veterans' service organizations (VSOs) that comprise the traditional veterans' lobby. We analyze the reasons for their declining membership, community presence, and political clout. We explain how inside-the-Beltway terrain shifted during the Trump administration and the old VSOs found themselves upstaged by a new veterans group backed by the Koch brothers. A series of legislative setbacks and the gravitational pull of the private sector have led some veterans' advocates to seek employment in the healthcare industry, in the same way that former military officers leave the Pentagon and go to work for arms manufacturers. Given the rising cost of VA outsourcing, this new revolving door is no more beneficial for taxpayers than the older one was. Plus, it signals further VSO surrender to the forces of privatization.

As Legion history confirms, there have been recurring generational conflicts between older and younger veterans over politics and postwar treatment of returning soldiers. In chapter 5 we introduce the "new VSOs," which are organized, funded, and led quite differently than the old ones. Whether engaged in nonpartisan advocacy or more party-aligned political work, these new players in the field of veterans affairs attract post-9/11 veterans. They are younger, more diverse in race and gender, and, in some instances, more critical of US foreign and military policy. Our survey of the post-9/11 "veterans' space" identifies who, organizationally and individually, has been occupying it influentially, for better or worse, in recent years. We also explore the personal and political tensions within this generational cohort that arise from differences based on race, class, gender, and ethnicity.

Chapter 6 chronicles VHA privatization, which began under President Obama and was greatly expanded under Donald Trump. As this trend accelerated, VSOs, old and new, failed to mount an effective challenge to bipartisan legislative threats and efforts to discredit the VA in the media. Besieged VHA caregivers, their unions, and supportive patients mounted a "Save Our VA" campaign, which suffered from its own divisions and distractions. In 2020, pandemic conditions slowed the pace of VA outsourcing, while also demonstrating the agency's critical capacity, when properly resourced and staffed, to act as a backup system during national public health crises or smaller-scale emergencies.

In politics, as we show in chapter 7, playing the veteran card is a venerable US tradition, one that has produced twenty-six presidents and, fifty years ago, a big majority of legislators on Capitol Hill. As the overall veteran population has shrunk, the number of House and Senate members with military experience has also declined, although veterans are still disproportionately represented. In recent years both major parties and allied groups have tried to reverse this trend. They've been actively recruiting, funding, and marketing a new generation of service candidates with backgrounds in the military, foreign service, or intelligence agencies. In this chapter we assess whether service candidate success at the polls improves the lot of other veterans or helps the US end "forever wars" and reorder its national priorities.

As chapter 8 reports, 2020 was also a year in which veterans could be found on opposite sides of the barricades in Black Lives Matter protests and presidential election campaigning. Democrat Joe Biden defeated Donald Trump with the help of disaffected active-duty military voters and more veterans than had favored Hillary Clinton four years earlier. Yet the election-year behavior of Trump's most zealous supporters—including some with military backgrounds, now wearing police uniforms, or both—did not bode well for peaceful resolution of domestic disputes in the future. Bipartisan opposition to Pentagon spending cuts that would have freed up billions of dollars for additional COVID-19 relief confirmed the continuing grip of the military-industrial complex, regardless of who occupies the White House or controls Congress.

The contested transition from one administration to another in January 2021 did create a political opening to reimagine veterans affairs. In our conclusion, we assess initial steps taken by President Biden to undo some of the damage done to the VA by Republican appointees under his predecessor. Unfortunately, reversing partial privatization of the VHA was not part of that reform agenda and is not likely to be, without far greater pressure on the White House from veterans, their organizations, VHA union members, and allies on Capitol Hill. During Biden's first term, he also had to contend with a MISSION Act–created panel charged with making binding recommendations about what VHA facilities to improve, expand, or close, decisions likely to have great impact on the agency's future. We end with a salute to men and women who went to war but now, with equal bravery, mount lonely challenges to the military-industrial complex, the source of so many veterans' problems and a never-ending drain on societal resources needed to address real national security threats, like global climate change and future pandemics.

1. A TOXIC WORKPLACE

The military is a collection of very dangerous occupations.
—RICK WEIDMAN, Vietnam Veterans of America

This isn't a regular workplace. You don't have rights.
People are being paid poverty wages to take abuse.
—PAM CAMPOS-PALMA, Vets for the People

On Veterans Day in 2019, the US Army launched a new online recruitment campaign. Its goal, according to the Army's Marketing and Research Group, was to "engage 17- to 24-year-old Gen Z youth, who live at the intersection of 'purpose' and pragmatism" but have "limited knowledge of the Army beyond its role in active combat." This effort represented a shift in strategy from a previous campaign called "Warriors Wanted," whose short ads featured mainly white, male Army Rangers fast-roping out of helicopters into hostile urban terrain in the Middle East as part of "a very modern, ready and lethal force."[1]

The new campaign—called "What's Your Warrior?"—was developed by DDB, a Chicago advertising firm with a $4 billion Pentagon contract. Its video content and high production values were worthy of a trailer for *Call of Duty*, with imagery borrowed from *Star Wars*, *The Matrix*, *Independence Day*, and *Game of Thrones*. Shot in Michael Bay style, in dusty sepia, yellow ocher, and burnished copper, "What's Your Warrior?" depicts the modern Army. The diverse cast of seemingly invincible creatures who flash by are male and female, Asian, African American, Latinx, and white. Some are still brandishing weapons or piloting sleek military helicopters through narrow mountain passes. But this is a different, more futuristic battlefield, where "a million experts" on "hundreds of career paths" create "one Elite organization" which can "take on anything"—by splitting cells, mastering the elements, learning to speak new languages, and commanding "the tools of tomorrow."[2]

Gen Z'ers interested in joining "the most powerful team on Earth" are directed to GoArmy.com. There they can match their own developing personal "skill sets"—as a "wordsmith, mechanic, techie, scientist, engineer, math whiz or problem solver"—with the right MOS, or "military occupation specialty." Not only does GoArmy showcase a dazzling array of available jobs; the site also advertises fringe benefits hard to find in the private sector: free healthcare, housing, and paid vacations while on active duty; and then, as a veteran, free higher education, hiring preferences, home mortgage loan assistance, and, if one becomes eligible, a military pension and VA health coverage. The message is clear: both now and later, "warriors" of this new type are well positioned "to impact the world, their community, and their own lives" in a positive way.[3] They will prevail not only on the battlefield but also in their subsequent civilian careers.

In *The Matrix*, one Hollywood inspiration for "What's Your Warrior?," Morpheus (the character played by Laurence Fishburne) famously warns Neo (Keanu Reeves) that the Matrix "is the world that has been pulled over your eyes to blind you from the truth." He challenges him to distinguish between that "dream world and the real world."[4] In the Army's version of this simulated reality, new recruits can fulfill their video game–fueled fantasies of being conquering heroes and bulletproof slayers of the enemy. At the same time, their enlistment decision augers a successful transition back to civilian life that will be uplifting and empowering, as it has been for some ex-military personnel.

Without a doubt, joining the military offers unique opportunities to escape dead-end jobs and high unemployment communities. There are few federally funded storefront offices, throughout the country, where young people can sign up to become union apprentices in the building trades or get free training to become a nurse, teacher, social worker, or public employee of any other kind. In contrast, the US military operates 1,400 recruiting stations, with almost 20,000 welcoming staffers. Young men and women who sign up with them can see the world, become part of a mission or cause larger than themselves, and mix and mingle with fellow Americans they might never have met or worked with outside of the military. "When we become civilians again, we carry with us our military experience and the things that we learned, including service to our country, dedication, discipline, and camaraderie," says Greg Cope White, a gay former Marine communications specialist, who became a TV writer/producer. "Had I not experienced those things I wouldn't be the person I am today."[5]

What newly minted "warriors" don't discover, until it's too late, is their risk of exposure to lasting mental or physical harm, due to multiple forms of preventable injury. This is true not only for those sent into combat but also for the vast majority of soldiers never deployed abroad. Even when hundreds of thousands of troops were being cycled through Iraq and Afghanistan at earlier stages of the bloody conflicts there, only about 40 percent of those who joined the military were deployed to a combat zone. Of those who were, only 10 to 15 percent ended up in actual combat.[6]

The military claims to be very safety conscious but is actually less so than many private-sector employers whose institutional disregard for workplace protections results in hundreds of thousands of job-related injuries and illnesses every year. Workers in private industry, whether unionized or not, have recourse to protective labor legislation like the Occupational Safety and Health Act, Fair Labor Standards Act, National Labor Relations Act, and Equal Employment Opportunity statutes. Where US unions still represent one-tenth of the workforce, they provide additional recourse, particularly in hazardous environments like firefighting, coal mining, or construction. In the military, workplace representation is nonexistent and legal rights are few. The Pentagon's focus on force readiness and its freedom from regulatory restraint can leave active-duty personnel extremely vulnerable. As Rick Weidman, executive director for Policy and Government Affairs at Vietnam Veterans of America (VVA), puts it, "The military is a collection of very dangerous occupations even for those serving in noncombat roles and far from any battlefield."

A TOTAL INSTITUTION

Men and women in the military first begin to sacrifice their health and well-being during initial training, socialization, and segregation from civilian society. Their new employer is the quintessential example of what sociologist

Erving Goffman calls, in his classic study *Asylums*, a "total institution."[7] Like a prison or traditional religious order, it's an organization that reshapes the thinking and behavior of new recruits by exercising total control over their minds and bodies. In this case the goal is normalizing the idea of taking human life in the name of the state, which involves a deep immersion in a culture of both violence and vulnerability. As former infantry officer Tyler Boudreau puts it in *Packing Inferno: The Unmaking of a Marine*: "Killing is not a by-product or some shitty collateral duty like peeling potatoes or scrubbing the latrine. It is the institutional point."[8]

Because there is—as Lieutenant Colonel Dave Grossman argues in *On Killing: The Psychological Cost of Learning to Kill in War and Society*—"an innate human resistance to killing one's own species," teaching people to kill requires an enormous amount of effort. This is why, as Grossman explains, armies over the centuries have all used similar "psychological mechanisms" to reduce that resistance to rubble.[9] Modern-day conditioning occurs during a carefully constructed indoctrination program that represents a "radical departure from the individual's prior experience" and results in changing the "individual's self-concept."[10] Dennis McGurk, Dave I. Cotting, Thomas W. Britt, and Amy B. Adler describe it as a process that is dependent on "separating the individual from prior contacts and by exposing the individual to a variety of stressors," whether as cadets at an elite military academy or lowly privates in basic training.[11]

In *Un-American: A Soldier's Reckoning of Our Longest War*, Erik Edstrom recalls that, upon arrival at West Point, his first-year class was immediately "isolated, separated from families and support networks. External contact during initial indoctrination was decidedly limited, sheltering us from anything that could temper or make us question military dogma."[12] As part of the process of getting "all-American swimmers, pious altar boys, cauliflower-eared wrestlers, nerdy class treasurers, and Eagle Scouts" ready for eventual deployments, cadets were marched in cadence to this edifying chant: "Left right, left, right, left right KILL! I went to the mosque where all the terrorists pray, I set up my claymore, AND BLEW 'EM ALL AWAY . . . I went to the store where all the women shop, Pulled out my machete, AND I BEGAN TO CHOP! I went to the playground where all the kiddies play, I pulled out my Uzi AND I BEGAN TO SPRAY."[13]

Cruz Gonzalez, the daughter of immigrants from Mexico, underwent this identity change after she joined the Army at age seventeen. Recruiters promised that "it would open doors for me, education-wise" as well as help her parents get citizenship.[14] She described basic training as a process in which the military tries to "degrade you way down so they can build you back up into the form of person they want you to be, so you perform the way they want you to perform." To accomplish this, her instructors were constantly demanding greater physical performance, imposing collective punishment, and using sleep deprivation to strip new recruits of "habits we had as civilians. If one person messes up, everybody's going to do pushups and sit-ups for an hour and a half so that you understand that this tiny little mistake can potentially end all of your lives."

Lack of sleep, Gonzalez recalls, was a very big thing. "You're allowed six hours of sleep, but that doesn't have to be consecutive. If they felt like it, they could let us sleep for an hour and then wake us up. It's exhausting." During her first three weeks of basic training, Gonzalez felt like "a walking zombie. I felt absolutely nothing emotionally and physically." Although things got better for her in Advanced Individual Training, the Cruz Gonzalez who entered the military was not the same person now ready for active duty. After attending her graduation, Gonzalez's brother no longer recognized his sister. "I don't know what they did to her, but that is not your daughter," he told his parents.

The military's mortification rituals often include serious, even lethal, personal assaults. Erik Edstrom came from a suburban public high school outside of Boston, where hazing and bullying were banned and could lead to disciplinary measures targeting either students or faculty. At West Point such behavior was part of the discipline. He saw cadets forced to watch or participate in rituals like guzzling liquids until someone suffered the humiliation of peeing in their pants. Cadets became terrified "of deviating from the herd" because that "brought social shame and the eviscerating notion that one was incapable of adapting" to a new culture of sacrifice and self-mortification.[15]

This happens not only inside elite military academies but also during basic training or boot camp. A report by the Department of Defense (DOD) Equal Opportunity Management Institute defines hazing as "any activity expected of someone joining a group (or to maintain full status in a group) that humiliates, degrades or risks emotional and/or physical harm, regardless of a person's willingness to participate."[16] Among the examples it cites are "water intoxication, public nudity, sleep deprivation, abductions and kidnaps."[17] The DOD report acknowledges that the military can be a breeding ground for such ritualized bullying precisely because of its "hierarchical structure/ high power distance between members, masculine culture, emphasizing discipline and deindividuation, authoritarian leadership, and stress associated with personal deployments."[18]

The "Hazing in the Military" report identifies real-life casualties like Private Danny Chen, who took his own life in 2011 after being brutally harassed and beaten in Afghanistan, and Corporal Harry Lew, who shot himself that same year following severe hazing by fellow Marines.[19] Authors of the report conclude that hazing is "a significant contributor to the cause of death of our most precious commodity, our military members." Among the fatalities not mentioned was Muslim Marine Raheel Siddiqui, who jumped to his death after being abused and humiliated at Parris Island, where several staff sergeants later faced court-martials for their cruel mistreatment of recruits.[20] The military culture of hazing or bullying is not unrelated to male-on-male sexual harassment and assault, as well as the male-on-female version of both. As VA reports confirm, while rates of military sexual trauma (MST) are higher among women, a significant number of male patients also seek treatment for MST.[21]

SEPARATE AND APART

Being in the military can also deprive soldiers of what Carl Castro, director of the USC Center for Innovation and Research on Veterans and Military Families, and Tiia-Triin Truusa call "civilian cultural competencies." As Castro points out, "Every service member has a job but the military goes beyond just providing employment to service members. It is structured so that every entry level position can lead to a career lasting 20 to 30 years until retirement." Service members who want to change careers do so in a very formal manner. Pay is standardized, with every service member getting paid exactly the same for the same job, no matter how brilliantly they shine or how extraordinary they are. There is no such thing as pay for performance in the military.[22] There is far less need to acquire skills like résumé writing or highlighting one's individual skills and accomplishments in a job interview, while in competition with other applicants. Nor do service members learn how to negotiate a better salary, promotion, better benefits, or an annual bonus.

Unlike civilian workers, service members have guaranteed medical coverage via their access to the military healthcare system. They receive subsidized food, housing, and daycare, plus a pension (after a twenty-year career) and access to free education and healthcare, if they qualify and have the necessary discharge status. However, not all benefits of what historian Jennifer Mittelstadt calls the "military welfare state" are as good as advertised.[23] Healthcare for service members and their families has been outsourced through Tricare, which comes with all the shortcomings of other private insurance networks. Base housing can be scandalously defective, as investigative reporter Haley Britzky has documented.[24] Management of many of the military's 134,000 housing units has also been privatized, resulting in unsafe conditions ranging from mice infestation to mold and lead paint exposure.[25] Across the country, soldiers "are choosing to live apart from their families for years at a time or, alternatively, quit the military altogether to avoid having to enroll their children in the underperforming schools surrounding some military bases."[26]

As the Center for a New American Security (CNAS) found, in its study titled "Lost in Translation: The Civil-Military Divide," service members and their families do "find many, if not all, needs met by military facilities: The commissary, exchange, schools, recreation centers, and hospitals provide cheap and convenient services within the boundaries of the base." The resulting social environment is similar to that of insular "gated communities," albeit without much upscale gloss.[27] With the rise of the all-volunteer military, these communities are no longer located everywhere in the country. Instead, they are mainly found in the South, the Southwest, and the Mountain states, where the local setting may be less reflective of national cultural diversity.

When deployed abroad, many service members experience gated community life on steroids. In a combat zone like Iraq or Afghanistan, soldiers rarely went off base to socialize or get to know local people, unless it was in the line of duty. Jeffrey McDowell,* a thirty-seven-year-old Iraq veteran who served in the Army as a geospatial intelligence analyst, recalls that when he was in Baghdad, he rarely ventured off base unless he had "a very good reason to, because it was too dangerous." An Arabic speaker, McDowell did get to know some Iraqis employed at the base in construction or other jobs but, as he recalls, "they were constantly guarded to make sure they weren't planning an attack."

When asked whether being deployed gave him a better understanding of foreign cultures, ex-Marine Alexander McCoy simply laughs. In his view, the notion that veterans have a deeper understanding of global issues because of their overseas service is like saying that college students who spend a semester abroad are now experts on international relations. A self-described Navy brat, McCoy grew up on US bases in Japan and England. In the Marines, he served as an embassy guard in Germany, Saudi Arabia, and Honduras. "When you're in the military, you may get more exposure to the rest of the world than the average American gets," McCoy says. "But you're not living out in the community. You may relate to local nationals, but they are usually deeply embedded in the US military and are not a representative sample."

"The military is very parochial," agrees Army Major Daniel Sjursen (ret.). It fails to give soldiers any genuine understanding of the people they are stationed among or their culture, even during prolonged occupations. "In Iraq, when we first got there, the military's lack of understanding of Iraq and Islam was so obvious—and even obscene—that it became a big source of embarrassment both in the media and Congress, and there was an effort to correct it." That course correction took the form of what Sjursen calls "a CliffsNotes version of cultural immersion." Soldiers received short Power-Point briefings that still prioritized battlefield skills rather than historical knowledge. The take-home message was "There are these Shia and Sunnis, and they hate each other, and it doesn't really matter why, but it goes back to the Prophet."

During his seventeen-year career, Sjursen noticed a distinct lack of curiosity about and even an aversion to all things foreign. Among both officers and enlisted personnel, the spectrum of opinion about "the wusses in Europe," including NATO allies, lurched between three main stereotypes. They were liberal (not good), socialist (even worse), or commie (the very worst). Even nations that did send troops to the Middle East—and suffered casualties there—were viewed as being less aggressive than the United States. According to Sjursen, the crass terms used to describe NATO forces on the same side (e.g., "pussies," "limp dicks") showed "how much concerns with masculinity and impotence play into views of foreigners."

FINANCIAL STRESS AND INSECURITY

A huge source of vulnerability for service members and their families is their financial condition. According to a number of recent studies and surveys, service members tend to have a debt-to-income ratio 10 percent higher than civilians. One 2016 article explained that, although the military expects service members to "keep up with their bills . . . the military lifestyle makes staying out of debt quite difficult." A recent survey found that 27 percent of service members had more than $10,000 in credit card debt. That's compared with just 16 percent of civilians. In addition, more than one-third of military families said they struggle to pay their bills every month.[28] Active duty service members are thus three times more likely than civilians to rely on payday loans; an estimated one in five patronize the payday lenders heavily concentrated around military bases, generating an estimated $80 million a year in fees for this exploitative industry.[29]

Service members struggle with debt for multiple reasons. The first is that military pay, although very reliable, is also low, particularly when one considers the risks of military service. It is tightly regulated and depends on rank, duty assignment, location, number of years in the service, and sometimes special skills. While promotions are also highly regulated, they tend to decrease in frequency as one moves up the ranks. Pay scales and allowances are applied collectively across the board and cannot be affected, as in the private sector, by individual deals or negotiations. Increases in military pay are also tightly regulated and based on the Bureau of Labor Statistics Employment Cost Index (ECI). Congress can also raise military pay, which it did in 2019 with a 3.1 percent pay raise, the largest since 2010.[30]

In 2020 base pay for the lowest-ranking officer—second lieutenant—started at $3,287.10 per month. After twenty years a full-bird colonel or Navy captain could earn $9,530.10 a month. A four-star general's monthly pay after the same amount of time was $15,546.[31] The most junior enlisted personnel earned $1,733 to $2,646 a month.[32] After twenty years a sergeant could earn $3,501.90, and the highest-ranking enlisted person $6,419.40. A private's annual pay ranged from $18,648 to $22,824.[33] Of course, these salaries were supplemented by combat or hazardous duty pay, housing and sometimes clothing allowances, free healthcare, and later educational or vocational training benefits.[34] Military pay may also be tax exempt when service members are deployed. After twenty years, service members are eligible for the kind of defined-benefits pension that has become extremely rare in the civilian sector.[35]

Nevertheless, military service often comes with other distinct financial disadvantages. In modern America most families cannot get by on just one income. The majority of civilian families can try to supplement one spouse's pay with another's income, but constant mobility makes it difficult for a nonmilitary partner in a military couple to "advance in a good paying job." Not surprisingly, the unemployment rate among military spouses is roughly 26 percent.[36] Constant mobility also exacerbates the problems of financial instability and stress. Because service members move so much, and often on short notice, it's harder for them to sell a home and then buy a new one. This forces service members to "pay mortgages on both their old and new homes in order to maintain good credit."[37]

Young men and women who join the military when they are eighteen have little financial experience. In 2013 Lieutenant Colonel Samuel R. Cook of the US Army Reserves studied the link between military suicide and financial instability. Entering the service at a very young age, Cook points out, means that soldiers lack what is known as "financial literacy." They suddenly have a steady paycheck but no "financial guidance or oversight" to help them learn how to manage money, make sound financial decisions, or plan ahead.[38] The financial resources available to them are often precisely the opposite of what they need. As ethnographer Kenneth MacLeish observes in his book *Making War at Fort Hood: Life and Uncertainty in a Military Community*, "Soldiers are a captive market for various semi-predatory retail enterprises that congregate in military towns, such as pawnshops, used car dealers, storefront lenders, credit cards, and other enterprises that seem to exist for the very purpose of destructive spending."[39]

Jose Caballero, who enlisted in the US Navy in 2004 when he was eighteen and served until 2010 as a nuclear reactor operator on the USS *Ronald Reagan*, has firsthand experience of how the cycle of debt consumes and sometimes destroys young sailors. "You enter the Navy at age eighteen and are immediately given a signing bonus of $2,000 back then, or up to $24,000 today. You're eighteen, and you've never seen so much money before—and believe me, the Navy is there to help you spend it." To do this, Caballero says, the Navy and US car dealerships have formed a partnership:

> When we were deployed in the Gulf, there were dealership kiosks set up inside the ship to sell expensive cars to kids who had a steady, guaranteed income and a signing bonus. Their pitch was that the car would be waiting for us in port when we got home. So, kids would get these really expensive cars and have these dramatic payments to make, even though, at that time, we were only making maybe $19,000 a year. By the time you finished your four-year enlistment, you would sit down with a Navy career counselor whose sole job is to get you to reenlist. The counselor would check out your debt-to-income ratio and go, "Wow, how are you going to make this car payment if you get out of the Navy? That's going to be really hard." They would then suggest that there was an easy solution—re-up for four or six more years. And since there is no safety net for new veterans when they get out of the service, people would do it.

In his study Cook found that after the economic recession of 2008, a great many Army families utilized food stamps and food banks. This has persisted well beyond the economic recovery. In February 2018 the Government Accountability Office (GAO) did a report on the use of these programs in the military and found that over twenty-three thousand active-duty troops used the Supplemental Nutrition Assistance Program (SNAP) in 2013, the last year for which such information was available. "About 751,000 food stamp transactions, or almost $80 million in purchases, were completed at military commissaries in 2015." Military families also use the Special Supplemental Nutrition Program for Women, Infants, and Children (WIC). They also qualify for the free and reduced-price lunch programs in on- and off-base schools and child development centers: "In 2015, 24 percent of 23,000 children in U.S. DoDEA schools were eligible for free meals, while 21 percent were eligible for reduced-price meals, according to the GAO."[40] During the recent pandemic, demand for help from food banks that help military families and veterans has dramatically increased.[41]

This reliance on food banks, food stamps, and payday loans not only confirms the difficulty of raising a family on military pay. Accessing off-base services allows service members to cope with financial distress without bringing it to the attention of superior officers. Although the military employs counselors who can help service members and their families deal with financial issues, the fear of losing face, a promotion, or a security clearance discourages many service members from getting such assistance.

A SAFETY-CONSCIOUS EMPLOYER?

The US military presents itself as an employer committed, like any other, to maintaining the highest safety standards. According to *Military.com*, all branches "ensure that safety is constantly focused on and regulations adhered to."[42] In reality the military has a long history of making top-level management decisions—about equipment use, training practices, or toxic exposures—that unnecessarily cause long-term damage. As a result, hundreds of thousands of veterans have developed service-related conditions that require lifelong care as well as partial or total disability payments. And, of course, citizens of other countries who end up in close proximity to US military operations or bases suffer from the resulting toxic environments with little or no compensation for the harm to their health or property.[43]

During his tour of duty as an Army medical corpsman in Vietnam, Rick Weidman of the VVA was one of several million US soldiers exposed, along with Vietnamese civilians, to the deadly herbicide Agent Orange. This left Weidman with diabetes, hypertension, and sometimes debilitating peripheral neuropathy and PTSD. Whenever Weidman, now retired, lobbied on Capitol Hill or talked to journalists about veterans' issues, he always presented them with a pocket guide titled *How to Take a Military Health History*, which is used by VA clinicians.[44] This brochure lists the hazardous exposures associated with each war or period of military service in the last eighty years so that related symptoms can be identified and treated. In addition to Agent Orange exposure in Vietnam, veterans who served during the Cold War found themselves involved in chemical warfare experiments, nuclear weapons testing, and base cleanups with little personal protection.

Between 1990 and 1991, an estimated 697,000 service members, exposed to widely used pesticides and/or releases of the nerve agent sarin, developed what's known as "Gulf War illness." As described in one VA advisory committee report, "This complex of multiple concurrent symptoms typically includes persistent memory and concentration problems, chronic headaches, widespread pain, gastrointestinal problems, and other chronic abnormalities not explained by well-established diagnoses." According to the authors of that report, "No effective treatments have been identified for Gulf War illness and studies indicate that few veterans have recovered over time."[45] As Gulf War veterans have pointed out, the Department of Defense and then VA has a long history of withholding or delaying the release of information on toxic exposures, including those involving depleted uranium.[46] They have also criticized the VA for failing to consider not only human but animal studies on the association of toxic exposures to a wide variety of illnesses.[47]

Infantry veterans from every era have developed later musculoskeletal problems due to the excessive strain placed on their necks, shoulders, knees, backs, and ankles by packs weighing sixty to one hundred pounds, as well as heavy protective armor that imposes a "grinding physical burden of simply moving around."[48] That's why younger veterans suffer from more chronic pain than their civilian counterparts.[49] Added to this, young men and women often survive wounds that would have proven fatal in prior conflicts because of the military's highly advanced methods of battlefield triage and fast transport to field hospitals. They may suffer from what is known as polytrauma— amputation, PTSD, burns, and a traumatic brain injury (TBI), or more— which leaves them burdened with chronic problems like severe pain and mental trauma, requiring extensive care and monitoring for decades, if not their entire lives. Chronic pain also increases the risk of suicide and can spur substance abuse. The rate of opioid overdose deaths among veterans is twice as high as in the civilian population.[50]

The Pentagon also puts service members at risk, even if they never leave an old or new military base. The DOD now lists 126 military installations where water "contains potentially harmful levels of perfluorinated compounds, which have been linked to cancers and developmental delays for fetuses and infants."[51] Fort McClellan, the primary basic training site for all Army women for decades, has been called "the most contaminated place in the United States."[52] Among other confirmed sources of chemically tainted drinking water were Marine Corps bases in North Carolina, including Camp Lejeune. Some soldiers have been exposed to contaminants on newer bases overseas, like Karshi-Khanabad Air Base in Uzbekistan. At this former Soviet military site, "a combination of uranium, jet fuel, and chemical weapons known as 'black goo' oozed from the soil," leaving veterans who served there with "a rash of rare and aggressive cancers."[53]

BURN PIT EXPOSURE

When hundreds of thousands of troops were shipped out after 9/11 to other newly created bases in the Middle East, the risk of poisoning came from the air itself. As former US Marine and Gulf War veteran Joseph Hickman documents in *The Burn Pits: The Poisoning of America's Soldiers*, over two hundred bases in Iraq and Afghanistan used open-air burn pits daily for disposal of thousands of tons of toxic material. These bonfires violated not only Environmental Protection Agency (EPA) air quality standards but the Pentagon's own regulations as well. They "were supposed to be used only as a temporary measure, until trash incinerators would be put in place," but "the Pentagon quickly approved their use . . . for the entire course of the wars." Soldiers regularly exposed to this never-ending "siege of smoke and ash" told Hickman that their only periods of respite occurred "when high-ranking generals or politicians came to visit their bases" and base commanders would put a temporary stop to the burning.[54]

Army Warrant Officer Daniel Tijerina tallied up the contents of burn pits operating near Camp Victory, just outside the Baghdad airport, while pointing an accusing finger at KBR, the Texas-based private contractor responsible for "burning vast quantities of this unsorted waste . . . with no safety controls." According to Tijerina, such waste included human corpses and animal carcasses, asbestos insulation, biohazard materials, cleaning supplies, hydraulic fluids, pesticides, human waste, lithium batteries, computer equipment, tires, trucks, polyvinyl chloride pipes, and many other hazardous materials. Making matters worse, when KBR hastily rebuilt some of the bases that later became burn pit sites, the company did so on land already contaminated by previous Iraqi military use. Rick Lamberth, a retired Army engineer who worked as a construction manager for KBR in Iraq and

Afghanistan, expressed concern about the lack of soil- and air-quality testing. In response, he later testified, "KBR management threatened to sue me for slander if I spoke out about these violations" and was "able to get away with this because the Army never enforced the applicable standards."[55]

In the course of researching his book, Hickman helped organize an academic study of the service records, burn pit exposure, and related health complaints of hundreds of soldiers who served in Iraq or Afghanistan. Seventy-four percent reported acute respiratory issues; the other 26 percent reported they were suffering from even more serious conditions, such as damaged bronchial tubes or throat, lung, or brain cancer. Hickman speculates that Major Joseph R. "Beau" Biden, the oldest son of President Joe Biden, might have been among those Iraq War veterans who later developed brain cancer from burn pit exposure. Major Biden was deployed as a member of the Army National Guard Judge Advocate General's Corps in 2009 after taking a leave from his position as attorney general of Delaware. He was deployed at two bases that "had multiple burn pits that operated around the clock, with no environmental restrictions." A previously physically fit forty-one-year-old, Major Biden suffered a stroke eight months after he returned, and in 2013 was diagnosed with the brain cancer that killed him two years later.[56] He was one of 3.5 million veterans that the VA estimates were exposed to burn pits since 1990.[57]

Unfortunately, in a September 2020 report for the VA, researchers from the National Academies of Sciences, Engineering, and Medicine found "insufficient evidence to determine whether US troops' exposure to burn pits in combat zones is linked to respiratory issues and said there needed to be further studies." Between 2007 and 2020, the Veterans Benefits Administration (VBA) approved only 2,828 burn pit–related disability claims out of 12,582 filed during that period. This 78 percent denial rate sparked mounting outrage among burn pit victims and their advocates. Under pressure from Congress and the VSOs, the VA announced, in August 2021, that it would consider asthma, rhinitis, and sinusitis as being presumptively related to exposure to particulate matter from burn pits in Iraq, Afghanistan, and other countries. These are, however, only a few of the many conditions that have been connected to burn pits. Critics also contend that, among other things, the VA has not considered animal studies when assessing links between these illnesses and burn pit exposure.

While more veterans pursue burn pit–related disability claims and legislation making them easier to prove, some are seeking monetary damages from KBR and Halliburton, its former parent company. In this ongoing litigation and related PR efforts, KBR has tried to shift responsibility for any wrongful injuries or deaths to the military, which can't be sued by service members or their families. During the first decade of the war in Iraq, KBR was awarded nearly $40 billion worth of military contracts, making it the leading corporate beneficiary of the US occupation. (Prior to helping President George Bush orchestrate the US invasion of Iraq, Dick Cheney served as Halliburton's chairman and CEO; when he left the company to become vice president in 2001, he received a $34 million severance package.)[58]

EQUIPMENT FAILURES

In their book *Shattered Minds: How the Pentagon Fails Our Troops with Faulty Helmets*, investigative reporters Robert H. Bauman and Dina Rasor describe a similar failure to protect service members in Iraq and Afghanistan from the risk of TBIS caused by improvised explosive devices (IEDS). According to Bauman and Rasor, the DOD refused to make additional helmet pads available as standard gear for members of the infantry, despite modifying such equipment for special forces troops. The authors estimate that properly engineered padding could have prevented between 300,000 and 400,000 TBIS. Instead, the military undermined a "helmet pad vendor's effort to provide a quality product to the military," which forced many soldiers to order state-of-the-art pads at their own expense or get help modifying their helmets from a nonprofit group called Operation Helmet.[59]

According to *Shattered Minds*, the Army provided adequate protection to "elite troops like special forces, who were," the Army deemed, "quite frankly, smarter" and decided that adding helmet pads to protect "the average troops" was too expensive and not worth the extra cost. This move ended up resulting in "enormous costs to taxpayers. As the Congressional Budget Office estimated, treating patients with brain injuries and PTSD cost the Veterans Health Administration an estimated $2.2 billion during fiscal years 2004 through 2009."[60]

Many veterans suffer from the kind of TBIS that have been linked to worsening tinnitus and hearing loss, problems with cognitive and social function, increased anger, irritability, and sometimes aggression, as well as PTSD. TBIS can cause long-term problems with daily functioning, including maintaining relationships and returning to work. They put people at risk for a host of other conditions like epilepsy, depression, and Alzheimer's disease and increase the risk of death.[61] TBIS can make it much more difficult for veterans to return to and succeed in school and hold on to a good job over the long term.

Due to the failure of personal protective equipment purchased by the Pentagon, two decades of military training and deployment for the occupations of Iraq and Afghanistan produced an epidemic of tinnitus and hearing loss. These two conditions are the reason most veterans, including many who served after 9/11, seek care from the VA, where about 2.7 million patients now have a disability rating for hearing loss or tinnitus.[62] Veterans generally are 30 percent more likely to have hearing problems than those who have never served in the military: every branch of the service, in its own way, subjects exposed enlisted personnel to high levels of noise.

In the case of troops sent to Afghanistan and Iraq, careful use of Combat Arms Earplugs Version 2 (CAEV2) was supposed to shield them from permanent hearing damage. These earplugs were designed by Aearo Technologies, a firm purchased in 2007 by 3M. This Minnesota-based Fortune 500 company has diverse product lines, including items related to fire protection, worker safety, and healthcare. Depending on which end you put in your ear, 3M-made earplugs had different functions: one to block sound, the other to block most battlefield noise while still permitting soldiers to hear one another as well as commands from their officers. Instead of working properly, they proved to be too short for some ears and lacked a protective seal. The fact that 3M knowingly defrauded the federal government when it supplied this defective equipment to the DOD was well documented in a qui tam lawsuit against the company, which was settled for $9.1 million. Now 3M, like KBR, is facing class-action litigation by veterans whose life and work after the military have been adversely affected by their exposure to workplace hazards that could have been reduced or eliminated by a military contractor.[63]

One of the 250,000 plaintiffs is Farid Hotaki, an Afghan American linguist who served two tours of duty in Afghanistan as a Marine and then returned there for another four years as a private contractor. He and his fellow Marine, Colonel Andrew Del Gaudio, explained the kinds of noise that were a constant both on the battlefield and off. In Afghanistan there are vehicles—mine-resistant ambush-protected vehicles (MRAPS) and Humvees—with Caterpillar 12 high-diesel engines, as well as fifty-three Echo Sikorsky helicopters, with their three 4,000-horsepower (for a total of 12,000 hp) engines. And then, of course, there is the noise of 500-pound joint direct attack munitions (JDAM) bombs, which have a huge blast and shock waves, as well as the roar of IEDs.

As ordered, Hotaki says, he and other Marines religiously donned their 3M earplugs, which, like IDs and dog tags, are "inspectable items." They had total faith "that these things work. To be honest, I had faith in every single thing that any one of my senior enlisted or officers would tell me to do or wear." In the heat of battle, Hotaki and other service members didn't necessarily notice their initial hearing difficulty. Once back home, the damage became more apparent. Animal noise or a simple conversation with one of Hotaki's friends or children became unbearable, leading to mounting irritation. "Every time someone talks, I would hear a pulsation and ringing, and I would say, 'Can you talk louder?' And people would say, 'You're telling me I'm talking too loud, and then you're telling me to speak up.'"

Hotaki struggled to find work and began isolating himself from his wife and three children. He sometimes blamed himself for the significant hearing loss in his left ear and the ringing in both ears that never ends. "Were we using the earplugs the wrong way?," he wondered. "Did we put them in wrong?" Then he began reading about the 3M manufacturing flaws and fraudulent practices that left him disabled and realized that a military contractor, hired to protect him and other soldiers from harm, was responsible. By late 2021, three out of four juries hearing bellwether cases against 3M agreed with that conclusion, awarding more than $16 million to just three veterans.[64] Farid Hotaki—and thousands of other plaintiffs in the largest multidistrict litigation ever—hoped that this process of determining the range of damages would lead to an overall settlement, sooner rather than later.

JOB-RELATED TRAUMA

Hearing loss is just one form of job-related trauma, with life altering impact. Between 18.5 and 42.5 percent of service members and veterans returned from Iraq and Afghanistan with some sort of mental health problem: over 18 percent were suffering from PTSD.[65] A number of research studies confirm that almost half of veterans have great difficulty adjusting to the civilian world, with a third "developing mental health problems including PTSD, anxiety disorders and depression."[66]

Some veterans suffer from schizophrenia and bipolar disorder as well as major depression and substance abuse disorders, which, some might argue, are encouraged by a military culture awash in booze. The military often tries to get out of paying for mental health problems acquired or exacerbated by service by claiming that a service member suffers from a "personality disorder" or schizophrenia. Because these may be viewed as conditions that existed prior to military service, the diagnosis may lead to not only a bad paper discharge but also, even if the term of enlistment is finished, a denial of treatment or compensation by the VA. As one report noted: "According to the Department of Defense (DOD), the military discharged 31,000 service members with a personality disorder diagnosis between 2001 and 2010. From 2001 to 2007, the military discharged over 4,000 enlisted service members per year for 'pre-existing personality disorders,' even though some of these veterans may have suffered from early stages of an acquired psychiatric disorder like post-traumatic stress disorder (PTSD)."[67]

All the mental and physical health problems soldiers and veterans experience affect their families and communities. Many of the children of soldiers who have been on multiple deployments—or even one—are also suffering from serious mental health consequences that the military has not addressed. One column by experts in military trauma estimated that more than 2 million children are dealing with the consequences of a parental deployment, injury, mental condition, or death. Between 22 and 35 percent of new recruits have had a parent who served in the Armed Forces.[68]

In 2020, Netflix released a documentary filmed over a ten-year period, which traced the adverse impact of one soldier's career on his two sons. *Father Soldier Son* tells the story of army sergeant Brian Eisch, a struggling single parent in upstate New York, who insisted on deploying to Afghanistan. His absence left his boys, who were sent to live with relatives, anxious and depressed. Eisch returned in excruciating pain from a shattered leg, which was later amputated. His disability made him angry, irritable, and difficult for his family to live with. In a bid to earn his father's favor and regain self-confidence, Eisch's older son, Isaac, enlisted in the army at age eighteen. There he developed behavioral problems of his own and was given an other-than-honorable discharge, which deprived him of the VA coverage his father needed and used.

EMBRACING THE SUCK

Not only does military service expose soldiers and, sometimes, their families to preventable harm; their military socialization discourages many from seeking help for any resulting physical or mental problems. As Carl Castro explains, "The worst thing that can happen to a soldier is 'being on profile.'" This occurs when a soldier is hurt and is put on what is called "temporary profile," which means they are excused from physical training. Rather than welcoming this potentially healing respite, soldiers experience it as a serious stigma. "You're considered to be a 'dirtbag,' a 'malingerer,'" Castro continues. "If you've got a good track record, it's not so bad. If you haven't established yourself, you're nondeployable and thus a shirker and risk not getting a good performance review and a promotion."

"The military magnifies broader cultural ideals about seeking help. No matter what their age, veterans say that they are discouraged from seeking help for even serious medical or mental health problems," writes anthropologist Erin Finley, who works at the San Antonio VA Medical Center. While some branches of the service are trying to address this issue, the message service members receive, Finley explains in *Fields of Combat*, "can run into direct conflict with the need to reach out for help when injured or unwell." She notes that "men may find it difficult to identify with the idea of being traumatized (which can carry the implication of being a victim) or may, when they experience uncontrollable emotion, see it as a threat to their sense of themselves as invulnerable and tough."[69]

This programming in help avoidance begins the moment a young man or woman enters the military. Consider, for example, the "Infantryman's Creed," which makes a clear connection between being a man, being in the military, and enduring pain and discomfort. "I am the Infantry. I am my country's strength in war, her deterrent in peace. I am the heart of the fight. I am what my country expects me to be. I yield not to weakness, to hunger, to cowardice, to fatigue, to superior odds, for I am mentally tough, physically strong, and morally straight."[70] The Marine Corps gives new recruits, known as "poolees," a T-shirt emblazoned with the slogan "Pain is weakness leaving the body."

During his first weeks as a Marine recruit, Michael Rickards began to experience what would become debilitating shoulder pain due to a nerve condition caused by punishing training regimens. The burning, tearing pain he suffered persisted throughout boot camp, combat training, and later classroom training to become a generator mechanic. "You just try to suck it up," Rickards said. "The general attitude was if you went to the medical, you were trying to get out of something, you were just faking it." He admits that he felt the same way about his fellow corpsmen. "Unless something dramatic happened, like someone twisted an ankle or broke a leg, it wasn't real."

If the problem was an emotional one, like alcohol abuse or depression, "it seemed like it could ruin your career," Rickards said. "The weird thing was, in the Marines, everyone seemed depressed. In general, it was just a normal thing, as was drinking." Unable to conceal his shoulder pain any longer, Rickards finally sought medical help. After a year of physical therapy at Walter Reed Hospital and then medical separation from the Marine Corps, he was able to get his symptoms under control. While upset about not being able to complete his expected four-year tour of duty, Rickards was relieved to be out of a situation in which he was constantly hurting himself.

Men aren't the only ones who become adept at sucking it up. While women in the civilian world are quicker to seek medical assistance than men, women trying to prove themselves in the military must be wary of displaying "weakness." After Air National Guard pilot Mary Jennings Hegar was badly injured in Iraq and returned home, she decided to seek help for PTSD symptoms. Because she was still on active duty, she initially hesitated to take this step because she "had always heard that getting help for this type of thing would ruin your career." But she had become fed up with a situation in which "we all had to hide our injuries from the flight doc and live in fear of being disqualified if we admitted to having nightmares." As an officer, she decided that "if I were half the leader I hoped to be, I should set the example and get some help."[71]

A HOSTILE WORK ENVIRONMENT

Women like Hegar now represent almost 20 percent of the active-duty Armed Forces.[72] According to a report by the Disabled American Veterans (DAV), they "must work harder to feel comfortable and accepted within a male-dominated, sometimes hostile work environment defined by archetypical masculinity and are less likely to feel supported by commanders, peers, and civilians alike."[73] Many female veterans—who now comprise 10 percent of the veteran population—are badly scarred by their military service.[74] Reflecting the toll military service takes on personal and conjugal relationships, data from the 2014 Veterans Population Projection Model showed that 19.3 percent of minority veterans were divorced, compared to 9.5 percent of nonveteran minorities.[75] According to the DAV, women veterans are more apt to be divorced than civilian women or male veterans and thus less "likely to have a support system that married military men enjoy." Their incomes are lower than those of male veterans, and more of them live in poverty and qualify for food stamps. Even homeless women veterans have problems unlike their male counterparts because many of them have custody of minor children. "Taken together," the report adds, "these circumstances mean women veterans have more economic stress than men and are more financially precarious."[76]

Women veterans utilizing VA maternity services are three and a half times more likely to have active PTSD, and five and a half times more likely to suffer from depression than civilian women. Pregnant women veterans with PTSD are at higher risk for complications like preeclampsia and gestational diabetes than their civilian counterparts and are more likely to deliver their babies before term. They also suffer from more mental illness and chronic diseases—arthritis and cancers—than civilian women. Plus, their risk for suicide "exceeds that of civilian women by two and a half times, and older women veterans are more likely to die of all-cause mortality than their civilian counterparts." When polled by the DAV, "60 percent of women who served thought their time in the military had negatively impacted both their physical and mental health."[77]

Mistreatment of women in and around the military is not a new phenomenon. Paul Cox, who served in the Marine Corps in Vietnam between 1968 and 1972, recalls that sexism and misogyny were not just part of the military culture but defined it. "If your superior officer thought you were whining or you couldn't hack it, you were a pussy." The few women then serving in the Corps were referred to as BAMS—"Broad-Assed Marines." In Vietnam, as well as Okinawa and Europe, Cox continues, one of the benefits of being part of an occupying army was access to prostitutes. "Your image of women was totally sexualized and defined by uber-masculinity, violent imagery, and disrespect."

Kevin Miller, who was deployed twice to Iraq and once to Bahrain between 2004 and 2006, served in a military that was more diverse. But during his active-duty years, Miller heard constant harangues against women and anyone who was lesbian, gay, bisexual, or transgender (LGBT), plus "a great deal of racist language against Latinos and African Americans, and Native American service members." According to Miller, "the worst thing wasn't being called a woman, it was that you were a queer or gay." While in Bahrain, he also witnessed the kind of misbehavior that would later erupt into a full-blown scandal involving "rampant sex trafficking, housing and pimping of female prostitutes in the Middle East."[78]

As reported by *Military Times* in June 2020, Navy personnel in Bahrain imported prostitutes from Thailand, housed them in taxpayer-funded apartments, and then sold their services to fellow sailors among the 7,300 based there. Navy officials eventually cracked down on this scandalous misconduct, which one admiral called "another black eye for the Navy." It wasn't the first of that sort. The reputation of both the Navy and Marine Corps took a similar hit three decades earlier, thanks to a drunken, off-duty rampage by officers belonging to the Tailhook Association. At "Tailhook '91," as it became known, eighty-three women and seven men were sexually assaulted in a Las Vegas convention hotel, with little or no later disciplining of those responsible.[79]

MILITARY SEXUAL ASSAULT

With many more women in uniform today, military convention guests aren't the only target of misogynist behavior. As the DAV explains, assaults on female soldiers "flourish in an environment where sexual innuendo, gender-based bullying, unfair treatment, low expectations and fundamental disrespect for women flourish."[80] According to the DAV, in 2016 alone, "1 in 23 military women survived sexual assault, 1 in 5 active-duty women reported they experienced sexual harassment or a sexually hostile work environment, and 1 in 4 women veterans reported they suffered sexual trauma while serving in the military. In fiscal year 2017, the military recorded a total 6,769 reports of sexual assault, an increase of nearly 10 percent compared to the 6,172 reports made in 2016."[81] Assaults are even more prevalent in the military service academies. In 2018, 28.5 percent of women and 5.8 percent of men experienced unwanted sexual contact, up from the numbers reported in 2016.[82]

As the issue has gained wider public attention, there have been even more reports of assault. In 2019 the DOD found there were 7,825 sexual assault reports involving service members as victims or subjects, a 3 percent increase over 2018.[83] Reports in which survivors confidentially disclosed an assault without starting an official investigation rose by 17 percent to 2,126.[84] No woman, no matter how high her rank, seems to be immune. Two former military women who became conservative Republican politicians have reported abuse by a superior or a spouse, which they were reluctant to reveal at the time. In 2019 newly appointed Arizona senator Martha McSally helped draw attention to MST by publicly disclosing that she was raped by a fellow Air Force officer.[85] Joni Ernst, an Army combat veteran and the highest-ranking woman in the GOP's Senate leadership, has cosponsored legislation to combat military sexual assault after disclosing past physical abuse by her ex-husband.[86]

The record of the military's response to the epidemic of MST is not reassuring—blaming the victim is the default position. "MST survivors are reluctant to report because it can lead to professional and social retaliation," writes Kristen J. Leslie. "For all survivors who seek redress through their chain of command, they can quickly discover how little they are valued. Reporting can harm one's promotion and ability to remain active duty. In other words, 'the rape was bad, but everything that followed was worse.'"[87] In its Military Assault Fact Sheet, the human rights group called Protect Our Defenders reports that 44 percent of victims of sexual harassment were encouraged to drop the issue, while 41 percent said that the person to whom they reported took no action. "Despite a 22% increase in unrestricted sexual assault reports since 2015, conviction rates have plummeted by almost 60% in the same time frame. In FY 2019, of the 5699 unrestricted reports of sexual assault, 363 (6.4% of cases) were tried by court martial, and 138 (2.4%) offenders were convicted."[88]

Brianna Holman came from a military family in Florida and long dreamed of serving herself, but never anticipated the price she would pay. She enlisted in the Air Force at age nineteen and was assigned to Peterson Air Force Base in Colorado. She served as a medical aerospace technician, working in family health screening patients who were coming in for medical appointments and reporting to and working with other healthcare providers. Holman had hoped to spend her entire career in the Air Force. But during her first year of duty, she was assaulted twice. The first incident occurred after she was offered a drink that was drugged. "During basic training the message was hammered in that, male or female, you trusted your buddies. They had your back, and you had theirs. So yes, I did take a drink from a stranger, but he was an airman, someone whom you were supposed to trust with your life."

Because she felt it was a classic "he said, she said" incident, and maybe even her fault, Holman did not report being raped. Then, a few months later, she started chatting on a dating app with a soldier stationed at nearby Fort Carson. When they finally met up, he too assaulted her. "What were the chances of someone being sexually assaulted twice within only four months—who would believe me?" she berated herself. Far from supportive friends or family, she sought help, admitting to a therapist that she was thinking of killing herself. Revealing details of the first assault, but not the second, she filed what is known as a "restricted report," which does not trigger an official investigation of the incident. After being hospitalized and given further treatment, she was put on a temporary-duty retirement list (TDRL) until the Air Force decided whether she was ready to return to active duty.

After a failed suicide attempt, she turned her report on the first assault into an unrestricted one, which triggered a belated investigation, which led to no action being taken against her assailant. Within three months of leaving the hospital, Holman was medically discharged. "I believe my discharge was politically motivated," she said. "The fact that the process took three months, when it usually takes between nine months to a year, I think was done to save the squadron commander and superintendent embarrassment. I was one of two airmen who had tried to die by suicide within three months."

Holman's experience is sadly familiar to survivors of sexual abuse and violence at one of the largest military bases in the world, Fort Hood, in Killeen, Texas. Since January 2016, there have been more than 159 noncombat deaths among soldiers at Fort Hood, including 7 homicides and 71 suicides. More troops have been homicide victims on and off the sprawling Army base than died in combat zones during the same period.[89] As US Army Secretary Ryan McCarthy was forced to publicly acknowledge, Fort Hood suffered from some of the highest rates of murder, sexual assault, and harassment anywhere in the Army.[90]

One of the most horrific cases involved Army Specialist Vanessa Guillen. Guillen's complaints about sexual harassment by a fellow soldier were ignored. Her assailant, who ended up shooting himself, finally killed her, hiding her partially dismembered body in a box, which was not discovered until two months later. Guillen's mother called for the creation of "an independent agency for members of the military to report sexual harassment and assault" because of the inadequacy of the Army's own response to her twenty-year-old daughter's complaint.[91]

In response to such demands, McCarthy created an independent panel to determine whether Fort Hood was living up to the Army's commitment to "safety, respect, inclusiveness, diversity and freedom from sexual harassment." The commander of the fifty-five thousand troops stationed there was removed and reassigned—and denied a pending transfer and promotion elsewhere. In December 2020, results of the Army's own internal investigation were released. According to Secretary McCarthy, there were "major flaws" at Fort Hood, and the base's command climate "was permissive of sexual harassment and sexual assault." Investigators interviewed more than five hundred female soldiers and found that ninety-three had credible accounts of sexual assault, but only fifty-nine had been reported.

As a result of their report, more than a dozen Army officials were fired or suspended.[92] Vanessa Guillen's death—and the larger Fort Hood scandal—spurred renewed congressional interest in passing legislation that would take sexual assault case investigations out of the hands of local commanders. "I hope it makes an impact, but I'm not sure," observes Ellen Haring, a retired Army colonel and research fellow at the Service Women's Action Network. "It doesn't get to the root of the problem, which is why are the assaults happening in the first place?"[93]

A SUICIDE MACHINE?

In her memoir about serving in Iraq as an Army linguist, Kayla Williams describes the moment in 2004, after she returned home, took a gun into the bathroom and considered killing herself. She writes eloquently about all the things in her life that she could not control: her memories of "men screaming, thrashing, bleeding on the ground"; her anger, which "flared up unexpectedly." Assailed by trauma, she could not imagine "going to the chain of command in my unit. . . . I couldn't admit these feelings of weakness in front of my leaders or—worse—my soldiers." What she could control, she thought, was her ending.[94]

Williams didn't pull the trigger on that fateful day, but many other service members have, making suicide a more serious threat than dying in combat. Although the military suicide rate has typically been lower than that in the civilian world, for the first time in history, American service members have had higher suicide rates than civilians. In 2012, after a decade of war in Iraq and Afghanistan, the DOD released statistics documenting that suicides had reached a then all-time high of 349 that year, up from 301 in 2011.[95] Those who had deployed only once accounted for most of the suicides. Those with two or more deployments were also among the statistics, but a third of those who died by suicide had never deployed at all. "This suggests," writes Kenneth MacLeish, "both that some cumulative effects of stress only surface with time, and that the pressures of protracted war taxed the full breadth of the military, not only those who have deployed to war zones."[96]

Despite $1 billion in DOD spending on the problem, the suicide rate, a decade later, was higher, not lower. In 2018, 541 service members in active-duty and Reserve units killed themselves. Within the active component, the suicide rate was 24.8 per 100,000 personnel. In the Reserves, the suicide rate for 2018 was 22.9 per 100,000, and in the National Guard, it was 30.6 per 100,000.[97] In 2017 there were 186 suicides among military spouses and dependents. In 2021, amid "continued war zone deployments, national disasters, and violent civil unrest," 580 soldiers died by their own hand, a 15 percent rise from the previous year.[98]

Suicide is also a significant problem after people leave the military. According to a comprehensive report conducted by the VA, veterans are 1.5 times more likely to die by suicide than nonveterans, and women veterans are 2.2 times more likely to die by suicide than civilian women.[99] A more recent report by Brown University's Costs of War Project, utilizing data from both the VA and the DOD, found "that four times as many men and women who have served in the US military have died by suicide than were killed in post 9/11 wars."[100] Costs of War researchers estimate that the total suicide toll among veterans and service members during the past two decades is more than thirty thousand.[101] As we've seen, there are multiple physical and mental problems that can lead to suicide, in the military and afterward. These include chronic pain—from the incessant ringing in one's ears to searing back, neck, shoulder, foot, and knee pain—and emotional problems like PTSD or MST, or those that result from a host of other physical ailments.

An additional factor is military socialization that helps soldiers overcome the fear of death, while discouraging them from seeking professional help for treatable mental health issues. As the authors of one study explain, "a lethal or near-lethal suicide attempt is extremely fear-inducing and often involves intense physical pain." Among people contemplating suicide who have past experience with "painful and provocative events," the fear and pain involved "may become less aversive and easier to tolerate." According to this study, current and former members of the military are more suicide-prone because their "combat exposure and training can cause habituation to fear of painful experiences, including suicide."[102]

Adding to this risk is the privatization of military healthcare and poor screening of transitioning service members. On military bases, there is a severe shortage of mental health personnel. Since 2012 the Military Health System (MHS) has sustained more than $70 billion in cuts, even as overall federal and private health spending showed steady growth. In 2020 the military budget, which was higher than ever before, included proposed cuts of some $2.2 billion to the MHS.[103] In 2019, thousands of uniformed MHS staff positions had already been eliminated.[104] In 2020 an audit by the DOD's inspector general found that the military had failed to address $552 million worth of unfunded requirements at sixty military medical treatment facilities (MTFs) and would, in the future, need to spend $14.8 billion to maintain health services necessary for force "readiness."[105] As overall DOD spending continues to rise, cuts in the budget for military healthcare can only be described as pennywise and pound foolish, due to the costs of treating these same underserved patients later on, when they become veterans. Of course, by then, it's a budgetary problem for the VA, not the DOD.

In 2018, the White House directed the DOD and VA to provide veterans with "seamless access to high quality mental healthcare and suicide prevention services as they transition, with an emphasis on the 1-year period following separation."[106] To accomplish this goal, the Pentagon was supposed to do a suicide risk screening and mental health assessment of every soldier undergoing a final "Separation History and Physical Exam" before mustering out. Instead, as the DOD's own Inspector General (IG) discovered three years later, the Pentagon screened only about one-third of transitioning troops—30 percent in 2019 and 34 percent in 2020—despite the fact that they face an overall risk of suicide that is three times higher than among active-duty military personnel. As a result of this lax approach, arranging "continuity of mental healthcare" became much more difficult for the DOD's downstream partner, the VA.[107]

BAD PAPERING

Helping former soldiers deal with physical or mental conditions acquired or exacerbated during their military service is far more difficult when they have "bad paper." Other-than-honorable discharges punish them for the very problems military service often creates. This results in veterans not getting much-needed help from the healthcare system best able to care for them. In civilian life, when a coal miner or construction worker gets fired from a hazardous job—for cussing out a supervisor, fighting with a coworker, or engaging in some other misbehavior—their loss of employment doesn't render them ineligible to receive state or federal workers' compensation for a documented job-related injury or illness, like black lung or asbestosis.

Yet in each branch of the US military, when you're drummed out for misconduct in uniform, the punishment is loss of similar benefits—including VA healthcare, disability pay, and access to GI Bill programs that make higher education and housing more affordable for those who have served. As noted earlier, about 575,000 former service members have been discharged under conditions "other than honorable," a determination too often made without benefit of any consistent application of standards across military branches or even individual commanders within the same branch.[108]

In the Vietnam era, many bad paper cases involved African American soldiers targeted for disciplinary action because of their role in the antiwar movement and its most militant protests. Between World War II and repeal of the military's "Don't Ask, Don't Tell" policy in 2011, an estimated 100,000 LGBTQ service members were discharged for alleged misconduct, leaving most of them with bad paper as well.[109] The men and women most adversely affected today are post-9/11 veterans who need specialized treatment for TBIS or PTSD acquired during repeated combat deployments or through military sexual assault. Service members who might have performed well before experiencing such physical and mental wounds often misbehave as a result of them—getting into fights, going AWOL, or abusing prescription drugs and alcohol. These veterans need VA help and, according to Swords to Plowshares, are "more likely to have mental health conditions and twice as likely to commit suicide."[110] It is very hard for a service member to receive a discharge upgrade from the military once they become a civilian, without a long legal fight.

Consider, for example, the case of thirty-six-year-old ex-Marine Tyson Manker, who became the lead plaintiff in a class-action lawsuit handled by the Veterans Legal Services Clinic at Yale against the Navy appeals board. This board considers bad paper cases and, according to Manker, denied discharge upgrades to veterans with PTSD diagnoses whose enlistments were terminated due to relatively minor misconduct. Manker started out with an exemplary service record. He was the top-rated Marine in his platoon, the first promoted to corporal, and then, during the 2003 invasion of Iraq, was put in charge of his own squad.

At the end of his combat deployment, he was given a one-page questionnaire to screen for posttraumatic stress. As reported by the *New York Times,* his completed form disclosed personal exposure "to nearly every type of trauma listed, including seeing dead civilians and Marines, killing enemy fighters and civilians, and experiencing nightmares and hyper vigilance."[111] There was no response from the Marines. Yet his commander acted much faster when Manker was caught smoking marijuana back in the United States, near the end of his enlistment period. His other-than-honorable discharge pitched him back into civilian life with none of the social supports that VA coverage and GI Bill benefits provide.

That's a fate that Manker shared with 125,000 other post-9/11 veterans, in part due to pressure on lower-level officers to rid the military of soldiers who cannot be quickly deployed. Daniel Sjursen, who commanded troops in Iraq and Afghanistan, explains the organizational mindset behind this: "We are in the business of war. We're not babysitters of problem children. So let's find the fastest way to get rid of everyone who's extraneous and not supporting the mission." If a junior officer is responsible for a unit with a "low readiness rate or too many disciplinary problems," that can damage his or her own career advancement. According to Sjursen, some commanders also use other-than-honorable discharges to send a message to service members they believe are shirkers. Their attitude, he says, is: "We're going to teach them a lesson. If you do X, Y, or Z, we're going to be tough—this will not just get you out of the Army; you're not going to have a good life."

Fortunately, Tyson Manker had supportive friends and family who cared about his well-being during a period of civilian misfortune that included a random, near-fatal stabbing attack. He was able to get costly private treatment for anger, depression, suicidal thoughts, and substance abuse caused by PTSD. With the help of student loans, Manker put himself through college and law school, and became a licensed attorney and business law professor in Illinois. In 2016 he became national coordinator of Veterans for Bernie and also ran for district attorney in a heavily Republican county in rural Illinois. His platform called for greater use of court diversion programs for veterans guilty of minor crimes. In late 2021, the class-action suit filed on Manker's behalf was settled favorably, on a preliminary basis. Subject to final federal court approval, the Navy agreed to review, on a case-by-case basis, discharges and status-upgrade procedures for thousands of former service members with behavioral or mental health conditions who are eligible to benefit from the settlement.

THE MARK OF CAIN

Kristofer Goldsmith is another veteran punished with a bad paper discharge. In his case, it was a general discharge under honorable conditions that did not deprive him of VA healthcare but did deny him access to GI Bill benefits. As a patriotic high school senior, Goldsmith idolized people in uniform. As soon as he could enlist, he joined the Army, and by January 2005 he was in Iraq, "trained to blow stuff up." His first forays into Sadr City, located on the outskirts of Baghdad, were quickly disillusioning. Two battalions before his had a casualty rate of 40 percent in that hostile Shiite neighborhood. Goldsmith became "pissed off at the Army for not letting us shoot back" more of the time and felt betrayed by his own "foolish belief that the Iraqis would be happy to have us there. . . . Hate isn't a strong enough term to describe what I was feeling for these people." Still a self-described "hyperconservative," he became increasingly angry about civilians back home not "appreciating what me and my buddies were going through."

Prior to enlisting, Goldsmith had generally refrained from alcohol and drug use because of addiction problems within his own family. But during his midtour leave, he began downing vodka like it "was a cleansing agent. I was cleaning Iraq out of me—the smell of dead bodies and sewage and oil fires." Burn pit exposure had so scarred and calcified his sinuses that he had to have surgery; his military doctor told him he "should never go back into the desert" and should seek a medical discharge instead. By January 2007 his life had become "drinking, getting into fights, and constantly contemplating suicide." And that was before President George Bush announced a troop surge in Iraq and his related "stop loss" policy, which suddenly aborted Goldsmith's plan to leave the military and return to school.

After hearing the news that he was about to be deployed again, even though his original enlistment contract was about to expire, Goldsmith began suffering panic attacks. He loaded up on the leftover Percocet from his sinus surgery, but was rescued in time and sent to the psych ward of a military hospital. Soon he was facing military discipline for malingering and not shipping out with his old unit. Eventually he was given a general discharge. The once proud, confident, and physically fit young man who had risen to the rank of sergeant found himself back home on Long Island, working with his younger sister as a part-time pizza delivery driver.

With help from the VA, Goldsmith spent five years putting his life back together. When he felt confident enough, he applied to school and got into Columbia University, taking out personal loans to finance his education. Like Manker, Goldsmith had the help of family and friends. Many other veterans aren't so lucky. Their struggle with painful legacies of military service can cast a long shadow over personal relationships and later civilian life and work.

2. LIFE AND WORK AFTER THE MILITARY

He was a war veteran. He was a Marine. He saw some pretty bad things, and a lot of people say he had PTSD, and that's a tough deal. . . . People come back [but] . . . they're never the same.
—PRESIDENT DONALD TRUMP ON IAN DAVID LONG,
a veteran he called a "sick puppy" after Long killed
twelve people in November 2018

The reality is veterans are incredible assets to any line of work.
—LIEUTENANT GENERAL MICHAEL FERRITER,
president and CEO of National Veterans Memorial and Museum

Any contemporary discussion of how millions of veterans are faring—at work, in the community, or in their personal lives—quickly leads to contested political terrain, where the fog of war is thick and confusing. Are veterans good workers, with disciplined habits and strong leadership skills, or men and women so traumatized by military life that as civilians, they have trouble finding housing, holding a steady job, paying their household bills, or completing their GI Bill–financed studies? Are they solid citizens, ready to start their own business, become corporate leaders, and then run for

Congress? Or do service-related conditions like PTSD, as President Trump once implied, make them more prone to harming themselves and others? Does their experience in civilian life vary depending on whether they had a twenty-year military career or served for shorter periods? Does belonging to the officer class help facilitate military-civilian transitions? Does being working-class, female, or nonwhite, from the enlisted ranks, make that same shift more difficult? Do veterans fare better in the more unionized public sector or the largely nonunion private sector?

In January 2019 the standoff between Democrats and Republicans in Washington triggered a federal government shutdown affecting 800,000 workers. It was accompanied by a media skirmish between two former military men, both on the federal payroll, which highlighted contrasting views of veterans. One combatant was Robert Wilkie, the Trump appointee in charge of the VA, and the other was Ed Canales, who suffered severe combat-related injuries during an Operation Desert Storm tank battle in 1991. During the federal shutdown three decades later, the VA—like the DOD—already had its funding in place. So the 300,000 staff members of the Veterans Health Administration (VHA)—a third of whom are veterans—were still reporting for duty, caring for patients, and getting paid as usual.

This was not the case for 150,000 veterans employed by other federal agencies, a third of whom had a service-related medical condition. Many were feeling the economic pinch, as were veterans and thousands of active-duty military families dependent on interrupted programs like Federal Housing Assistance, food stamps, or WIC—the nutritional program for women, infants, and children. As the shutdown dragged on, Canales, a veterans' liaison officer at the Bureau of Prisons, started getting more calls from fellow members of the American Federation of Government Employees (AFGE) who were upset or depressed about the growing financial pressure on their families. In his capacity as an AFGE local union president, Canales told NBC News that the federal government furloughs were a "shameful" slap in the face of "every veteran who has served their country" in uniform or as a civilian. "If this shutdown does not stop," he predicted, "we're going to have fatalities. We're going to have suicides."[1]

This elicited a stern rebuke from the top federal official responsible for the health and welfare of 19 million veterans. In an official VA press release brimming with indignation, Secretary Robert Wilkie accused Canales of "employing insulting and misleading stereotypes about veterans" that were particularly damaging to "those attempting to enter the civilian workforce following their service." He demanded that the AFGE apologize for its lack of "proper respect for our nation's heroes" and stop trafficking in "shopworn canards" that "veterans and their advocates are continuously fighting." According to Wilkie, "The notion that most Veterans are so fragile from their service that the slightest hint of hardship can push them to the brink of mental breakdown or even self-harm is preposterous"—part of the "veteran as victim myth." He proceeded to enumerate "the true character traits of those who've worn a military uniform," including being "models of civic engagement, holding stronger ties to their communities and volunteering and voting at higher rates than their non-Veteran counterparts."[2] According to the VA leader, the 2019 unemployment rate among veterans was far "lower than the national average" precisely because companies hire so many of them "for complex and demanding jobs" due to "their leadership ability and work ethic."

One irony of Wilkie's dressing down a fellow veteran for stereotyping other veterans was the fact that his own boss had recently stigmatized former soldiers in far more dramatic fashion. In November 2019, after twenty-eight-year-old Ian David Long walked into a country music bar in Thousand Oaks, California, and fatally shot twelve people, President Trump quickly pronounced him "a very sick puppy." With little actual knowledge of Long's medical history, Trump confidently explained, "He was a war veteran. He was a Marine. He was in the war. He served time. He saw some pretty bad things, and a lot of people say he had PTSD, and that's a tough deal. . . . People come back—that's why it's a horrible thing, and they're never the same."[3] On that occasion Trump's comments elicited no reproach from Wilkie but did stir criticism from veterans, across the spectrum, who objected to their being described as damaged goods.

Over the years such negative labeling has been critiqued by sociologist and Vietnam veteran Jerry Lembcke in several books, including *PTSD: Diagnosis and Identity in Post-empire America* and *The Spitting Image: Myth, Memory, and the Legacy of Vietnam*. In the latter he argues that "by broad-brushing Vietnam veterans as crazy, prone to violence, and otherwise disabled by the war, all veterans were stigmatized and pushed to the margins of American consciousness."[4] Former Marine Anuradha Bhagwati, who was featured in a 2021 PBS documentary called "American Veterans," defended her generational cohort against similar stereotyping. She describes the military as "an extraordinary institution that draws so much talent." In her role as a training officer, Bhagwati was "just completely wowed by my Marines every day. It's remarkable, the level of excellence, the level of initiative, and of problem solving. I just don't see that in everyday civilian life."[5]

Similarly, Kristen Rouse of the NYC Veterans Alliance argues that former soldiers will bring "energy, talent, and discipline to any organization." As she told a group of human resource directors at a TD Bank–sponsored event in New York City, twenty-three years of military service provided her "with essential leadership, team-building skills, and job training." She assured her audience that most post-9/11 veterans are similarly adept at "navigating complex systems, rules, and procedures," plus many know how to "step into leadership roles that go well above their rank and assigned position."[6]

THE OFFICER CLASS ADVANTAGE

No matter how many leadership skills they mastered in the military, few veterans, among the 10.1 million in the US workforce, become captains of industry or high-ranking managers, unless they served as officers. The social structure and job stratification that veterans encounter in civilian life is no different than that of the military itself, which West Point graduate Andrew Bacevich reminds us "is a hierarchy, a class society, with the working class in the enlisted ranks." Within that hierarchy, military training and indoctrination of enlisted personnel is much focused on developing what another retired officer calls "a capacity for two tasks—comply and execute."[7] As David Vine, author of *Base Nation*, notes, even the layout of military bases highlights the distinctions between officers, who issue orders, and those trained to follow them. "A form of class segregation is strictly enforced in on-base housing," Vine explains. "Rank and pay grade determine the size and quality of one's quarters, and officers are usually housed in different neighborhoods or residential complexes from the enlisted troops. Officers also often have their own clubs, dining halls, and even gym changing rooms."[8]

Officers, who comprise just 18 percent of the military, are far more likely to land white-collar jobs in business or government than any enlisted man or woman.[9] As retired Army major Danny Sjursen observes, "when officers get out, jobs come looking for *them*. . . . Corporate headhunters sign up many young officers—especially West Point grads—for good-paying, upwardly mobile, middle-management jobs in New York, LA, Houston, or Chicago. Military service . . . is seen by employers as a positive, a stepping stone to future management positions." Sjursen's own peers could be found "working for Texas oil firms, managing a Walmart, trading stocks on Wall Street, and finishing up an MBA at Harvard." The soldiers who served under him in Iraq and Afghanistan had more limited employment opportunities. When those "average Joes got out, they searched desperately for civilian work," because "delaying college to drive a Humvee or kick in doors isn't exactly a plus on most job applications."[10]

In contrast, officers who served as highly trained pilots in the Air Force or Navy long had a smooth glide path to well-paid unionized jobs in commercial aviation.[11] Among them was former fighter pilot Chesley Sullenberger (aka Captain Sully), a leading member of the Air Line Pilots Association who gained international fame in 2009 when he landed a crippled US Airways plane in the Hudson River, with no injuries to passengers or crew. Other officers leave the military and lay claim to a disproportionate share of leadership positions in corporate America. A 2010 study published in the *Harvard Business Review* found that "former officers attain chief executive officer positions in major corporations at three times the rate of their representation in the male population."[12] FedEx, Coca-Cola, and USAA, the financial services provider for veterans and military families, are among the big-name firms that have installed former officers in their top ranks and embraced military leadership principles.

Navy veteran Ralph J. Roberts founded Comcast and built it into the largest cable TV provider in the nation; his company is now part of the media giant known as Comcast/NBCUniversal, which continues to prioritize veteran hiring.[13] Former Army captain Robert McDonald became one of the most successful Fortune 500 executives with a military background during his thirty-three years with Procter & Gamble. After he retired in 2013, he returned to government service as secretary of Veterans Affairs. In a 2019 House speech, West Point graduate Mark Green, a medical doctor and Republican congressman from Tennessee, paid tribute to the career success of others who graduated with him. Green's not-atypical cohort at the academy included, of course, nearly twenty generals, active or retired, but also judges, state legislators, university administrators, and "22-plus presidents and CEOs of major corporations."[14]

After his own retirement with the rank of major, Green also became a CEO, heading up a company that provides emergency room staff for hospitals. Danny Sjursen's more critical look at Green's graduating class confirms that it produced "influential leaders in Congress, corporate America, the Pentagon, the defense industry, lobbying firms, Big Pharma, high-end financial services, and even security-consulting firms."[15] Many of these corporate leaders, like Green, not only promote VA privatization but also adamantly oppose any serious attempt to reproduce the military or veteran healthcare system or educational benefits in the civilian sector. Determined to make sure that former enlisted men and women never get a chance to experience socialized services outside the military setting, he argued on Twitter that "socialized medicine will not only entail a massive government expansion into the private life of every American: It will also place a tremendous burden on the backs of American taxpayers."[16]

Few members of the class of '86 wielded more influence in the Trump era than Mark Esper, Trump's last secretary of defense, and Mike Pompeo, who first served as CIA director and then became secretary of state. Pompeo transitioned to the Trump administration after his position as a Kansas congressman much favored by Koch Industries. Esper made good use of the revolving door in Washington, DC, that enables former officers to gain lucrative employment with Pentagon contractors and, in his case, return to the DOD as Army secretary and then its top civilian manager. He worked at the Heritage Foundation and performed staff jobs on Capitol Hill and at the Pentagon. Prior to his nomination by Trump, Esper spent six years as Raytheon's vice president for government relations, making him the top lobbyist for the third-largest defense contractor in the world. At his Senate confirmation hearing, Esper refused to recuse himself from participating in DOD decisions involving his former employer and was asked not a single question about ongoing military operations in Afghanistan and Iraq. The Senate approved his appointment by 90 to 8.[17]

As the Project on Government Oversight (POGO), a nonpartisan research group, documented in 2018, nearly four hundred former high-ranking Pentagon staffers, like Esper, took contractor jobs in the previous decade; nearly a quarter of them landed at Lockheed Martin, Boeing, Raytheon, General Dynamics, or Northrop Grumman. In these new positions, POGO found, they utilize relationships with former colleagues to help conflate "what is in the best financial interests of defense contractors—excessively large Pentagon budgets, endless wars, and overpriced weapons systems— with what is in the best interest of military effectiveness and protecting citizens."[18]

Personal transitions often have the seamless feel of Colonel Dan Sauter's move from one wing of the military-industrial complex to another. When Sauter retired as chief of staff for the Thirty-Second Army Air and Missile Defense Command, he didn't go to work for Walmart, Amazon, or any other veteran-friendly firm hiring thousands of low-wage workers. He made a beeline for Lockheed Martin, which manufactures the same Terminal High Altitude Area Defense (THAAD) system that his old unit used. His new employer soon tasked him with overseeing its installation in Saudi Arabia, after that nation's $1.5 billion equipment purchase. Al Lee, director of quantitative analysis for the salary website Payscale.com, explains such moves thus: a key skill of former military people transitioning to top aerospace companies and weapons makers "is that they understand how to work with the government and the military."[19]

The West Point classmate of Sauter, Esper, and Pompeo who helped the latter two land in Trump's cabinet is David Urban, a football player at the academy who was later awarded the Bronze Star during Operation Desert Storm. After serving in the military, Urban became a corporate lawyer and then chief of staff for a US senator. For the last twenty years, he's been a high-priced lobbyist for clients including Comcast, Walgreens, Hewlett Packard, and Raytheon. Urban was an early backer of Trump's 2016 presidential campaign, served as a senior campaign adviser, and helped his candidate become the first Republican to carry Pennsylvania in three decades. After promoting his former classmates for Trump cabinet positions, Urban was particularly well positioned to help Raytheon—his major client and Esper's former employer—sell weaponry to Saudi Arabia and the United Arab Emirates, a deal Congress tried to block.

In 2019 that $8 billion deal received an emergency waiver from the State Department, despite the Saudis' past deadly use of Raytheon missiles and bombs against civilians in Yemen. This action followed a one-on-one meeting between Pompeo and Raytheon's CEO Thomas Kennedy, who the year before had correctly observed that Trump's first term was "the best time that we've ever seen for the defense industry."[20] The resulting waiver sought by Kennedy was defended by Pompeo as being absolutely necessary "to keep America safe." When the secretary of state was queried about Urban's behind-the-scenes role, he denied any improprieties and instead vouched for his former classmate's sterling character as "an American patriot."[21]

A WORKING-CLASS WORLD

Blue-collar veterans who have been trained to drive a vehicle, maintain equipment, or provide security rarely end up at the nexus of politics and business inside the Beltway. When they leave the military, they usually return to hourly employment in the private or public sector. According to the Pew Research Center, 7.2 percent of employed veterans work in installation, maintenance, and repair occupations, versus 3 percent of employed nonveterans. Veterans are also five times as likely as nonveterans to work in the federal government or the defense industry.[22] The top twenty public and private employers of former military personnel are concentrated within the defense and aviation sectors.[23]

A Census Bureau study of how veterans fared after discharge between 2000 and 2014 found a small number working in mining and an even smaller percentage landing jobs in finance and professional, scientific, and technical services (where, after ten years, they might be earning as much as $110,000 a year). Far more veterans find employment in the retail sector, hospitality and food services, transportation, warehousing, and manufacturing, where salaries might start at $17,000, $22,000, or $24,000 a year and rise to $32,000, $43,000, or $47,000 after ten years.[24] These pay ranges show why, according to the Economic Policy Institute, an estimated 1.8 million of the 9 million veterans in payroll jobs—that's one in five—in 2017 would have benefited from an increase in the federal minimum wage from $7.25 to $15 an hour. This study of veteran employment outcomes also confirmed that "the federal government is consistently one of the better paying employers" of veterans due to salary levels two or three times higher than those in the private sector. The average income for those who had worked in the federal government for ten years was over $85,000 a year.[25]

Charles Szypszak, a professor at the University of North Carolina at Chapel Hill and a former Marine, estimates that about 14 percent of all public service employees are veterans. This makes them "a major part of the rank-and-file of functioning government," even if they "are rarely found in public policy making positions." According to Szypszak, "Veterans are especially well represented within federal agencies. More than 600,000 are employed in the executive branch, about 30 percent of its total employees. They comprise a large segment of civilian employees in the Department of Defense, Veterans Affairs, Homeland Security and Transportation, and many are employed in the Interior and Justice Departments and the General Services Administration."[26] Since World War II, the federal government has given hiring preferences to qualified veterans, which does not guarantee a job but does give an applicant with military experience priority in the appointment process.[27] As a result, about one-third of the 300,000 staff members of the VHA are veterans working in jobs ranging from nurse, physician, nursing assistant, and therapist to clerical worker and building maintenance. As described in chapter 6, this helps create a unique culture of empathy and solidarity between patients and providers that has no counterpart anywhere else in the US healthcare system.

The US Postal Service, with a workforce that is one-fifth Black, employs 113,000 veterans and counts military service as prior employment.[28] This means that, unlike in the private sector, the postal service considers military work to be legitimate work experience, so a veteran doesn't start with a blank slate in a new job.[29] As William Burrus, the first Black president of the American Postal Workers Union (APWU), points out, "The post office has permitted millions of African-Americans to better themselves" in stable employment, which today provides an average salary of $55,000 a year.[30]

Keith Combs, the president of APWU's 1,500-member Detroit local, comes from a family of veterans and is among those African Americans who took this route after leaving the military. In his view, "military values like hard work, showing up on time, and taking pride in your work sets you up perfectly for postal jobs." In addition to the preferential hiring treatment veterans get when they apply, Combs explains, veterans who are disabled, "like many I work with in Detroit, get special consideration too. And once they get here, they get the hard-won benefits of our union, including generous medical leave and benefits, including Wounded Warriors leave."[31] This is separate from postal service sick leave and enables veterans with a disability rating of 30 percent or more to take time off, at full pay, to undergo medical treatment for a service-related condition.

Before 2021, more than 20,000 veterans, with the help of a transition assistance program called Troops to Teachers, found employment as K–12 teachers in public, charter, and Bureau of Indian Affairs schools. At a cost of just $15 million per year, this twenty-eight-year old initiative provided up to $10,000 in financial support and helped job seekers connect with school officials with vacancies to fill. In 2021, however, Pentagon officials "announced they were ending the program completely and shifting resources to 'higher priority programs' more closely aligned to the National Defense Strategy."[32]

THE VET-TO-COP PIPELINE

Policing is the third most common occupation for men and women who have served in the military. Unlike teaching, it's an employment choice widely encouraged by career counselors in the military and veterans' organizations like the American Legion. Under the Obama administration, the Department of Justice (DOJ) provided local police departments with tens of millions of dollars to fund veterans-only positions. As a result, several hundred thousand veterans are now wearing a badge of some sort. Although veterans comprise just 7 percent of the US population, they represent 19 percent of all law enforcement personnel. This disproportionate representation is due, in large part, to preferential hiring requirements mandated by state or federal law. In addition, as the Legion points out, "some police departments have programs that waive initial degree requirements and allow veterans to serve as a police officer while earning their degree part-time."[33]

Hiring preferences were first enacted after World War II, when returning veterans represented a much larger cross section of the population. Today, as revealed by the Marshall Project in a 2017 report, "When Warriors Put on the Badge," this combination of hiring preferences and special funding has "tended to benefit whites disproportionately and make it harder to build police forces that resemble and understand diverse communities."[34] Take the case of Boston, which has a population more than half nonwhite but a police department that is still two-thirds white. Several recent Boston police commissioners, including Kathleen O'Toole—the first woman to hold the position—and William Evans, both tried to hire more African American and Latinx officers in order to change the culture of the department and promote "community policing." But as the Marshall Project found, under state law any "honorably discharged vet skips to the top of police hiring lists, which makes it more difficult to hire both women and minorities" because almost nine out of ten Massachusetts veterans are white.[35] Without veteran status, competitors for a Boston Police Academy slot needed a near-perfect score.

When O'Toole was commissioner—before becoming Seattle's police chief—she worked with many vets who were "great cops," but she also needed to attract people with very different skill sets. "We are facing complicated issues with people who are in crisis every day," she said. "Why wouldn't I want people who majored in human services? Or psychology or sociology?"[36] In an attempt to bypass veteran hiring preferences in Massachusetts, Evans recruited young Bostonians from minority backgrounds into a police cadet trainee program. After a two-year period, these new cadets became eligible to serve as full-time cops.

In response to nationwide protests over the June 2020 killing of George Floyd by Derek Chauvin, a former military police officer, law enforcement officers of all types were deployed in paramilitary uniforms with body armor, automatic rifles, bayonets, and grenade launchers. Their other cast-off Pentagon equipment included armored vehicles and surveillance drones. This triggered a renewed public debate about overly militarized policing in many cities and calls for "defunding" the police. But even before that ongoing controversy developed, a series of studies showed that hiring too many people with experience in actual war zones may not be the best way to prevent the US from becoming one as well.

For example, the Marshall Project looked at officer-involved shootings in several cities, including Albuquerque. Its police force had been cited by the Justice Department for a high level of unjustified officer-involved shootings. "Of the 35 fatal shootings by police between January 2010 and April 2014 . . . nearly one-third were by military veterans." In the course of litigation over the killing of an unarmed Albuquerque motorist, it was revealed that the officer involved was an Iraq War veteran whose PTSD caused flashbacks, nightmares, and blackouts. Nevertheless, as the Marshall Project discovered, he was "assigned to patrol a high-crime area of town known as 'the war zone.'"[37] In Boston and Miami, officers with military experience generated more civilian complaints of excessive force.

Another study by researchers at the University of Texas School of Public Health in Dallas found that one-third of the 516 Dallas officers involved in shooting incidents during a ten-year period were veterans. Those who had been deployed overseas were nearly three times as likely to have fired their weapon; those who had not been deployed were still twice as likely to be involved in a shooting. The study concluded that some veterans employed by the Dallas Police Department lacked "critical thinking skills" when confronted with "high stress scenarios." The researchers called for additional studies on the relationship between veteran status, deployment history, combat experience, and officer-involved shootings. Future research, they argued, should help "differentiate the effect of combat exposure, number of deployments, traumatic brain injury, mental health and substance use problems on shooting involvement among LEOs [law enforcement officers]."[38]

A 2009 report by the International Association of Chiefs of Police and the Bureau of Justice Assistance also assessed the strengths and weaknesses of post-9/11 combat veterans serving in law enforcement roles as compared to previous generations of returning soldiers. Former military personnel got high marks, of course, for their physical fitness, weapons-handling experience, habituation to discipline, and leadership qualities. Yet the report warned that past deployments in Iraq or Afghanistan "may cause returning officers to mistakenly blur the lines between military combat situations and civilian crime situations, resulting in inappropriate decisions and actions, particularly in the use of less lethal or lethal force." The report also noted that combat veterans who suffer from PTSD and related "depression, anger, withdrawal, and family issues" may have a greater propensity for "inappropriate use of force."[39] Some chiefs felt that veterans under their command came back "ill prepared for the civilian world" because their PTSD left them with "exaggerated survival instincts" and "a low tolerance for civilian complaints."[40] As historian Kathleen Belew suggests, some former service members steeped in violent military culture may also bring racist, white supremacist attitudes to their new jobs as police officers.[41]

An additional concern is that veterans who trade one uniform for another will be more vulnerable to well-known occupational hazards of police work, such as substance abuse, divorce, and high rates of suicide. Blue HELP, a mental health advocacy group for police officers and their families, reports that far more cops died by their own hand (228) in 2019 than were killed in the line of duty (132).[42] Fred Fuller,* an Iraq War veteran interviewed for a previous book, suffered from severe PTSD but nevertheless found work as a deputy sheriff in Hawaii. His mental health condition made juggling the demands of domestic life and his new job increasingly difficult. Finally, Fuller's wife threatened to leave him if he didn't seek professional help. Desperate to keep his family intact, Fuller did two stints in a residential PTSD program. When he left the program the second time, he realized that he could not move forward if he remained in law enforcement. "I don't like gray areas," he confessed. "If I'm in for a penny, I'm in for a pound. What that means is I can play cop, or I can play family man." That mindset made him overly aggressive, angry, and irritable—all the behaviors he was trying to overcome. The VA provided Fuller with $25,000 worth of vocational rehabilitation services, and he was able to transition into a new career as a skilled construction worker.[43]

As the Marshall Report found, some law enforcement agencies "employ the use of administrative interviews and psychological evaluations to assess how veteran officers will perform the essential functions of their position, while other agencies revert to their department medical officer, or lack any policy at all." Without more rigorous psychological screening, potential employers are less likely to detect the severity of service-related conditions like Fuller's that may adversely affect future job performance. On the level of broader public policy, the Justice Department under Presidents Obama and Trump displayed little interest in systematically tracking the job performance of recently hired veterans or sponsoring further research on how their military background might affect their behavior vis-à-vis the public. As former DOJ official Ronald Davis told Marshall Project researchers, "I reject the notion that a returning veteran, who has seen combat, should cause concern for a police chief. I would even hire more if I could."[44]

According to one former VA staffer, who has helped other veterans find civilian jobs, career counselors in the military also steer soldiers in the direction of the private security industry. Instead of telling them, "you may have been an infantryman, but there's a whole world of other things out there you can do that may have nothing to do with guns," there is much encouragement to trade one uniform for another—in the private sector. According to this former VA official, the Pentagon's many post-9/11 partnerships with private security firms gives recruitment by these contractors the virtual "imprimatur of the United States Army." As he told us, "a lot of people, particularly if they have kids, would feel, 'How can I let this opportunity pass me by?' So, they would sign up to be everything from glorified mall cops to providing armed protective services to elite billionaires."

Such enticing career options owe much to what Peter Singer, in his book *Corporate Warriors*, calls the "unprecedented . . . wholesale outsourcing of U.S. military services since the 1990s."[45] As William Hartung from the Center for International Policy reports, most "independent contractors" employed in war zones—more than 60 percent—"are now engaged in support services such as serving meals, doing laundry, maintaining and repairing vehicles, or transporting fuel and equipment." A critical minority use their active duty experience to score jobs "guarding embassies, serving as bodyguards, protecting oil pipelines and other infrastructure and doing training."[46]

One popular employer, then called DynCorp, was paid more than $20 billion by the Pentagon and State Department to train local police in Iraq and Afghanistan, with not great results. By 2016, private contractors represented one-quarter of the armed personnel supporting the US occupation of those two countries.[47] According to Hartung, while an armed contractor with a background in the Marines could earn $200,000 per year in Iraq, the bulk of contract employees working there were poorly paid, much abused immigrants from countries like Nepal and the Philippines.

Privatized military firms (PMFS) now supply workers from all over the world to do everything from logistics and technical support to "maintaining, fueling, and arming most of the sophisticated weapons systems like the F-117 stealth fighter."[48] As Singer notes, not everyone is pleased with this trend, because "PMF's use public funds to recruit on the basis of higher pay," while getting the benefit of "all the human capital and investment that the military originally paid for." When individual soldiers look at the many roles taken over by these firms, some wonder "whether the loss of these professional skills and functions will hamper the military in the future."[49] More to the point, limiting the range of noncombat jobs available in the military, by outsourcing so much work previously performed by active-duty personnel, means more men and women leave the service with a limited resume, rather than a broad one reflecting a wide range of transferable skills.

SMOOTH CAREER TRANSITIONS?

Thus, for many veterans, finding employment, outside of law enforcement or PMFs, is not as easy as military recruiters and counselors promise. Military service does not necessarily translate into what civilian employers consider useful on-the-job experience. As one advice column for veterans observes, "It's not always easy to explain why the medals and rankings you've earned are relevant, or how leading troops through dangerous conditions, or being in charge of millions of dollars' worth of machinery can benefit the company you're applying to."[50] Even a highly accomplished former officer like Daniel Gade, who left the military with several advanced degrees, experienced "the most painful and difficult period" of his life after retiring from a twenty-five-year Army career. "The next day," he recalls, "I realized to my horror that I was waiting for the phone to ring. My whole life I had been the leader, the problem-solver, the 'answer man.' All of a sudden, I wasn't that man anymore. Nobody needed me. Nobody was going to call."[51]

As one 2018 survey of 5,000 veterans found, "more than half struggle to find work in their desired fields because civilian employers want experienced and educated candidates."[52] According to a Center for a New American Security study, even managers and supervisors in large corporations, with a professed commitment to hiring veterans, don't "know how to adequately account for both the hard and soft skills that veterans bring to the workplace."[53] Veterans in earlier eras could find more private-sector opportunities for on-the-job training as newly hired employees. Over the past thirty years, fewer employers have been willing to invest in that kind of training, even in industries like construction where union apprenticeship programs were once the norm. One national survey of employers found that between 2001 and 2009, there was a 28 percent decline in company-provided training.[54]

Employers with a high turnover workforce have the least incentive to spend money on training because they won't recoup their investment.[55] Cruz Gonzalez's experience seeking entry-level jobs is a case in point. An Army recruiter blithely promised her that companies would put her at the top of their list when she applied for a job. She quickly learned that some employers did just that, but for positions she didn't want, like being a swim instructor or a retail clerk. "I gained all this experience in helping the nation be protected from threats and hazards," she said with frustration. "I could use it working for a utility company, or the nuclear power industry, or in the chemical industry dealing with toxic hazards." But none of her assigned duties in the military seemed, on paper, to prepare her for such work. Instead, being a veteran helped her jump the queue and get a customer service job at Sam's Club. After quitting that position, she sought part-time work so she could use her GI Bill benefits to take college courses that would make her more marketable.

Many other veterans have discovered a similar unexpected need to get recredentialed. As CNAS explains, "While the military trains well for military jobs, it doesn't provide the licenses or certifications needed for civilian jobs of the same caliber."[56] Someone who entered the military with only a high school education and served as a truck driver or medic—the equivalent of a nurse—or, like Gonzalez, was the equivalent of a nursing assistant or even licensed practical nurse needs further education to get a license or two- or four-year degree and then perhaps graduate school. "There are several instances where military experience directly translates to civilian skills," CNAS reports, "but the requisite licensing or credentialing required to legally perform such roles slows the veteran transition to the civilian sector."[57]

Forty-five-year-old Bridget Lattanzi became a skilled heavy equipment mechanic during her nineteen years in the Illinois National Guard. When she got back from deployments to Iraq in 2004 and 2005, she assumed her military service would help her get hired. It didn't. "I couldn't get anything," she said. Employers feared that she would have to take too much time off for Guard duty or that she would be redeployed. One employer insisted she find a replacement when she was unavailable to work, due to weekend training. She finally stopped putting anything about her military service on her job applications.

She also had to downplay her service-related health issues. "I injured my back, my shoulder, my knee, and have chronic migraines. Most employers don't understand your health problems," she explains. "Even in places where an HR manager is supportive, I got resentment from coworkers. I was working in retail, and I got treatment for my back and couldn't bend or lift for a month. The people I worked with would say I was useless. They thought I was trying to get out of something." Lattanzi encountered customers who were verbally abusive, behavior that she found particularly offensive in light of her past sacrifices on their behalf. Fortunately, Lattanzi was able to improve her job prospects with help from the VA's vocational rehabilitation program. She has returned to college to pursue a career in human resource management, a field giving her future opportunities to assist other veterans in the workplace.

No group of veterans ends up with bigger barriers to employment than those who are unhoused or incarcerated. According to a 2019 report, on a single night in January 2019, there were 37,085 veterans who were homeless—or 8 percent of all then homeless adults. The vast majority—90.3 percent—were men, and 24 percent were chronically homeless.[58] Homeless veterans have served in all of America's recent wars, and over 90 percent are male, according to the National Coalition for Homeless Veterans. Another 1.4 million veterans, although not currently homeless, are deemed at serious risk of being without housing "due to poverty, lack of support networks, and dismal living conditions in overcrowded or substandard housing."[59]

A 2019 report to Congress highlights the impact of homelessness on African Americans, who comprise "one-third of veterans experiencing homelessness (33%) and a quarter of veterans experiencing unsheltered homelessness (25%). African Americans were considerably overrepresented compared to their share of all U.S. veterans (12%). While a majority of veterans without housing were white, they were underrepresented compared to their share of all U.S. veterans (82%). . . . Hispanic or Latino veterans experiencing homelessness were twice as likely to be in unsheltered locations as in sheltered locations (17% vs. 8%)."[60] Although the number of homeless veterans has dropped since 2018, this decline largely reflects a decline in white veteran homelessness.

Adding to their job and housing woes, some former soldiers end up with criminal records as well. Between 8 and 10 percent of those incarcerated in the United States are veterans, and 70 percent of them are serving time for nonviolent crimes. According to one study, "On average, veterans in jail have had five prior arrests, and 45 percent had served two or more state prison sentences. More than half of those who were incarcerated had mental illness or substance abuse disorders." Of veterans who had served in Iraq or Afghanistan, 43 percent had an alcohol use disorder and 37 percent a drug use disorder. Thirty percent had a history of homelessness. Fifty percent of homeless veterans have had some kind of encounter with the legal system.[61]

A special report from the DOJ's Office of Justice Programs estimated that "a greater percentage of veterans (64%) than non-veterans (48%) were sentenced for violent offenses. Forty-three percent had four or more prior arrests, 77 percent had discharges that were honorable or under honorable conditions." The report also noted that combat veterans who were in prison or jail were more likely than incarcerated noncombat veterans to have been diagnosed with a "mental disorder."[62]

THE PROBLEM OF MORAL INJURY

Veterans can be scarred by their military service, even if they are later able to attend college, find decent jobs and housing, and stay out of prison. One less visible wound of war has been identified, with some controversy, as "moral injury." The concept was first popularized by VA psychiatrist Jonathan Shay in his 1994 book *Achilles in Vietnam: Combat Trauma and the Undoing of Character* and further elaborated in *Odysseus in America: Combat Trauma and the Trials of Homecoming.*[63] According to Shay, warriors from Homer's time to ours have experienced the "violent rage and social withdrawal when deep assumptions of 'what's right' are violated."[64]

Moral injury, Shay argues, occurs when there has been a betrayal of what is morally right by someone who holds legitimate authority in a high-stakes situation—in this case, war, which produces "lethal danger and the fear of it. . . . When a leader destroys the legitimacy of the army's moral order by betraying 'what's right,' he inflicts manifold injuries on his men."[65] Subsequent iterations of this concept focus on the injury to an individual's moral conscience that occurs, for example, when a soldier goes to war to save the world from weapons of mass destruction only to discover that they did not exist (in Iraq at least). Not surprisingly, race impacts the incidence of problems like PTSD, which is closely connected to the experience of moral injury.[66] Studies have shown that veterans of color have higher rates of mental health issues like PTSD compared with white veterans, even when controlling for where they were deployed and the pressures of returning from war.[67]

However one chooses to categorize the result of exposure to violence and vulnerability during military service, what veterans experience in war is far outside the civilian norm, at least in Western industrialized societies during peacetime. According to statistics collected in 2003, during the early stages of the occupation of Iraq and Afghanistan, 32 percent of troops in direct combat reported that they were responsible for the death of an enemy, 20 percent reported being responsible for the death of a noncombatant, and 60 percent encountered women and children in need of medical aid, which they were unable to provide.[68] Plus, as we've seen earlier, service members themselves were exposed to bullying, hazing, and military sexual trauma

(MST). For those who have experienced sexual trauma, the sense of betrayal and loss of trust becomes what is known as a secondary, or even tertiary, assault. Sexual assault, writes Kristen J. Leslie, "devastates a survivor's ability to trust others and the military culture that committed to honoring them. The increased sense of vulnerability can be jarring and morally abhorrent to a service member who has been told that vulnerability is a sign of weakness and failure."[69]

For Brianna Holman, whom we met in the previous chapter, it has taken years to recover from serial rape involving fellow soldiers she had trusted. Her healing was aided by the wonderful therapist she found at the VA and a revival of her religious faith. Holman has delved into the literature on toxic masculinity and sexism in the military and now views her experience through the lens of institutional betrayal, which she considers a secondary trauma on top of her assault: "From the moment you hit boots on the ground in basic training, you're immediately broken down to rely on each other as a team to get through training. It's instilled in you that you've got to have your brother's back. You're told, 'Who cares what you think of him or her? You've got to have their back.' You're training for combat and to trust this person who you may eventually be in a foxhole [with], and they turn around and assault you—what do you do now?"

To make sure this does not happen to other women, Holman became a counselor with the Service Women's Action Network (SWAN). She also returned to school to get a social work degree, so she can work with survivors of MST as a sexual assault response coordinator and advocate for DOD policy changes that would better support them.

The feeling of institutional betrayal experienced by Holman, or a bad paper victim like Kris Goldsmith, focuses on the military. In other veterans it can morph into more diffuse anger at the government and authority figures in civilian workplaces. In this disgruntled vet mindset, writes Shay, "The boss who hires and fires him, writes recommendations for him, raises or lowers his pay, and otherwise disposes of his destiny is nothing but a soft civilian. . . . While the veteran was risking his life for his country, the boss and the foreman were having an easy time of it."[70]

Different veterans, of course, experience this postwar sense of mistreatment in different ways. After the Vietnam War, some who were drafted or enlisted concluded they had been lied to about the nature of that conflict. Like members of Veterans for Peace, whom we will meet in later chapters, they turned not only against that military intervention but war in general. Other veterans felt betrayed by civilian leaders who failed to do what was necessary for victory in Vietnam. There is the same range of veteran opinion about Iraq and Afghanistan today, including over whether the chaotic evacuation of Afghan allies should arouse "feelings of shame and betrayal" because some were left behind to face Taliban retaliation in August 2021.[71]

ALIENATION FROM THE CIVILIAN WORLD

Whether the wars they waged were won or lost, veterans' reentry into the civilian world can be a personal challenge for many. As noted earlier in this chapter, some manage this transition well, particularly if they are not hampered by service-related conditions and have the benefit of prior higher education, officer status, and related social connections. Other former military personnel experience a panoply of problems that may include a feeling of alienation from, and sometimes even hostility toward, civilians. This phenomenon can be more pronounced among those who've served in the era of the all-volunteer force. Because the burden of post-9/11 military service has been shared by such a small portion of the US population, some newer veterans harbor resentment toward the many fellow citizens who did not serve. Often, as the Center for a New American Security notes in its report "Lost in Translation," these two populations do little mixing or interacting, thus reinforcing a "civil-military divide" which creates new "transition challenges" for modern-day veterans.[72]

Former military personnel have been shaped by a process of indoctrination and socialization whose very raison d'être is to create a radical separation—what Erving Goffman calls a process of "deculturation"—from the civilian world. Once back in that world, veterans can be as confounded by it as foreign immigrants who find themselves in a baffling new culture.[73] To better navigate this new terrain, veterans have to unlearn behavior that was functional in military culture but may be misunderstood or even frowned upon outside it. In very personal terms, Ari Sonnenberg, a thirty-one-year-old recently returned Iraq and Afghanistan veteran, described this challenge to an audience of civilians at the Commonwealth Club in San Francisco. After fourteen years in uniform, Sonnenberg was still wearing a military-style buzz cut and speaking in rapid-fire bursts, even though he works as an artist now. In the military, he explained, "I learned all my values, all my morals, all my skills—everything I needed to stay alive. And it kept me alive in all these combat tours. And it's funny because all those skills are now . . . all wrong. Here, in the civilian world, if you communicate loudly, you're called aggressive. If you're always watchful and you're always making sure you're not sitting with your back to the door, you're being hypervigilant. Basically, my whole life now is being turned upside down."[74]

Jeffrey Kixmiller, a clinical psychologist, hears similar stories from participants in the Post Deployment Assessment Treatment Program (PDAT) he directs at the VA in Martinez, California. PDAT is a residential program for Iraq and Afghanistan veterans who suffer from mild TBIs and PTSD. As they prepare to reenter the civilian life, some have to learn what others their age figured out how to do when they left home after high school (but not to join the military). "They don't know how to go grocery shopping, cook a meal, shop for clothes, not to mention write a résumé, go in for a job interview, or ask for a salary increase," Kixmiller says. Furthermore, the communication style they've acquired in the military is less useful outside it. "You don't speak until spoken to, you don't offer your opinion, you follow orders. There is a very, very specific way of communicating that is short and sweet and takes turns and is hierarchical. This doesn't work well in civilian life."

Veterans also struggle to fit into a society which values individual competition, achievement, and performance far more than collective action and accomplishment.[75] Some feel that this new environment lacks the superior values of military culture, which teaches soldiers to be self-sacrificing, loyal, and responsible for the fate of others around them. "Here, people only think about themselves," one newly returned Iraq veteran complained. "In the military there is always accountability. Where is the accountability here?"

Similarly, Sasha Best, a psychologist who has worked with PDAT, stresses the difficulty of adjusting to a world suddenly lacking in camaraderie and mutual trust. "One of the wonderful things about military service," she points out, "is the deep and powerful connections that are developed between members of the team. These are very powerful connections that many veterans find hard to replicate in the civilian world."

Alienation from the civilian world may also be fostered by veterans' perception that civilians are largely clueless about the "real world," as they've experienced it overseas. As a troubled teenager from South Milwaukee who needed to get his life together, Jerome Serdinsky joined the Army at nineteen in 1999. He did maintenance work, served in the Reserves, and in 2005 was deployed to Iraq. When he returned from the Middle East, Serdinsky found that civilians didn't understand "that the world is dangerous and dark. I saw how horrible the world is and I am alone in this knowledge." To make matters worse, people were "bitching about all this trivial shit, and you want to tell them, 'Hey, don't you realize it's a privilege to have a toilet or running water?'"

Jeffrey McDowell* grew up in rural New Hampshire and joined the Army when he was nineteen, in large part because he needed GI bill help to attend college. When he returned from Iraq, he moved to New York City to attend the School of Visual Arts. Founded by a World War II veteran, the school markets itself as being "Military Friendly," offers special counseling for veterans, and participates in the Yellow Ribbon Program, which "helps pay for higher out-of-state, private school, or graduate school tuition that the Post-9/11 GI Bill doesn't cover."[76] Nevertheless, McDowell confesses, "I felt alone and lost in this huge city. When I began thinking about why I was so depressed, I realized it had to do with the depth of relationships I had formed in the military. I was twenty-three and was in a private art school with a lot of younger kids from very affluent backgrounds." Joining the military to pay for a visual arts education was not something his nonveteran classmates ever had to consider, nor had they experienced any life-or-death situations routine in a combat zone.

THE "ANGRY VET" PHENOMENON

A combination of emotional and physical problems, readjustment, and cognitive issues can simmer below the surface or regularly erupt, adversely affecting veterans' relationships with friends, coworkers, or intimate partners. Whenever there is a high-profile incident involving an angry, violent veteran, VSOs and other advocacy groups are quick to reassure the press and public that most men and women who served in the military are not unhinged or dangerous. Unfortunately, such efforts to dispel negative stereotypes about all veterans can have the unintended effect of downplaying service-related problems that are real and need to be addressed for the benefit of those who are at risk of hurting themselves or others.

As David Grossman explains in *On Killing*, the military is well aware that "the loss of comrades can enable killing."[77] One of the most effective ways of overcoming resistance to taking life is to channel anger, frustration, or grief over combat casualties into a vengeful response that is mission driven. But for many of the veterans treated for combat-related PTSD by Jonathan Shay, their grief was replaced "by rage that has lasted for years and became an entrenched way of being."[78] As one Iraq veteran recalled his experience of being on the front lines: "They're lobbing mortars at you all the time. You can't get a full night's sleep. You go to eat, and you can't eat because they've shot off a mortar round. You just get irritated. Can't I just fucking eat my dinner, please? Really?" And then, of course, your friends are getting killed, and you may have just narrowly escaped death yourself. "Eventually," he told us, "you just get permanently pissed off."

According to Edgardo Padin-Rivera, who served in Vietnam and later as chief of psychological services at a VA hospital in Cleveland, soldiers are trained to react to, rather than reflect on, what is going on around them. "They learn what we call a behavioral—not a negotiated—reaction." Whether they saw combat or not, Padin-Rivera believes, service members learn to live in a state of high arousal. "Many of these men and women become very reactive, with hair-trigger responses, and may roll right from pain to anger." The problem of veteran anger has been well documented. In his study of military training and personality traits, Washington University psychologist Joshua Jackson found that "military training was associated with changes in personality. Compared with a control group, military recruits had lower levels of agreeableness after training. These levels persisted for five years, even after participants entered college or the labor market."[79]

Another 2010 study surveyed 18,305 members of full-time military and National Guard units. Of the soldiers who had returned from combat in Iraq and Afghanistan, half had problems with alcohol use and aggression, some of which increased over time.[80] Researchers at the VA Puget Sound Health Care System in Seattle, Washington, found that among Iraq and Afghanistan veterans, anger was "independent from, albeit related to, PTSD." Veterans who had been diagnosed with PTSD or "subthreshold PTSD" reported increased levels of anger, hostility, and physical aggression, particularly in their intimate relationships.[81]

According to VA psychologist Jeff Kixmiller, such anger has made it difficult for some Iraq and Afghanistan veterans afflicted with PTSD or TBIS to hold a steady job. Even navigating their day-to-day dealings with family members, friends, or other social contacts can be very challenging. When such patients first entered his treatment program, Kixmiller found them to be "beyond irritable. Irritable was their baseline, and they would flare up from there. They told us about their 'man caves,' the places they holed up in, where they could go so everyone would leave them alone."

INTIMATE PARTNER VIOLENCE

One by-product of such isolation and anger is "intimate partner violence" (IPV). As a 2013 report by the VA explains, "military service has unique psychological, social, and environmental factors that may contribute to elevated risk of IPV among active duty servicemembers and Veterans. Multiple deployments, family separation and reintegration, demanding workloads at home and while on duty, histories of head trauma, mental illness, and substance abuse can contribute to partner conflict and elevated risk of IPV among active duty servicemembers, Veterans, and their intimate partners."[82]

VA researchers conducted a broad analysis of peer-reviewed literature on the topic of IPV. They concluded that 25 to 33 percent of partners of active-duty service members experienced some physical violence, while between 14 and 18 percent experienced severe physical violence.[83] In the veteran population, estimates of IPV "perpetration" ranged from a low of 15 percent to a high of 60 percent.[84] Not surprisingly, many of the male veterans who were perpetrators of violence had PTSD, depression, or adjustment disorder.[85]

According to one study of Vietnam veterans who had served in combat and had PTSD, 33 percent had engaged in physical violence toward a partner. In another study of Iraq and Afghanistan veterans referred for behavioral health evaluations, 60 percent reported some domestic abuse perpetrated on partners.[86] Studies suggest that 35 percent of female veterans experienced some IPV. In yet another study, 33 percent of women veterans, versus 23.8 percent of nonveteran women, reported that they had been subjected to IPV at some time in their lives, and 48 to 86 percent of women who use the VHA for primary care reported IPV.[87]

The spouses of military personnel and veterans are often reluctant to report domestic abuse. In a 2017 survey, 87 percent of military spouses suffering abuse did not report it, either because they minimized the impact or feared that their partner's job or chance of promotion would be jeopardized. Among the spouses of veterans who had been abused, an even higher percentage did not take action out of personal embarrassment or concern about possible loss of financial support or benefits.[88] No veterans advocate has done a better job of documenting this dynamic in military families than Stacy Bannerman, author of *Homefront 911: How Families of Veterans Are Wounded by Our Wars*.

Bannerman's former husband, Lorin, served two tours in Iraq, returning with PTSD and a TBI. During their fifteen years of marriage, he tried to strangle her while he was on active duty. Nevertheless, she did not join the 20 percent of all spouses of active-duty service members who end up divorcing them. Nor did she report the assault to military authorities because "it would be the end of his career, the end of us."[89] Her role, she writes, was "to be resilient, cheerful, patriotic, and uncomplaining. My job was to stand behind the Blue Star flag, with a smile on my face, and keep my suffering to myself."[90]

After Bannerman's husband left the service, she still stuck with him, desperately trying to cope with the fact that "Lorin had weaponized his trauma so that it became a deadly tool." After her husband became addicted to crystal meth, his bullying and verbal abuse continued. Making matters worse for Bannerman was "the profound isolation that exacerbates behavioral health issues for military families, particularly Guard and Reserve, who lack the formal and informal supports and services available to active-duty families residing on or near post."[91] According to Bannerman, this separation between service members and the rest of society, combined with "warrior culture" stigmatization of mental health treatment, creates a major barrier to seeking and getting care.

Bannerman's own deteriorating situation, as a caregiver, led her to contemplate suicide. One night she found herself sitting in her home, a glass of wine, a bottle of pills, plastic bag, and duct tape by her side, ready to end it all. Only then did she realize that she could no longer help her husband and had to help herself. "I called a divorce attorney the next morning and told him to get divorce papers ready to file. I would lose my life to keep it."[92]

The aggressive behavior of a small subset of veterans, particularly those with substance abuse or mental health problems, poses a danger not only to family and friends but also to their VA caregivers. In January 2015 a VA psychologist was killed by an angry veteran employee in El Paso.[93] In December 2016 a seventy-seven-year-old veteran went to an appointment with a nurse practitioner at the Denver VA Medical Center. As soon as he entered the small exam room, he pulled out a handgun, threatened her, and held her hostage. Fortunately, the nurse—as well as VA security—de-escalated the situation, and no one was hurt. A subsequent investigation revealed that the veteran, who brought extra ammunition with him, planned to shoot at the ceiling, thereby attracting return fire from VA police so he could commit "suicide by cop."[94]

In Suzanne's many years of interviewing VA patients, she has been struck by how often the VA becomes a convenient target for veterans' anger. The trigger may be a VHA psychologist suggesting that a patient try talk therapy rather than medication, a VA hospital administrator who doesn't have room to admit a suicidal veteran because of understaffing and underfunding, or a VBA compensation-and-pension examiner who delays or denies a claim for service-connected disability because of missing paperwork. While private-sector medical providers have much freedom to "fire" angry, aggressive patients, the VA does not have the same ability to turn troublesome people away. So, in recent years, it has developed a rigorous program to teach frontline staff how to deal with patients who are verbally or even physically abusive.[95]

A MASS SHOOTER CONNECTION

No profile of "our veterans" would be complete without taking note of the sad fact that a small number have played a disproportionate role in mass shootings. As David Swanson, author of *War Is a Lie,* has documented, more than a third of all US male mass shooters between the ages of eighteen and fifty-nine have been veterans. While veterans represent only 15 percent of US men in the same age range, 36 percent of mass shooters served in the military. According to Swanson's analysis, "a mass shooter is well over twice as likely to be a veteran."[96]

The gunmen involved in three of the ten most deadly mass shootings in modern US history had military backgrounds.[97] In 1995, Gulf War veteran Timothy McVeigh used a car bomb, not guns, to kill 168 people and injure 680 others at the Federal Building in Oklahoma City, the second-worst terrorist attack on US soil. (As Kathleen Belew reports in *Bring the War Home,* McVeigh was part of a broader network of white supremacists with combat experience who joined paramilitary groups after the Gulf War.[98]) In November 2018 Marine Corps veteran Ian David Long (Trump's "sick puppy") killed twelve people in a bar in Thousand Oaks, California. Eight months earlier, Albert Wong, an Army veteran, shot himself and three mental health professionals at the Pathway Home in Yountville, California. Pathway's nonprofit residential treatment for veterans with PTSD and other mental health problems gained national attention via David Finkel's book *Thank You for Your Service* (and a 2017 Hollywood movie based on it). Wong was a Pathway patient who proved so disruptive that he was asked to leave the program. In response he took five people hostage and then killed three women who were Pathway's primary clinicians—one of whom was thirty-two weeks pregnant.[99]

In such cases, the veterans involved often have psychological problems that should have been an obstacle to enlistment. For example, Long had a history of aggressive behavior in high school. But friends and neighbors didn't report their concerns about the teenager because they didn't want to endanger his dream of joining the military to "kill for his country."[100] Wong too had a troubled record. But Army recruiters welcomed him for the usual reason—their need to meet recruitment quotas.

By 2006, the growing unpopularity of the Iraq War and a more robust economy created a major recruitment crisis. As one Princeton study documented, "The number of volunteers declined sharply, leading to a corresponding decrease in overall quality of the Army's recruits and an increase in ethics violations committed by recruiters." The Army relaxed its standards on drug testing and granted waivers for felons.[101] In 2017 it waived a previous ban on the recruitment of soldiers who had a history of "self-mutilation, bipolar disorder, depression, and drug and alcohol abuse."[102]

The anger, alienation, and aggression of some veterans has made them prime recruitment targets for white supremacist groups. In recent years current and former service members have been linked to the Atomwaffen Division, the Proud Boys, and the Boogaloo movement.[103] A neo-Nazi group known as the Base hopes to take advantage of an "impending societal collapse" by recruiting and training ex-military people in both the United States and Canada.[104] Ed Beck, a former Marine who tracks extremism among veterans, told us that he's watched once-close friends from the service become radicalized and isolated online. "Joining the military is in some ways a radicalization process, albeit to patriotic ends," he explained. "You are conditioned to become comfortable with violence and doing extreme things. There's also a rush to that edginess, and I think some vets want to reclaim that after they get out."

As the Pathway Home tragedy illustrates, serious misbehavior by veterans poses a particular challenge to private groups helping them readjust and succeed in civilian life. As noted above, the VA utilizes—although not always successfully—strict protocols for protecting veterans and their caregivers. When a dangerous or lethal incident occurs at the VA, one facility may be affected but the whole system does not shut down as a result.[105]

In contrast, after the March 2018 killings at the Pathway Home, that much acclaimed treatment program was forced to close its doors amid an avalanche of costly litigation. Smaller nonprofits serving veterans do not have the same scale, institutional resources, or resiliency as the VA, particularly during public health emergencies and related economic downturns.

VETERANS AND THE PANDEMIC

The need for reliable and effective support for veterans became even more critical during the COVID-19 pandemic. The veteran unemployment rate had shown a promising decline from 4.5 to 3.5 percent in 2018. But some of the labor market sectors hardest hit two years later—mining, oil, gas extraction, transportation and warehousing, employment services, travel, leisure and hospitality, and construction—employed a significant number of former military personnel.

In the spring and summer of 2020, amid the economic fallout of the pandemic, 12 percent of all veterans were left jobless. A March 2020 report by the Bob Woodruff Foundation (BWF) predicted that unemployment among veterans could reach 14 percent and that the negative impact on their families and communities would take years to reverse.[106] Half of veterans between the ages of twenty-five and fifty-four "had less than $3000 to $4000 in their combined checking and savings accounts—not nearly enough to cover the three to six months of living expenses to cope with unplanned job loss."[107] The Woodruff report warned that some would fall deeper into debt because of greater reliance on predatory loans and credit cards.

Even former members of the officer class, used to much higher incomes, were adversely affected. Pilots who served in the Air Force or Navy have long been able to use their specialized training and skills to become crew members of commercial air carriers. In August 2020 the union that represents many of them, the Air Line Pilots Association, reported that eleven thousand pilots had received furlough warnings at major airlines as business travel and tourism dwindled.[108] Without further federal assistance, total job cuts in the airline industry were projected to reach fifty-five thousand or more. In October 2020, United and American Airlines announced they were cutting thirty thousand jobs.[109]

As another ripple effect of COVID-19, state and local governments faced huge budget shortfalls due to reduced tax revenues. So veterans employed in the public sector experienced job insecurity as well, just as they had when government employment dropped by 600,000 after the recession of 2008–9. Higher levels of unemployment and related evictions and home foreclosures were likely to exacerbate problems described above—like homelessness, incarceration, depression, and even suicide. Amid widespread civilian unemployment, there were strong incentives for enlisted men and women to remain on active duty. But those who left the military in 2020–21 had even more reason to use the GI Bill to obtain degrees that could improve their postpandemic job prospects.

Those in need of mental health care, counseling, and other services were likely to become more dependent than ever on the VA and a host of private charities. Unfortunately, as the Woodruff Foundation noted, "the vast majority of veteran-serving organizations are small: they are among 88 percent of American nonprofits that spend less than $500,000 annually for their work." Like half of all nonprofits, most have less than one month of cash reserves on hand, which makes them as "vulnerable to financial uncertainty" as the people they serve.[110] As we report in the next chapter, some private philanthropies raising money for veterans—along with for-profit colleges chasing their GI Bill dollars, healthcare startups promising to cure them, and big companies seeking to hire them—are less veteran-centric than they claim to be.

3. STOLEN VALOR

Soldiers and veterans don't need priority boarding, 10% discounts
at gimmicky chain restaurants, or a few crinkled bills stuffed into a
charity's coffee can. What they need is a nation that can find
the courage and conviction to stop misusing their service.
—ERIK EDSTROM, former platoon leader and author of
Un-American: A Soldier's Reckoning of Our Longest War

Among the writers chronicling the aftermath of America's post-9/11 wars,
no one does a better job of lampooning commercial valorization of military
service than Ben Fountain, author of *Billy Lynn's Long Halftime Walk*.[1] In this
novel, later turned into a film directed by Ang Lee, the main character is a
nineteen-year-old Texan from a troubled family. Billy Lynn is pressured to
enlist when a high school legal jam lands him between the proverbial rock
and a hard place. Once in the hard place (aka the US Army), Billy ships out
to Iraq and wins a Silver Star for exceptional heroism in a firefight caught on
film by *Fox News*.

The footage of Billy and seven other Bravo team members goes viral. This
inspires someone in the White House to bring the unit home for a two-
week "victory tour" to help revive lagging public support for the war. Wined,

dined, interviewed, and profiled—even wooed by a Hollywood producer eager to turn their story into "the next *Platoon*"—Billy and his comrades begin to feel like circus animals, surrounded by well-meaning but essentially clueless civilians. And that's before they become the special guests of the Dallas Cowboys.

During a pregame reception, the team's super-patriotic owner, who never served in the military, introduces them to his wealthy pals from the Texas real estate, oil, and gas industries. These high-rolling fans and their arm-candy wives fawn over the boys from Bravo, who are plied with drinks and asked no end of embarrassing questions. The squad is then paraded out on the field—along with the team's famous cheerleaders—as part of a star-spangled halftime show headlined by Beyoncé. During a locker room tour, Billy also meets some pumped-up NFL gladiators, "who seem much more martial than any member of Bravo." They pepper him with questions about gear that can knock down all opponents, for good. Like shoppers at a gun show, they want to know what it's like to handle an M4 standard semiautomatic assault rifle, or an M240—a weapon that's fully automatic and capable of laying down 950 rounds per minute—or, better yet, manning a .50-cal on the top of a Humvee. SPC Lynn answers all their technical queries, including those about AK-47s, the insurgent weapon of choice. But he's taken aback when several Cowboys ask how they could, like Bravo, do some "extreme things" in Iraq with all that high-powered weaponry. Would it be possible to arrange a live-fire USO tour so they could "bust up some raghead ass"?

Billy is "tempted to think they're all punch-drunk from years of taking too many blows to the head." But, remaining polite, he just agrees, "We could use the help." He does point out, however, that doing anything "extreme" would require enlisting first, and then the Army would "be more than happy to send you to Iraq." This suggested career change is met with loud snorts and derisive laughter. "We got *jobs*," one Cowboy reminds him. "This here is our *job*, how do you think we going quit our *job* to join some Army? Go on, now."[2]

On February 2, 2020, an estimated 100 million Super Bowl watchers discovered that Fountain's fictional rendition of patriotic halftime displays wasn't that exaggerated.[3] On this particular Sunday, in lavish fashion, the NFL was celebrating its own hundredth birthday, an event seemingly disconnected from military service, past or present. Yet who was there to have that service recognized on what football commissioner Roger Goodell called "the country's largest stage"? Four hardy survivors of World War II who also happened to be one hundred years old. Right before kickoff time, these veterans were driven out on the field at Hard Rock Stadium in Miami in front of sixty-two thousand screaming fans. Their convoy of golf carts was stationed behind a red, white, and blue barrier surrounded by flags. A detachment of active-duty troops took the barrier down, leading to a dramatic roll call of the names, ranks, and battlefield decorations of the four centenarians.

Such utilization of veterans as political props is, of course, a venerable American tradition, dating back to the post–Civil War era, when Grand Army of the Republic survivors were often deployed in Republican campaigns in the North, while the not-so-victorious sons of the Confederacy were trotted out—sometimes in white robes and hoods—to support revanchist Democrats. As ex-Michigan congressman Dave Bonior, a cofounder of the House Veterans Caucus in the 1970s, told us, "The plaudits that modern day veterans regularly receive in NFL and MLB stadiums are a weak attempt at national absolution by the 97 percent of citizens whose connection to war and our military has, for four decades, now been severed. There ensued a huge disconnect between the realities of the war at home and the war abroad." Bonior questions whether "these momentary attempts at gratitude carry any weight for those whose lives and the lives of their families have been so brutally damaged." For post-9/11 veterans, he says, "the contrast is more than just surreal, it is heartbreaking. For many, being a hero is not possible given the bloody and ghastly nature of their military service and their later struggle to live with its physical and mental scars."

STOLEN-VALOR PHONIES

America's feverish post-9/11 valorization of combat veterans has led some soldiers to embellish their own, more ordinary service records, with often embarrassing results. In the public mind, this practice is most commonly associated with nonveterans, who award themselves veteran status or military laurels they never earned. But, as the *New Yorker* discovered in its exploration of the stolen-valor phenomenon, résumé embellishers have even included Chris Kyle—the legendary marksman played by Bradley Cooper in *American Sniper*, the highest-grossing war movie in American history.[4] In Kyle's 2012 autobiography, which sold a million copies, the much-decorated Navy SEAL gave himself an extra Silver and Bronze Star on top of the one Silver Star and three Bronze Stars he did earn. This news broke two years after Kyle was killed at a gun range by a mentally disturbed fellow veteran he was trying to help.[5]

If the former sniper had survived, he might have had some explaining to do or a public apology to make, like Hollywood actor and ex-Marine Brian Dennehy after he was outed for falsely claiming to have been wounded in Vietnam,[6] or US Senator Richard Blumenthal of Connecticut, a former Marine Corps reservist who claimed to have served in Vietnam, when, in fact, he was never deployed there.[7] Even Robert McDonald, a West Point graduate with Army Ranger training and a distinguished record as an Eighty-Second Airborne Division officer, found himself stepping on the same PR land mine. In January 2015, not long after Barack Obama appointed him VA secretary, McDonald engaged in a televised exchange with a homeless veteran who reported that he had served in the special forces. "Special forces? What years? I was in special forces!" McDonald told him. When this claim was broadcast in a CBS News report, a few angry viewers with specialized knowledge ignored the good news about VA assistance to homeless veterans. As *Huffington Post* reported, they fixated instead on the fact that graduating from Ranger School is not the same thing as serving in a Ranger battalion or any other special operations unit. Like Dennehy, McDonald was soon issuing apologetic clarifications, which, fortunately for him, passed muster at the White House.[8]

Other cases reported by the *New Yorker* involved much less well-known vets. All did some version of the same off-the-cuff résumé inflation while speaking to schoolchildren, preaching in church, or running for public office—as two Army veterans did against each other in a Texas sheriff's race in which both claimed to have taken "a bullet for my country" but neither had.[9] Since 2012, Congress has "made it illegal to fraudulently wear medals, embellish rank, or make false claims of service in order to obtain money or some other tangible benefit." Violators of the Stolen Valor Act can be prosecuted and, if found guilty, fined or jailed, although most just end up doing community service in some form.

Offenders are usually outed by what is now a small army of amateur detectives and whistleblowers who have military backgrounds of their own. They operate message boards, Facebook groups, and websites like Military Phonies and StolenValor.com. The results of their investigations of veterans and nonveterans who have allegedly inflated or invented military credentials is widely shared and publicized. One wishes there were a similar volume of YouTube outrage directed at a bigger and more influential crowd of phonies, namely the individuals and institutions who loudly proclaim their love and support for veterans while actually being more concerned about gaining "money or some other tangible benefit" for themselves. As this chapter confirms, there is far less public shaming or legal sanctioning of for-profit businesses, philanthropists, corporate lobbyists, or industry front groups that engage in this form of stolen valor, which adversely affects far more veterans, particularly those using GI Bill benefits.

GI BILL DEFRAUDERS

When the Department of Defense began building an all-volunteer force in the early 1970s, military recruiters soon discovered that education benefits were a major factor in the enlistment decisions of nearly 80 percent of their new recruits. In the decades since then, enrolling in private colleges and even state universities has become so costly that federal student debt now amounts to $1.5 trillion, a crushing burden made even heavier by the pandemic-driven economic downturn in 2020.[10]

Since 9/11, more than a million men and women who left the military have been able to return to school at taxpayer expense and, in theory, without having to join the ranks of our nation's 43 million student debtors. Unfortunately, the twenty-first-century terrain of higher education in America is much changed since the more generous benefits of the original GI Bill enabled millions of World War II veterans to attend trade schools, colleges, and universities of all kinds seventy-five years ago. One problematic feature of the current landscape is the existence of far more for-profit educational institutions, which have been vacuuming up nearly 40 percent of GI Bill tuition and fee payments in recent years.[11] As the Student Veterans of America (SVA) and others have warned, the risk of fraud, waste, and abuse is "exceptionally high at for-profit schools," which have left too many veterans with worthless degrees, course credits they can't transfer, exhausted GI Bill benefits, and student debt that their military service was supposed to help them avoid.[12]

Over the last two decades, the big post-9/11 increase in veteran utilization of GI Bill benefits has not been accompanied by effective regulation of educational service providers. The election of Donald Trump in 2016 and his appointment of fellow billionaire Betsy DeVos as education secretary made a bad situation worse as DeVos began "eviscerating student protections and quality controls," according to the SVA.[13] This left a whole generation of student veterans, often from communities of color, at the mercy of firms more concerned about private profit than quality education.

Based on their own résumés, Trump and DeVos were predictable architects of a deregulatory fiasco. Among his many past hustles and scams,

Trump lent his name to the fraudulent venture known as Trump University, an unaccredited for-profit institution that used misleading sales pitches to recruit students. That "swindling of thousands of Americans out of millions of dollars," as one state attorney general described it, triggered multiple investigations, consumer complaints, and lawsuits.[14] Trump University was eventually shut down. After years of class-action litigation, Trump settled all claims against him for $25 million.

Before joining Trump's cabinet as top administrator of a federal agency created to support public education, DeVos was a leading conservative critic of public schools and proponent of a voucher system to replace them. In her home state of Michigan, she succeeded in greatly expanding the role of charter schools in Detroit.[15] The millions of dollars she spent on privatization efforts there and elsewhere led to a further drain on the resources of already-troubled inner-city schools. Public oversight of their for-profit competition, which often failed to produce the better outcomes promised by DeVos, was also weakened.

With Trump and DeVos turning a blind eye or tipping the scales in their favor, for-profit institutions that were already problematic for veterans under the Bush and Obama administrations faced little pressure to clean up their act in the Trump era. As a result, student veterans and other alumni of notorious outfits like Capella, Corinthian, ITT Tech, Ashford University, and the University of Phoenix ended up paying a heavy personal price.

Tasha Berkhalter is a Black Army veteran who exited ITT Technical Institute with her GI Bill benefits exhausted, huge personal debt, and a degree from a now-defunct institution that, she says, no employer takes seriously. As Berkhalter summarizes it, "That school completely smashed my dreams." Before ITT collapsed in 2016, fifty-two-year-old David Boyer, a Navy veteran, borrowed money to get an ITT degree in electrical engineering that cost more than his GI Bill benefits would cover. After graduation he was only able to secure minimum-wage work repairing soda machines and microwave ovens in convenience stores. He stopped listing his tainted degree on his résumé, now teaches in a trade school, and someday would "like to have a degree that means something."[16]

Shawn Cooper is an Air Force veteran forced to sue Capella over needless prolonging of his and other students' doctoral programs, which left him with $100,000 in student loans to repay. "At the end of the day, I feel like it's all just a facade on their end," he told the *New York Times*. "Get people in, take their money and get them out, usually without anything to show for it."[17] Richard Baca, a former National Guard medic, was forced to give up his dream of becoming a doctor after racking up debt and learning little at Ashford University, which Iowa senator Tom Harkin denounced as "an absolute scam," way back in 2011.[18]

As such accusations and complaints mounted over the years, the for-profit college industry spent heavily on Capitol Hill lobbying, while lawyering up Trump University–style to defend its business model in court. It hired lobbyists with good connections to federal agency officials installed by Trump. For example, Bridgepoint Education Inc.—Ashford's former parent company—deployed Matt Smith, the VA's former deputy assistant secretary of public affairs, to lobby on GI Bill–related issues. Three officials with past Bridgepoint ties actually joined the Trump administration. And one, Robert Eitel, became a senior aide to Secretary DeVos at the Department of Education.[19]

Bridgepoint also became a corporate sponsor of the Enlisted Association of the National Guard of the United States, one of the few veterans' groups not committed to reforming what's known in Congress as the "90/10 rule."[20] This rule required that for-profit colleges get no more than 90 percent of their revenues from federal student aid. But conveniently for them, GI Bill payments did not count as such aid, which provided such schools with a powerful incentive to recruit as many student veterans as possible, with any kind of sales pitch. During the Obama administration, organizations like the SVA and Veterans Education Success (VES) demanded that Congress amend the 90/10 rule to reduce misleading marketing practices.[21] But Republican friends of for-profit schools, flush with campaign cash from them, blocked this change until early 2021, when Democrats won control of both the House and the Senate.[22]

Obama appointees did establish a GI Bill complaint system and an online tool for easier consumer comparisons of schools wooing veterans. Obama's new Consumer Financial Protection Bureau (CFPB) also created an office dedicated to protecting service members, veterans, and military families from predatory lenders. In 2016 the CFPB fined Bridgepoint $8 million and directed it to discharge $23.5 million in student loans because of its deceptive practices. Before leaving office in 2017, Obama promised that tens of thousands of student vets would get some measure of debt relief after his Department of Education determined that such deception was widespread.[23]

Once DeVos became secretary of education, she made reversing this policy a high priority. She issued a new federal rule, effective July 1, 2020, that required debt relief applicants to file a claim within three years of any alleged deception and supply more evidence of how they were personally misled and financially harmed. On the eve of its implementation, veterans' groups won broad congressional support for a resolution calling on the Trump administration to rescind DeVos's proposed new rule. As American Legion Commander James Oxford reminded the White House, "This type of deception against our veterans and service members has been a lucrative scam for unscrupulous actors."[24] President Trump ignored such appeals and vetoed the House-Senate resolution.

During Trump's four years in office, other Obama-era initiatives were thwarted with less public outcry. Among them was a 2012 executive order requiring closer collaboration between the Departments of Defense, Veterans Affairs, and Education on ways to better measure educational outcomes for student veterans. The CFPB was itself gutted, which left its office serving veterans and active-duty military personnel understaffed and suffering from high leadership turnover. Crippling the CFPB limited its consumer education function and weakened enforcement of the Military Lending Act, which caps interest rates for active-duty service members.[25]

Under Trump, the VA was similarly reluctant to use its own regulatory powers to sanction educational institutions guilty of deceiving veterans. In 2018 the Government Accountability Office (GAO) found that an annual allocation of $21 million a year was insufficient for effective VA oversight, including more site visits to schools and proper tracking of the flow of GI Bill dollars to them.[26] That same year, the VA's own inspector general estimated that if oversight was not ramped up significantly, $2.3 billion in GI Bill funds could be funneled to potentially ineligible academic programs over the next five years, putting the educational outcomes of more than seventeen thousand student veterans at risk.[27] Nevertheless, it took the VA another two years to suspend GI Bill payments to the University of Phoenix and other outfits accused of "erroneous, deceptive, and misleading enrollment and advertising practices." As investigations by the Center for Investigative Reporting and others have documented, Phoenix ran "recruitment drives disguised as résumé workshops" and utilized "military insignias in school marketing without the required permissions."[28]

The VA's belated action occurred shortly after the Federal Trade Commission reached a $191 million settlement of its own charges against the University of Phoenix for deceiving active-duty service members, veterans, and military spouses. After a four-month suspension of VA funding of Phoenix and fellow offenders, the Trump administration found they had taken "adequate corrective actions" and were once again eligible to receive tuition reimbursement payments under the GI Bill.[29] This slap on the wrist occurred just as COVID-19 was driving millions of students, including veterans, into various forms of distance learning. For-profit providers of online classes, including schools with graduation rates no higher than 25 percent and sometimes in the single digits, were well positioned for market growth in this new environment. "In times of economic downturn, that's when the for-profit colleges start to thrive," says Eileen Connor, director of Harvard Law School's Project on Predatory Student Lending. According to Connor, online colleges "have a running start, especially when there's an economic downturn keeping people in their homes. That is a perfect storm for the thing that they're trying to do."[30]

MENTAL HEALTH MAGICIANS

In addition to for-profit educational institutions trying to hoover up GI Bill money, the healthcare industry is also flush with startup firms focusing on the veteran market. Utilizing Republican Party connections and donor access to the Trump administration, these firms have tried to capitalize on the VA outsourcing trend described in the next three chapters.

Unlike in the VA, where adoption of new treatments is evidence-based, there is less quality control in the world of private-sector mental health care. Dr. Matthew Friedman, a clinical psychiatrist and cofounder of the VA's National Center for PTSD, is one of many experts in the field worried that "self-proclaimed magicians" are getting the green light to peddle their wares to desperate veterans and, in some cases, partner with the VA itself. "If it hasn't been proven, it's not something the VA should endorse," Friedman argues. "They should live by the same rules other treatments live by; they should be tested in rigorous, randomized clinical trials. That's the coin of the realm. And if they haven't done that . . . stay away, baby. Stay away."[31]

Instead, during Donald Trump's presidency, Congress and the VA were heavily lobbied to authorize taxpayer funding of questionable offerings by for-profit providers. Among these treatments are havening, which claims to be a "system of scientific procedures" involving eye movements and touching people on their arms; hyperbaric oxygen therapy, wherein veterans are placed in a total body chamber with intense air pressure; and equine therapy, a favorite of Congressman Andy Barr, a horse-loving Republican from Kentucky who believes that horse-rider interaction can provide long-lasting therapeutic benefits.[32]

In similar fashion, the Carrick Brain Centers, founded in 2012 by North Texas businessman Ken Beam, had a local Republican booster in the form of Rick Perry. Then governor of Texas and later energy secretary under Trump, Perry helped Carrick get a $2.2 million state grant. His enthusiasm was shared by some former Dallas Cowboys suffering from concussions and possible TBIs, like many combat veterans. At Carrick such patients were strapped into a gyroscopic chair that spun them around to increase blood flow to damaged parts of their brain and alleviate related symptoms. But an in-depth investigation conducted by the *Dallas Morning News* in 2015 found little evidence of the treatment's effectiveness.[33] Not long after that media exposé, Carrick shut down its Texas operations. But in Colorado another firm, called Revive Treatment Centers, continued to market the same controversial gyroscopic chair rides to veterans.[34]

Like Perry in Texas, Senator Dean Heller from Nevada was so enthusiastic about a firm offering experimental treatment that he sought a government contract for it. This company, named CereCare, used electromagnetic brain stimulation on patients with addictions or PTSD. CereCare just happened to be a business partnership with close ties to Glenna Smith, Heller's former aide, who became a VA public affairs officer in Reno. So, as *ProPublica* reported, Heller cosponsored a bill mandating that the Reno VA medical center utilize CereCare's procedure in a local pilot program designed to get it adopted throughout the country. One of CereCare's nonphysician partners "participated in drafting the legislation," which authorized "no additional funding, so the pilot program would come at the expense of other VA treatments that are already proven to be effective."[35]

Heller's bill drew a strong rebuke from the Veterans of Foreign Wars (VFW), which agreed that VA patients were better served by "therapies that have shown promise or have a proven track record." His boosterism for CereCare was also questioned by the American Federation of Government Employees (AFGE), the largest VA union and a critic of VA privatization, which backed the Nevada Democrat who defeated Heller when he ran for reelection in November 2018.[36]

One of the biggest private mental health initiatives for veterans is the brainchild of Steven Cohen, who donated $1 million to Trump's inaugural committee in January 2017, along with twenty-four other Republican billionaires. Now owner of the New York Mets, Cohen first achieved Wall Street acclaim as founder of SAC Capital Advisors, which left him with a personal fortune worth about $14 billion. Cohen's son served in the Marines, leading him to develop a personal interest in PTSD and related mental health challenges facing veterans. In 2016 Cohen invested $275 million in the modestly named Cohen Veterans Network (CVN), a group of private clinics offering short-term therapy for veterans with mental health conditions like PTSD, anxiety, and depression. His initial plan was to have twenty-five clinics up and running by 2021, with the capacity to treat thousands of patients around the country. In pursuit of this goal, CVN wielded an ample checkbook to poach experienced staff from top academic and healthcare institutions, including the VA, and launched its own related research venture, Cohen Veterans' Bioscience, which hopes to identify a biomarker for PTSD. The CVN board included Admiral Mike Mullen (ret.), former military adviser to Barack Obama and George Bush; and Joe Lieberman, a senator from Cohen's home state of Connecticut.[37]

Skeptics about Cohen's veteran-related ventures note that they were launched during his two-year Securities and Exchange Commission ban from managing other people's money because of his involvement in one of the largest insider trading schemes in US history. Between 2013 and 2016, eight of Cohen's former hedge fund colleagues pleaded guilty to or were convicted of related charges. SAC Capital Advisors itself paid a total of $1.8 billion in fines imposed by federal prosecutors and securities regulators.[38]

"You have to wonder where [Cohen's] sudden burst of eleemosynary instincts came from," says Rick Weidman, the former executive director for policy and government affairs at Vietnam Veterans of America (VVA). "This guy was in hot water, he was . . . swindling people through his hedge fund, and he made billions. And suddenly he thinks, 'Okay, let me figure out what to do to up my image,' and he starts the Cohen Veterans Network."

In 2018 CVN hired two legislators-turned-lobbyists to expand its reach within the Trump administration. They helped the network secure a major partnership with the VA to "increase veterans' access to mental health resources." Cohen's bioscience venture has also joined forces with a number of pharmaceutical groups to create the Coalition to Heal Invisible Wounds. This consortium successfully lobbied the VA to support clinical trials of experimental new drugs, including antipsychotic medications and muscle relaxants, which have been found to have potentially dangerous side effects. This occurred just as the VA was making progress in reducing patient reliance on potentially addictive painkillers and had achieved a 41 percent reduction in opioid-prescribing rates.

What worries Weidman and others is CVN's emerging goal of replacing, rather than just supplementing, VA mental health care services—and with treatments that would be less well tested and more expensive. The understandable appeal of CVN services, as originally marketed to veterans, was that they were free—and not limited to the veteran population eligible for VA care. But by becoming part of the VA's community care network, CVN is now being partially reimbursed with taxpayer dollars coming out of the VA budget, not surviving on the widely advertised largesse of its Wall Street founder.

HELPING VETERANS OR THEMSELVES?

Organizations assisting wounded warriors have also become the charities of choice for corporate America, influential law firms and foundations, and wealthy individuals with lower net worth than Steven Cohen. Today there are more than forty thousand nonprofits providing services to veterans. Many are well intentioned and well run, utilizing dedicated staffers and volunteers working under the direction of conscientious board members. But in some of these charities, as the donations started flowing in, people doing good for veterans have succumbed to the temptation to feather their own nest as well.

Like similar high-overhead "boiler room" operations making heart-rending telemarketing appeals for police or firefighters, the worst of these offenders have been outfits like the Circle of Friends for American Veterans, forced to shut down in 2019 after a news report found it was directing nine out of every ten dollars raised to pay staff.[39] Another bad actor was the Coalition to Salute America's Heroes. Founded by Roger Chapin, a veteran of the US Army's Finance Corps, the coalition paid out millions to Chapin and his wife in salaries, bonuses, and expense reimbursements. Charity dollars also bought the lucky couple a $440,000 condominium and a $17,000 golf club membership.[40]

During the last decade, Wounded Warrior Project (WWP) was the most infamous poster child for this problem, until damaging publicity forced a leadership shake-up followed by better handling of annual revenue now amounting to more than $226 million.[41] WWP was founded as a small venture in 2003 by John Melia, a Marine veteran wounded in a 1992 helicopter crash in Somalia. In the group's early days, Melia distributed backpacks of supplies to patients at military hospitals. Originally a subsidiary of the United Spinal Association (USA), WWP became a separate entity in 2005 thanks to a nearly $3 million grant from USA. The charity began to attract sufficient big-donor interest to support new programs related to veteran mental health and employment. As the organization grew in scale, it acquired a new CEO—Steve Nardizzi, an attorney who had represented disabled veterans. Nardizzi took a far more aggressive and entrepreneurial approach to WWP fundraising, which enabled the group to pay him nearly $500,000 a year by 2014.

By 2016, however, only 60 percent of WWP revenue was being spent on programs helping veterans; the remaining 40 percent went to overhead costs. *New York Times* and CBS News investigators found that millions of dollars were being spent on luxury travel, fancy hotels, expensive dinners, and "team-building" events for WWP employees.[42] At a staff retreat, for example, all five hundred flew to Colorado Springs and stayed at the five-star Broadmoor Hotel, which has three swimming pools, five tennis courts, and twenty restaurants. To Jesse Longoria, a Marine combat veteran who left the organization, it seemed like "where the money was going" was "a big lie."[43]

Embarrassed by this bad publicity, WWP board members fired Nardizzi and another top executive. They hired an outside law firm to conduct an independent review of the charity's finances and installed a new CEO, Lieutenant General Mike Linnington (ret.).[44] He cut executive pay in half and reduced other administrative costs. In the wake of these reforms and a renewed focus on services to veterans, WWP was removed from Charity Navigator's watch list, and the Better Business Bureau found that the group's spending was once again "consistent with its programs and mission."[45] Unfortunately, the lessons of the WWP scandal seem to have been lost on others in the field of veteran philanthropy.

In the Trump era, a well-endowed charity called the Independence Fund (TIF) emerged as the latest example of both questionable practices and politicization of the field. TIF raises money to help severely wounded veterans and their caregivers. It is best known for giving away all-terrain wheelchairs to selected disabled veterans before large audiences at country music concerts. Sarah Verardo, a TIF board member and its CEO, first got involved in its work as caregiver to her husband, Mike, a two-time Purple Heart winner and survivor of multiple IED blasts in Afghanistan. The now-defunct Donald J. Trump Foundation donated $15,000 to TIF in 2013, the same year that *Fox News* star Bill O'Reilly became TIF's highest-profile supporter. O'Reilly promoted the charity's work on his prime-time show and in newspaper columns. TIF soon amassed a long list of other wealthy or influential admirers, including country music stars, corporate executives, and prominent Republicans like Thom Tillis, a senator from North Carolina, who made a promotional video urging all veterans to "get involved with the Independence Fund."[46]

The charity's tax status prohibits it from directly or indirectly backing political candidates. But six days before the 2016 election, Mike Verardo's endorsement of Trump was highlighted in a front-page *New York Times* story about veteran support for him.[47] During that presidential campaign, TIF's chief advocacy officer, Bob Carey, served as the GOP's top coordinator of veteran voter turnout. A pugnacious Navy veteran with his own one-man consulting firm, Carey then took on a number of new corporate clients looking for an in with veterans. TIF's influence in veterans' policy circles grew after Carey's political ally Robert Wilkie became Trump's second secretary of veterans affairs. Leading figures in TIF, like the Verardos, in turn praised President Trump for having the most pro-veteran administration in US history.

With big donations flowing in from brand-name firms like American Airlines, UPS, and Wendy's, TIF was able to transform itself from an all-volunteer operation taking in just $600,000 a year in 2012 to one collecting tens of millions of dollars. With those resources it has provided 2,500 wheelchairs to veterans and helped more than two thousand vets and military families pay their rent and other costs during the 2020 pandemic. But as a *Mother Jones* investigation found that same year, some TIF insiders have been taking even better care of themselves, leading other staffers to quit the organization and speak out. "Rather than helping veterans, the charity has basically become the Sarah Verardo Fund," one ex-employee complained. "Sarah's spending was breaking the organization," reports another. "She travels like a Fortune 500 CEO," according to Paul McKellips, TIF's former chief communications officer. "She stayed at fancy hotels, flew first class most of the time, and wanted Town Car service, while myself and others were hunkering down at Hampton Inns and car-pooling in sub-compacts."[48]

Charity Watch, a nonprofit oversight group, found it difficult to gauge the actual extent or effectiveness of TIF's work because so much of its charity was dispensed via vaguely recorded cash disbursements. In 2015, for instance, TIF listed nearly $12 million in amorphous "benefits paid to or for members." That same year, an internal audit document revealed that the charity did not maintain standardized sets of financial statements or a general ledger. That audit further suggested that TIF's nonaccounting of funds "could have an effect on the organization's tax-exempt status." Numerous TIF financial transactions involve companies with ties to its staff or board members. The charity also spent more than $400,000 on treatments of questionable worth at a hyperbaric oxygen center in North Carolina. At least one caregiver whose husband used that particular center reported that his eardrums were damaged as a result of faulty operation of its equipment.

Despite these warning signs, TIF continued to be an inside-the-Beltway player during the Trump years. Sarah Verardo's relationship with high-ranking VA officials like Keita Franklin, who once served as the agency's chief suicide prevention officer, paid off in the form of a new VA partnership with Operation Resiliency, TIF's own suicide prevention program. As the 2020 election approached, TIF lobbied in favor of a new VA grant program (described further in chapter 6) for nonprofits like itself serving troubled veterans and their families. Working with equine therapy fan Andy Barr, TIF was able to ensure that charities offering "non-traditional and innovative approaches and treatment practices" would have equal access to the fund that Congress allocated for this five-year program. The Trump administration official responsible for dispensing this grant money, at least before January 2021, was none other than Secretary Robert Wilkie, TIF's good friend and ally at the VA.[49]

VETERAN-FRIENDLY COMPANIES?

The problem of veteran suicide has also provided corporate America with many chances to demonstrate its concern for the health and well-being of the nation's 20 million veterans. In 2020 the US Chamber of Commerce Foundation declared its support for a Trump administration suicide reduction initiative. Called "Prevents," its objective was building "a public/private partnership to strengthen emotional well-being in the workplace." Amazon, Walmart, Starbucks, Comcast, Sprint, T-Mobile, and financial services company USAA were among the first twenty-five "forward looking employers" to sign a related "Hiring Our Heroes Employer Challenge Pledge." For Walmart, this represented a renewed commitment to being veteran friendly. In 2013 the nation's largest private employer announced plans to hire 100,000 former military men and women over the next five years, in addition to the 100,000 already on its payroll of 1.5 million. Walmart has lauded veterans as "team players" and "quick learners," and, of course, each one hired enables the company to claim a federal tax credit of up to $9,600.[50]

In addition to hiring more veterans, corporate signers of the Employer Challenge Pledge also agreed to develop "best practices in the workplace for strengthening mental wellness and preventing suicide."[51] The pledge notes that their "employee populations," including veterans, may have certain risk factors, such as "financial stress, emotional stress, and substance use and abuse." To reduce these risk factors, the companies agreed to "promote a safe, inclusive work environment and leverage employee resource groups" to "create communities of support."[52]

Despite signing the Employer Challenge Pledge, neither Walmart nor Amazon—two of the most antiunion firms in the nation—is known for its "best practices in the workplace." In fact, labor rights advocates have long criticized the pay scales, benefit coverage, and scheduling policies of both companies.[53] Amazon, in particular, has come under fire for its overly intrusive employee surveillance systems. As the Open Markets Research Institute reported, management "uses such tools as navigation software, item scanners, wristbands, thermal cameras, security cameras and recorded footage to surveil its workforce in warehouses and stores." This is designed both to boost output and to closely monitor employee involvement in any workplace organizing activity.[54]

Amazon was founded by Jeff Bezos, now the world's richest man and a patron of the With Honor Fund, which tries to elect more veterans to Congress (as we report in chapter 7). His company pledged to hire twenty-five thousand more veterans and military spouses by 2021, who would then be encouraged to join one of its Warriors@Amazon affinity groups. As coronavirus-related stay-at-home orders generated a huge increase in Amazon's online order flow, shareholder value increased by nearly $500 billion, to more than $1.4 trillion. By mid-2020 Bezos's personal net worth rose to nearly $190 billion. To handle the surge of new business that generated such great wealth, the company hired thousands of new warehouse workers to replace those like Navy veteran Seth King, who quit after three months.

In a town hall meeting hosted by Senator Bernie Sanders, King described Amazon's employment model as "a revolving door of just bodies that they're throwing at the floor." Telling a now-familiar Amazon tale, he recalled working long hours under the pressure of demanding productivity standards, with few chances to sit down or take a bathroom break. As King drove to work every day, it "was exhausting just thinking about having to come in and start another ten-hour shift, being on my feet the whole time." At a company supposedly sensitive to risk factors for suicide, King felt like he "didn't want to be alive anymore if that was the future that I had to look forward to. I was in the Navy for eight years, and there wasn't a single day that I felt as miserable or isolated as I did at Amazon."[55]

Even veterans hired to be Amazon warehouse managers have made similar unfavorable comparisons. One, an officer still active in the Reserves, reported that his warehouse was understaffed and overheated due to insufficient air-conditioning. When mistakes occurred, he said, he'd usually get chewed out by one of his bosses. "I didn't get treated as bad in the [military] in basic training," he said. "You screw up—it's a screaming, cussing, yelling tirade on the floor." Like several other warehouse supervisors interviewed by CNET, this veteran faced pressure to leave the military because, he was told, a "manager wouldn't be able to advance at the company if he continued to serve both the military and Amazon." When queried about these alleged violations of the Uniformed Services Employment and Reemployment Rights Act (USERRA), which protects service members from job discrimination or denial of promotions due to their absence from work for military commitments, Amazon proclaimed its commitment "to supporting our military and veteran employees and providing opportunities for their long-term career growth and success."[56]

An exposé in the *New York Times* documented the degree to which Amazon actually "intentionally limits upward mobility for hourly workers." One top executive torpedoed a proposal from HR to "create more leadership roles for hourly employees, similar to non-commissioned officers in the military." Instead, "guaranteed wage increases stopped after three years and Amazon provided incentives for low-skilled employees to leave." Such policies reflected Amazon founder Jeff Bezos's belief that hourly workers who stayed too long at the company would become lazy, disgruntled, and entrenched, putting Amazon on what he called "a march to mediocrity."[57]

In response to mounting public criticism in 2020, Amazon highlighted its hiring of veterans who lost their jobs due to the pandemic and made some COVID-19–related workplace changes.[58] Management announced what proved to be a temporary wage hike for warehouse workers, whose starting pay is $15 per hour. The company also modified its leave policy to permit employees with virus symptoms to stay home for up to two weeks with pay. Workers later contended that this policy was not fairly or consistently implemented.[59] By the 2020 holiday season, Amazon was acting like the pandemic was over, according to Courtenay Brown, an employee in New Jersey. Bezos, she noted, had "made $70 billion since March when the pandemic started," but the company still "canceled the measly $2 bonus back in June." Meanwhile, "Amazon calls us heroes in their commercials, they call us essential, but it feels like we are expendable." Brown was among the Amazon workers who joined forces with Walmart employees in a national campaign called "Five to Survive." As she explained, its five demands included "$5 per hour in essential pay, safety on the job, and real protections from retaliation if they speak out about working conditions or health hazards."[60]

Unfortunately, as former Amazon vice president Tim Bray pointed out in a *New York Times* op-ed piece, the company's "productivity targets" continued to make the "already stressful work of those who sort, package, and deliver Amazon goods even worse." Workers who participated in protests over working conditions faced continuing threats of disciplinary action, including dismissal. According to Bray, only unionization will ensure better treatment of the company's hourly workers, including the 18,400 veterans, military spouses, and part-time military personnel among them.[61] In early 2021, a group of Amazon workers in Bessemer, Alabama, took Bray's advice and sought a National Labor Relations Board (NLRB) election in a warehouse with six thousand employees.[62] After an aggressive antiunion campaign, management persuaded a majority of those voting to reject union representation.

CORPORATE RHETORIC VERSUS WORKPLACE REALITY

Even with collective bargaining rights, veterans and their coworkers have noticed big gaps between corporate rhetoric and workplace reality. "At job fairs, companies like to say they're hiring a lot of vets because of their organizational and leadership skills from the military," says ex-Marine Ray Rodriguez, secretary-treasurer of Communications Workers of America (CWA) Local 6222 in Houston. "But they never mention they're letting them go out the back door." Such separations from the payroll can occur, en masse, when there is an across-the-board reduction in telephone technician jobs, a not-uncommon occurrence in a rapidly changing telecom industry. They can also occur in individual cases where a CWA member's difficulty readjusting to civilian life— or job performance issues related to PTSD, anxiety, or depression—results in disciplinary action, particularly if they work under "a stressed-out manager who doesn't know how to deal with a veteran of Iraq and Afghanistan."

Rodriguez reports past union jousting with phone company management over such issues as giving veterans time off for a doctor visit at the VA, where he himself is a patient. And he has been involved in disputes over management attempts to reduce disability benefit coverage for union members with a partial disability rating from the VA and related entitlement to federal benefits from that source. Veterans and their coworkers at "union free" companies like Amazon, Walmart, or T-Mobile have no one like Rodriguez who can challenge personnel policies that turn out to be not so veteran friendly. In all three of these firms, plus partially unionized but bitterly antiunion Comcast, many workers have been fired, suspended, harassed, or otherwise discriminated against by management, as documented in dozens of NLRB cases over the years.

One contributing factor to veteran suicide is, of course, financial distress. That condition became far more common among veterans who lacked well-paying union jobs or employer-provided medical coverage after COVID-19 disrupted the economy, produced high levels of unemployment, and killed at least 375,000 Americans in 2020. Under the CARES Act, financial institutions like Texas-based USAA helped distribute federal stimulus money to families in need, those with incomes of less than $75,000 a year. Treasury Secretary Steve Mnuchin had the authority to exempt these payments from debt collection by banks, but Mnuchin, a former Goldman Sachs executive, refused to do so. If any company should have refrained from such dunning on a voluntary basis, it was USAA, a Hiring Our Heroes pledge signer. Much of its customer base of 13 million consists of military families, and its corporate credo—"Many Faces. One Mission"—could easily be mistaken for an Army recruiting slogan.

However, as the *American Prospect* reported, USAA put profit before patriotism by garnishing the checks of customers with existing debts. After reviewing text messages from USAA to many angry customers, *Prospect* executive editor David Dayen discovered that the company had sent them all the same "boilerplate statement to respond to customer complaints about taking their payments." In veteran circles the social media and political backlash against this debt collection was fast and furious.[63] Adam Weinstein, a journalist and Navy veteran, tweeted a threat to cancel his USAA membership and urged his friends to do so as well. Common Defense, the progressive veterans' organization, called USAA's seizure of stimulus payments "absolutely unacceptable" and urged Congress to "make it illegal."

USAA quickly reversed course, assuring the public that any seized funds would be returned to customers in need so they could have "access to their full stimulus payment to help cover the costs of rent, food and other important necessities." In the meantime, a twenty-two-year-old mother of two from Minnesota whose disabled husband was injured on active duty was one of many distressed customers whose confidence in USAA was deeply shaken. Her family's fortunes had recently taken a turn for the better when she landed a new job in childcare and found a new apartment. Suddenly she was laid off due to stay-at-home orders, leaving CARES Act money as the only "chance to stay on top of the bills." After her family's total payment of $3,400 was initially seized, she confessed to Dayen that she didn't "know where the rent is going to come from" or who was "going to help my 18-month-old get her meds. . . . I'm at a loss for words, they don't care."[64]

A RENT-A-VET STRATEGY

Too often veterans' organizations have regarded wider social access to government benefits like free higher education or universal healthcare as a threatening encroachment on what should be, now and forever, a veterans-only entitlement. This narrow and ultimately self-defeating mindset has led some VSOS down a not-so-valorous path. In California, the point man for these tawdry expeditions has been a state capitol insider known as "Mr. Veteran." Until his retirement, Pete Conaty spent two decades as president of Pete Conaty & Associates, a lobbying firm that boasted about its involvement in "over 500 legislative bills dealing with military and veterans' issues." Among these bills were one that made it easier to prosecute "stolen valor phonies" and a law that designates every March 30 as "Welcome Home Vietnam Veterans Day" in California.

Conaty was decorated for his own combat role in Vietnam. He remained in the Army until 1986, when he retired as a lieutenant colonel. After leaving the service, he joined the staff of a newly elected State Assembly member, later becoming his chief of staff and then chief consultant to a key Assembly committee. After Conaty opened his Sacramento lobbying shop in 1996, he signed up, as clients, VSOS directly representing over 800,000 veterans in the state, who belonged to more than 1,000 local posts of the Legion, VFW, and other groups. Conaty's well-advertised connection to this grassroots network enabled him to devise a "rent-a-vet" strategy that's been a big money-maker for his firm and a winner for corporate clients in several high-profile California referendum campaigns.[65]

Win or lose, Conaty's rallying of veterans behind ballot measures or legislation has repeatedly put them—without most even knowing about it—at odds with labor, consumer, and tenant groups, whose membership also includes many veterans. In 2012, for example, Mercury Insurance and its wealthy CEO, George Joseph, wanted to deregulate auto insurance in California and roll back consumer protections previously approved by voters in the state. The big auto insurer spent $17 million to get Proposition 33 on the ballot. However, to win voter approval, backers of the measure needed a display of public support from outside the insurance industry.

Among those willing to be Mercury's beard for a fee was Conaty. As Jamie Court, a Prop. 33 foe and leading California consumer advocate, reports, he made a paid appearance on behalf of Mercury in the state capitol "wearing his veterans' cap and brass." Then, says Court, Conaty's "veteran clients were trotted out across the state in order to falsely drape an American flag on an anti-consumer measure" that would allow firms like Mercury "to charge low-income drivers, including retired military personnel, more if they had a lapse in their auto insurance coverage." Fortunately, Court's own organization, Consumer Watchdog, and allied groups were able to defeat Prop. 33, even though they were outspent 200 to 1.

Four years later, Conaty had more success going to bat for asbestos manufacturers and their attorneys around an issue directly affecting Navy veterans. About 30 percent of all those who have died from asbestos-related lung cancer served in the military during the era when this flame-retardant material was used in naval vessels and buildings on bases. After years of litigation about their liability, the firms that produced asbestos—and long denied that it was hazardous—were forced to set up compensation funds that have paid out more than $17 billion to about 3 million victims, most of them civilian workers.

In 2016, however, lobbyists for the industry persuaded Blake Farenthold, a conservative Republican from Texas, to file a House bill mandating public sharing of sensitive personal information about veterans and other asbestos fund claimants under the guise of reducing fraudulent claims. Then–Democratic minority leader Nancy Pelosi challenged Farenthold's own claim that the Republican majority was only interested in assuring greater "transparency." According to Pelosi, their bill was designed to "support asbestos companies and intimidate victims."[66]

In a letter to the House leadership, fifteen national veterans' organizations all agreed with Pelosi. They denounced the bill as an "offensive invasion of privacy to the men and women who have honorably served" and pointed out that it did "nothing to assure their adequate compensation or to prevent future asbestos exposures and deaths." Back in Sacramento, however, Conaty responded to a request for lobbying help from the US Chamber of Commerce by getting state officials of VVA, the Military Officers Association of America, the American Legion, and three other groups to send a letter to Congress backing Farenthold's bill, even though their national organizations were all opposed to it. The House proceeded to pass Farenthold's bill anyway, despite President Barack Obama's veto threat.[67]

Later that same year, Conaty assembled an even bigger coalition of state veterans' groups on behalf of Big Pharma. This time, his efforts were not disavowed by any of their parent organizations, including the VVA. Both Conaty and local veterans' organizations were financially rewarded by an industry that spent more than $90 million to defeat Proposition 61, the California Drug Price Relief Act. According to Consumer Watchdog, Conaty's firm received $5,000 a month, and then $10,000 monthly as part of this "vote no" campaign; local veterans' groups received thousands of dollars for Prop. 61–related "meetings and appearances."[68]

Backers of Prop. 61, like the California Nurses Association, collected hundreds of thousands of signatures to place it on the November 2016 ballot so future bulk purchases of prescription drugs by the state would be tied to prices paid by the VA for the same drugs. The VA is empowered by federal law to negotiate better drug prices for its 9 million patients, so it pays less for pharmaceuticals than any other public agency in the US, including the state of California. In 2017, for example, the VA "paid an average of 54 percent less for prescription drugs than Medicare did."[69] Prop. 61 promised California taxpayers similar "drug price relief" to the tune of $1 billion per year by lowering the cost of prescriptions for millions of people covered by the state's Medicaid program.

Prop. 61 in no way undermined the better deal on drug prices that veterans get as VA patients. If approved by the electorate, Prop. 61 would have greatly benefited lower-income Californians who are people of color. But voters in Richmond, California, a majority minority community, would never have known that from the billboard that suddenly appeared on Twenty-Third Street, just several blocks away from the city's Veterans Memorial Hall. Paid for by Big Pharma, the billboard depicted an older African American wearing a generic veterans' organization cap. His message to local voters, courtesy of Pete Conaty, was that Prop. 61 was a threat to veterans and their healthcare. Billboards like this, with images adjusted to local demographics, popped up all across the state.

In 2018 similar messaging helped sway voters against Proposition 10, which was defeated after $74 million worth of negative advertising. This time, millions of California voters got glossy mass mailers from "a coalition of veterans" that relied on "major funding" from the California Association of Realtors and two big real estate investors. Among the groups listed were Pete Conaty's usual VSO clients, like the American Legion, VFW, and the American Veterans organization (AMVETS), along with their lesser-known cousins like the American GI Forum, the Women Veterans Alliance, and Jewish War Veterans. In one mailer Richmond voters were told by Latino veteran Frederick A. Romero from the GI Forum that "Prop 10 will eliminate homeowner protections and could reduce average home values by $60,000." In the same mailer, there was a full-page photo of Colonel Lorna Griess (ret.), a veteran of twenty-six years in the Army Nursing Corps, who is holding a framed display of her service decorations. Says Griess: "I was a veteran in Vietnam. Prop 10 will make housing less available for homeless and struggling veterans."

What was Prop. 10 really about? As housing activist Amy Schur explained, it would have removed "a state impediment to municipal action against rent gouging and skyrocketing rents" by repealing a state law that limited local rent regulation to housing built after 1995 and allowing big rent hikes when tenants move out of rent-controlled units. Prop. 10 had the support of the state Democratic Party, the city councils of San Francisco and Los Angeles, and major unions representing state employees, teachers, nurses, and other hospital workers.

In November 2020, Conaty enlisted his vso clients in the business-backed "Californians for Responsible Housing / Vote No on Prop. 21 Coalition." Like Prop. 10 before it, Proposition 21 tried to expand the scope of local rent regulation so more tenants could be protected from unreasonable increases at a time when millions of Californians faced loss of their rental housing due to pandemic-related unemployment. As one fellow veteran and former Sacramento lobbyist told us, this measure "would not harm veterans. It's going to absolutely help veterans who need a leg up, who are elderly, or just coming back from military service." Nevertheless, Prop. 21 was defeated by roughly the same 20 percent margin as Prop. 10.

Among the prominent Californians on the losing side was ninety-year-old Dolores Huerta, a longtime social justice advocate and cofounder of the United Farm Workers. She and Cesar Chavez braved beatings, death threats, picket-line arrests, and jailing when they struggled to improve housing conditions and workplace protections for immigrant farmworkers. In tribute to those valorous efforts, Chavez's name now adorns countless schools, streets, and community buildings throughout California. Thousands of units of low-income housing have been built or renovated by a foundation named after him. But thanks to Conaty, one of the most famous names in Latino labor history popped up on the "Vote No" side of the Prop. 21 campaign. Among the eighteen veterans' groups opposed to making housing more affordable in the Golden State was the Cesar Chavez Chapter of the American GI Forum in Sacramento.

4. LAST STAND OF THE LEGION POST?

We did some great things over the last one hundred years.
—AMERICAN LEGION NATIONAL COMMANDER
BRETT T. REISTAD, January 2019

We used to be a leader—now we ride coattails.
—ANONYMOUS LEGION HEADQUARTERS
STAFFER, summer of 2019

On a chilly night in January 2019, as the American Legion entered its centennial year, a convoy of black SUVs with tinted windows made its way up Pacific Avenue in San Francisco, California. The vehicles were accompanied, front and back, by a squad of SFPD motorcycle cops with their lights flashing and engines gunning. This VIP escort suggested that a visiting dignitary was making a stop in Chinatown as part of an official itinerary. And sure enough, the lead vehicle stopped right in front of New Asia, a cavernous banquet hall at 772 Pacific beloved by tourists and locals alike.

Waiting dutifully by the front door was a small group of men and women in red shirts, eager to greet their out-of-town guest. He stepped out of the car into the cool, foggy night and headed toward them. They quickly ushered him inside, past hundreds of young San Franciscans attending a dinner tribute to four newly elected members of the city's left-leaning board of supervisors. In a much smaller banquet space, sectioned off in the back of New Asia's second floor, about seventy-five men and women, mainly middle-aged, were already seated at round tables or clustered near a cash bar.

By their dinner dress alone—distinctive headgear, buttons, and badges—and their flag-bedecked podium, it was obvious they belonged to a different tribe than the one downstairs. The guest of honor, Brett P. Reistad, was a tall, stocky Virginian, not a local politician. He was a conservative retired police officer and, at the time, national commander of the American Legion. His entourage looked the part as well, consisting mainly of paunchy, older white males of Vietnam-era vintage.

Nevertheless, Reistad's local hosts defied popular stereotypes about the Legion. Their Cathay Post 384 was founded in 1931 by veterans who had been excluded from other San Francisco Legion affiliates after World War I because they were not white.[1] To this day, Asian Americans still comprise the majority of the Cathay Post membership, which now numbers about 150. Its recent leaders have included Nelson Lum, who served in the 101st Airborne Division; Helen Wong, a retired Army lieutenant colonel; and Roger Dong, a former Air Force colonel.

Thanks to their energetic recruitment efforts, Post 384 has attracted some younger veterans of wars in the Middle East who became students at San Francisco State on the GI Bill. Unlike many Legion affiliates, this one has no bar in its building, preferring to maintain a "family atmosphere" instead. Present day members of the first all-Chinese Boy Scout troop in the US meet there on a regular basis. The Cathay Post also provides scholarships to cadets in Reserve Officers' Training Corps (ROTC) programs at local colleges and high schools. Its members march in Memorial Day and Veterans Day parades, and feed active-duty naval personnel during San Francisco's annual Fleet Week.

As the program for the evening got underway, Legion protocol was observed with a salute to the colors and a POW/MIA recognition moment. These were followed by the Pledge of Allegiance and recitation of a section of the Legion's national constitution, which commits every member "to foster and perpetuate one hundred percent Americanism."[2] A visiting Legion official briefed the crowd on their guest speaker's personal history. After four years in the Army, Brett Reistad spent three decades in local law enforcement, retiring as a police lieutenant. Before becoming national commander in 2018, he rose through the Legion's ranks in Virginia and helped coordinate its lobbying with other veterans' groups so they could "speak with one voice" in Richmond, the state capital.

When the mike was handed to him, Reistad lauded Nelson Lum, a retired police officer, for having "the kind of pull" necessary to arrange such an impressive motorcycle escort. The affable and loquacious Legion commander then reported on his recent trip to the Far East, followed by other stops in California, where Legionnaire Pete Conaty had just helped landlords thwart a statewide expansion of rent regulation. While overseas Reistad visited US troops on Okinawa and conferred with their commanders about "national security issues." After landing in Taiwan, he met its president, various Taiwanese military officials, and members of a local veterans' council. He had assured these US allies that when he returned home, he was going to "put all 2 million members of the American Legion behind lobbying efforts on their behalf."

The major challenge Reistad wished to discuss in what proved to be a forty-five-minute talk was domestic, rather than foreign, and internal to the Legion. To continue doing "all the great things we've done over the last hundred years," he said, the organization had to stop a continuing loss of membership, which added up to eighty thousand lapsed dues-payers in just the previous year. He invited his listeners to become part of the Legion's "Team 100"—active recruiters of new members—and proceeded to tick off highlights of the Legion's hundred-year history that might be useful selling points.

Reistad reminded his audience that one founding purpose of their organization a century ago was "creating an infrastructure to take care of comrades who came back wounded and maimed, to take care of widows and orphans left behind." One of its first legislative victories was securing federal funding for hospital construction and consolidated services for World War I veterans under a single US Veterans Bureau, predecessor of today's VA.[3] Similarly, after World War II, the Legion helped line up a key congressional committee vote to secure passage of the Servicemen's Readjustment Act of 1944.[4] As Reistad noted, some members of Congress believed that paying for college tuition and other benefits for 15 million returning soldiers would be too costly. As it turned out, that bill "didn't break the treasury and fostered prosperity like we've never seen before."

By the fiftieth anniversary of its founding, the Legion was, in Reistad's recounting, going to bat for a new generation of veterans in need. "The American Legion worked hard on behalf of our Vietnam veterans who began suffering health issues that were attributed to the defoliant Agent Orange," he said. "The VA was dragging their feet in providing healthcare treatments and compensation, and the Legion ended up suing the federal government to get them to take action." As a result, he proudly reported, "our Vietnam veterans . . . were granted healthcare and compensation."

In Reistad's view, the Legion was still a key "stakeholder" in the VA and an always-alert "watchdog" over its leadership. "When they do good," he explained, "we pat them on the back. And when they stray off course, we're among the first in line to help get them back on course and do what they need to do for our veterans." Among the Legion's top priorities for the 116th Congress was passage of a bill called the Blue Water Navy Act, written so seventy thousand former sailors could more easily pursue VA benefit claims related to their offshore exposure to Agent Orange during the Vietnam War. Six months later, this bipartisan legislation was passed by Congress and signed into law by President Trump, notwithstanding some initial complaints about its cost impact by some Senate Republicans.[5]

Reistad noted disapprovingly that the VA was, once again, insisting that "all sorts of scientific studies be done first. And you know what happens then, they drag on, and our fellow service members suffer because they don't receive the compensation and they don't receive the treatment." He failed to mention any DOD culpability for the original workplace exposure five or six decades ago or any Republican foot-dragging that might have contributed to this delay.[6] Nor did he ever drop the name of President Donald Trump, whose political appointees were running the VA and, by early 2019, aggressively pursuing privatization of the agency, which the Legion itself had argued was not beneficial for 9 million VA patients.[7]

Preferring to end on a happier note, Reistad praised Congress for authorizing a special American Legion centennial coin, to be minted in several different precious metals. "Once available for sale," he predicted, "they will be great keepsakes, will increase in value, and, if all are sold, will earn $9 million toward our programs and our charities." This income boost was, he warned, no substitute for signing up new Legionnaires "to stop this drain of membership we've been experiencing."

Reistad was, by now, running out of time to entertain any questions from his hungry audience. To get the Legion's recruitment drive in the Bay Area off to a rousing start, he asked everyone to rise and join a call-and-response. He explained that members' role in this exercise would be shouting out, on cue, the second half of the Legion's official Team 100 campaign slogan: "We Are Team 100." Three times in a row, the national commander led off, in a resounding voice, with "We are . . ." Each time, his now-standing audience shouted back in unison, "Team 100!" With that drill dutifully completed, Cathay Post 384 members, spouses, and invited guests could finally dig in to their long-delayed New Asia fare.

SPEAKING WITH ONE VOICE?

Replete with uniformed pomp and circumstance, comforting organizational ritual, reverence for rank and the memory of departed comrades, this veterans' dinner in San Francisco displayed both the surviving strengths and the glaring shortcomings of traditional veterans' service organizations (VSOS). The Legion is the largest and best known of this constellation of advocacy groups. Other members of the "Big Six," as they're known in veteran circles, include the Veterans of Foreign Wars (VFW), AMVETS, the Disabled American Veterans (DAV), the Paralyzed Veterans of America (PVA), and Vietnam Veterans of America (VVA). As national organizations formed after particular late nineteenth- or twentieth-century conflicts, all followed in the footsteps of a Civil War–inspired predecessor known as the Grand Army of the Republic. Founded by Union veterans in 1866, the Grand Army had local posts throughout the North and didn't disband until 1956, when its last surviving member died. Its counterpart among the defeated was United Confederate Veterans, which similarly aged out of existence.

In the aftermath of the Spanish-American War, the group now known as the VFW was established—and has continued to replenish its ranks, thanks to a never-ending series of foreign wars. Veterans of World War I formed the Legion and the DAV. The latter focuses on problems of former soldiers who've been injured, as does the PVA, created in 1947. AMVETS, which claims 250,000 members today, was started by World War II veterans but later opened its doors to any honorably discharged person who served on active duty, in the Reserves and National Guard, in any era. The VVA is a Vietnam-era veterans' project, now in danger of extinction as its generational cohort dies out. There has long been membership overlap between the big umbrella groups, like the Legion and VFW, and much smaller outfits organized around ethnicity, past officer rank, or branch of service, like the Jewish or Italian American War Veterans, the Military Officers Association of America, or the Marine Corps League.

Like US unions during their post–World War II heyday, the Big Six gained and wielded considerable political clout by being membership organizations with millions of dues-payers. VSOS have both elected national organization leaders and professional staff members in Washington, DC. They have state and national conventions where elected delegates vote on organizational policies and positions. In the case of the Legion and VFW, they maintain a grassroots network of local affiliates with their own elected officers, membership base, buildings to meet and socialize in, and community service programs like scout troops, sports leagues, and scholarships for local young people. Because of its concern about substance abuse among veterans, the VVA distinguished itself by not operating clubs with bars; for many years, it opened thrift shops instead. In thousands of US communities, local posts or chapters of the Legion or VFW have long been part of the infrastructure of working-class life for members, their families, and guests, which often include individuals or groups renting meeting or party space for nonveteran use.[8]

At the local level, VSOs are a vehicle for expressing, in ways both positive and negative, a shared veteran identity. They foster a culture of solidarity, mutual aid, and protection for their members, just like well-functioning, community-based trade unions do. In a fashion very important to the millions of veterans with service-related health problems, they function much like associations of injured workers always have throughout the history of American labor, by pursuing individual and collective claims for better compensation and treatment.[9]

While the VSOs often lobby together for VA funding and benefit expansion, veterans themselves have rarely "spoken with one voice"—either about the VA or their former employer, the US military, which tends to get far less blame for any service-related problems than the VA does for real or imagined failures to fix them. The actual history of the Legion, as opposed to the anodyne version offered up at Cathay Post 384 by Commander Reistad, is replete with ideological conflict and jousting with other organizations. During recurring periods of postwar turmoil, the two main VSOs—the Legion and the VFW—were so slow to respond to the needs of their primary constituency that militant veterans were forced to take direct action. They created grassroots protest movements or new progressive advocacy groups to influence Congress, the White House, and public opinion in different and more effective ways.

Issues related to class, race, gender, or foreign policy have long created deep fault lines among former soldiers, from the founding of the Legion to the present day. And long before post-9/11 veterans started their own alternative groups, as described in the next chapter, there were other political voices and organizational forces trying to woo veterans away from Legion-defined "one hundred percent Americanism" and its narrow defense of veterans' interests. The Legion, meanwhile, has continued to play a conservative role in American society as a bulwark of the status quo and pillar of the political establishment. In fact, the role it played as a modern-day foe of consumers' and tenants' rights today in California, as recounted in the previous chapter, merely reprised its alliance with big business a century ago.

TAKING CARE OF OUR OWN?

As Secretary of State Mike Pompeo told Legion members, when addressing the organization's national convention in 2019, "'Americanism' means taking care of our own."[10] From the moment of its birth, that Legion watchword signaled that its political agenda would be broader than just lobbying for disabled comrades. World War I officers, rather than enlisted men, dominated the Legion's founding meetings in 1919. Labor unrest at home and abroad—in revolutionary Russia—was very much on their mind.[11]

The Legion's first national commander, Franklin D'Olier, was a millionaire textile manufacturer from Philadelphia. As such, he was well positioned to raise money from other employers to help fund an organizational counterweight to insurgent native-born workers and foreigners of suspect loyalty. During the same year that nearly 1 million former soldiers and sailors joined the Legion, D'Olier was able to supplement the Legion's membership dues income with generous donations from big business, a fundraising strategy pursued by veterans' organizations, including the Legion, to this day.[12] The Legion quickly became a source of management muscle, much applauded in the mainstream media, during a period of deepening political reaction.

James Maurer, president of the Pennsylvania Federation of Labor, recalled this thuggery as follows: "Constitutional rights were flagrantly violated, free speech was throttled, public and labor union meetings were mobbed, labor schools, labor union headquarters, and the offices of labor and progressive publications were invaded by mobs composed of American Legion members, disbanded sailors and soldiers, deputy-sheriffs, state police and just plain hoodlums."[13] Alvin Owsley, who commanded the Legion in the 1920s, was an admirer of Italian dictator Benito Mussolini, who was favorably profiled in the Legion's national magazine. "Do not forget," Owsley said, "that the Fascisti are to Italy what the American Legion is to the United States."[14] In 1930 the Legion even tried to get Il Duce to speak at its national convention. By then Wall Street had crashed and the Great Depression was underway.

This left many World War I veterans impoverished and angry about waiting until 1945 to receive promised postwar bonuses.

A few hundred set out from Portland, Oregon, to petition Congress for immediate payment; their numbers swelled to twenty thousand by the time they reached Washington, DC, in May 1932. President Herbert Hoover, a conservative Republican, refused to meet with them and rejected their main demand. His position was backed by the Legion, which feared that earlier payment of veterans' bonuses would place "unnecessary financial burden upon the nation."[15] The Bonus Marchers created a huge encampment along the banks of the Anacostia River, not far from the Capitol. The crowd included women and children and was multiracial in an era when both the military and veterans' organizations were segregated. Roy Wilkins, who became president of the National Association for the Advancement of Colored People (NAACP) and a reporter for its newspaper, was so impressed that he "saw it as a model for integration in the United States."[16]

All the major veterans' organizations were dismissive of the protest: the VFW's deputy commander claimed that the "'Bonus Army' was doing all veterans all over the country great harm." The national commander of the DAV disavowed any connection to it. Legion headquarters remained aloof as well, due to Hoover's red-baiting of the Bonus Marchers and his false claim, in a letter to Legion members, that "less than half" of them had "ever served under the American flag."[17]

After a two-month standoff, Hoover ordered active-duty troops—led by future World War II generals Douglas MacArthur, George Patton, and Dwight D. Eisenhower—to eradicate this threatening display of "lower-class veteran solidarity."[18] Using cavalry, tanks, tear gas, and fixed bayonets, the regular Army destroyed and burned the Bonus Army's campsite, driving its inhabitants from the city. Two veterans were killed and a thousand wounded. Like a smaller-scale and less violent confrontation in Lafayette Park eighty-eight years later, this distressing spectacle did much damage to the reelection chances of an incumbent Republican president. In 1934, after Hoover's electoral defeat, Congress finally authorized payment to World War I veterans in the form of bonds, which most cashed in immediately to survive the Depression. When the Legion began pushing for passage of the Servicemen's Readjustment Act of 1944, the memory of the Bonus March was a valuable lobbying tool. Legion commander Henry Colmery reminded Congress about all "the men who wore uniforms" on different sides in World War I and then tried to overthrow their own governments.[19]

COLD WAR DISSENTERS

After World War II, the Legion was eager to reprise its post–World War I role as a patriotic foe of labor and the left. Its leadership strongly opposed any efforts to reduce Cold War tensions between the US and its former ally, the Soviet Union. Instead, both the Legion and the VFW backed the costly and dangerous nuclear arms race that soon commenced between the two postwar superpowers. To ensure that the "subversive activities" of any Americans critical of the Cold War were closely monitored and reported to the FBI, the Legion offered the volunteer services of its eleven thousand local posts.[20]

By 1947 nearly 100,000 returning veterans who were more liberal minded or peace oriented had joined the American Veterans Committee (AVC) instead of the Legion. AVC's organizational motto was "Citizens First, Veterans Second."[21] Unlike the Legion and the VFW, the AVC welcomed women and nonwhite men as full members and had racially integrated local chapters in southern states even before the civil rights movement began. The organization was heavily red-baited during the McCarthy period and conducted its own divisive purge of veterans linked to the Communist Party. After that, AVC membership shrank even further, but the group soldiered on into the 1960s and 1970s, advocating for civil rights, civil liberties, and nonwhite veterans who were discharged unfairly. In 1965, former *Stars and Stripes* columnist June Willenz became its executive director. She was the first woman to head a veterans' organization, and she remained at the AVC's helm until it disbanded in 2003. Willenz lobbied the VA to create its first advisory committee to assess the needs of female veterans and urged Congress to upgrade benefits and expand career opportunities for women in the military, a cause later embraced by the new VSOs profiled in the next chapter.[22]

By the early 1970s, the older VSOs were all dominated by World War II and Korean War veterans. Their top officials and local post leaders were generally in favor of the US intervention in Vietnam and not welcoming to returning veterans who questioned the war. The latter responded by forming their own organizations—Vietnam Veterans Against the War (VVAW) and then the VVA, which worked closely with a like-minded congressional caucus of Vietnam-era vets who were similarly critical of old-guard VSO behavior. The VVAW was forged by militant protest movements inside and outside the military. While still on active duty, draftees and volunteers opposed to the Vietnam War were able to find validation, solidarity, and support via the GI Coffeehouse network, which was part of the broader antiwar movement.

Dramatic expressions of Black pride and power by African Americans in uniform were a key part of this resistance in Southeast Asia and on military bases at home. While student demonstrators and draft resisters drew more mass media attention at the time, many active-duty soldiers and recently returned veterans turned against the war with equal fervor and often with greater impact.[23]

During its period of peak membership—twenty-five thousand—and activity in the late 1960s and early 1970s, VVAW sponsored a series of high-profile antiwar actions while also "providing information on GI resistance, lobbying for GI rights and benefits, organizing on campuses, and running a recruiting ad in the February 1970 issue of *Playboy*, which brought thousands of new members."[24] As Vietnam veteran and VVAW member Jerry Lembcke recalls in *The Spitting Image: Myth, Memory, and the Legacy of Vietnam*, President Richard Nixon tried to counter huge antiwar demonstrations in the fall of 1969—and the increasing support for them among military personnel—by rallying "the VFW and American Legion as players in the street politics of the Vietnam War."[25]

In April 1971, a thousand VVAW members set up a Bonus March–style encampment in Washington, DC. Their planned Capitol Hill lobbying took place amid a tense legal battle—which reached the Supreme Court—over VVAW's right to camp overnight on the Mall. As lawyer and Air Force veteran Brian Wilson recalls that standoff in his 2018 memoir, *Don't Thank Me for My Service*, "Many Congresspersons and Senators publicly supported the veterans, but traditional groups like the American Legion and Veterans of Foreign Wars harshly condemned them."[26]

Before VVAW members dispersed peacefully, hundreds of them approached the steps of the Capitol and, one by one, threw their medals over a fence erected around the building. This became one of the most moving and dramatic rejections of the Vietnam War ever captured on film or in news coverage. At a congressional hearing inside, a VVAW member named John Kerry was invited to speak on their behalf before the Senate Foreign Relations Committee. There the Yale graduate and Navy veteran helped launch his own political career by asking the famous question "How do you ask a man to be the last man to die for a mistake?" Kerry and the VVAW soon went their separate ways; the latter descended into "sectarian strife" that left it "seriously undermined" by 1972.[27] Kerry went on to become lieutenant governor of Massachusetts, then its US senator, a Democratic presidential candidate in 2004, and secretary of state in the Obama administration. As Kerry explained in his autobiography, "VVAW was divided over issues of class . . . between opposition to the war in Vietnam and opposition to all wars, between those who believed that America could be put back together and those who thought the whole system was rotten to the core. I was decidedly in the camp that wanted to set the country right."[28] Other VVAW alumni, more left-leaning than Kerry, went on to create Veterans for Peace (VFP). Its thirty-five-year-old network of four thousand veterans continues to oppose war and imperialism with a multigenerational membership base. Although notable for its fractious internal debates and political disputes, the VFP—unlike newer veterans' organizations—has dues-paying members, local chapters, and a democratic internal structure, including regular elections of its national leadership.[29]

THE VIETNAM VET CHALLENGE

Much definitely needed to be done for the nation's 9 million Vietnam-era veterans, about a third of whom served in or near Vietnam. Their postwar unemployment rate was high: an estimated 30 to 50 percent of all disabled veterans were unable to find jobs, even though Congress passed legislation—not effectively enforced—that gave ex-soldiers preferential hiring consideration for public-sector employment and jobs with federal contractors. Vietnam combat veterans had readjustment problems, including drug and alcohol abuse, that landed some in jail.[30]

Several hundred thousand received bad paper discharges that deprived them of any VA benefits and "severely damaged their employability for the rest of their lives."[31] Adding insult to injury were presidents who "spent billions of dollars per week prosecuting the war each vetoed or threatened to veto proposals for the war's veterans on the basis of expense."[32] Under Lyndon Johnson, Vietnam GI Bill benefits authorized by Congress in 1966 were so paltry that the percentage of veterans who became students was lower than after World War II or Korea, and few could attend elite private universities because only a fraction of their higher tuition costs was covered. More than 40 percent of Vietnam veterans who went to college had to work part-time to survive financially, which made it harder for them to complete their studies and get a degree. During his first term, Republican Richard Nixon—a World War II veteran—balked at GI Bill benefit increases proposed by Congress. Amid worsening conditions in overcrowded veterans' hospitals—depicted most memorably in the book and film *Born on the Fourth of July*—Nixon vetoed an appropriation bill because it contained $105 million more than he had requested for the VA medical system.

Nixon and his Republican successor, Gerald Ford—also a World War II veteran—were not the only executive branch obstacles to making progress on behalf of Vietnam veterans. Their hopes for a better deal under Democrat Jimmy Carter, a Naval Academy graduate whose son was a Vietnam veteran, were slowly crushed as well. As a presidential candidate in 1976, Carter told the Legion that Vietnam vets "have been a victim of government insensitivity and neglect" and declared that he would shake up the "incompetent, inefficient, and unresponsive" federal bureaucracy that was failing them. But even with Max Cleland, a disabled Vietnam veteran, serving as its VA secretary, the Carter administration was notable "for the slowness of its response," according to Dave Bonior, an Air Force veteran elected to Congress in 1976. Bonior helped form a new Capitol Hill caucus composed of Vietnam-era veterans, including Al Gore from Tennessee and John Murtha from Pennsylvania. Their eleven-member group rallied support for a proposed Vietnam Veterans Act of 1979, which addressed the need for "jobs, education, reform of the GI bill, compensation for Agent Orange poisoning, mental health counseling, and upgrading discharges."[33]

According to Bonior, "The traditional veterans' establishment wanted nothing to do with our effort," which helped ensure that any of its legislative gains in the next few years would be piecemeal and incremental. As Bonior notes in his memoir, *Whip: Leading the Progressive Battle during the Rise of the Right*:

> The three largest vets advocacy organizations—the American Legion, with 2.5 million members and an auxiliary of 930,000; the Veterans of Foreign Wars, with two million members and 700,000 in the auxiliary[;] and the Disabled American Veterans (DAV) had the size and power to block us. The Veterans Administration . . . was led by an older generation of officials intent on protecting benefits for their fellow World War II vets. . . . An arch-conservative Democrat from Texas who chaired the Veterans Affairs Committee, a naval veteran of World War II and Korea, displayed allegiance only to veterans from his generation and never held a single day of hearings on bills introduced to aid those who'd served in Vietnam [because he saw such legislation] as inevitably diminishing programs on which older veterans relied.[34]

To prevail over this "iron troika that stood in the way of progress," the Vietnam veterans in Congress worked closely with the VVA. Originally known as the Council of Vietnam Veterans, VVA was cofounded in 1978 by Bobby Muller, a disabled former Marine lieutenant. Within five years, VVA had thousands of members and hundreds of local chapters. After Carter's loss to Republican Ronald Reagan in 1980, VVA and Bonior had to defend recently authorized funding and VA staffing of a nationwide network of Readjustment Counseling Centers—known as Vet Centers—created to expand community-based treatment for PTSD, an approach initially opposed by the Legion.

Although Reagan remained popular with the VFW and other veterans' groups because of his hawkish foreign policy views, his administration opposed expanded Vietnam vet access to GI Bill benefits, small business loans, and employment programs. Even legislation backed by the VVA, which sought VA healthcare and compensation for victims of Agent Orange exposure, was not enacted until 1991 because of undermining by the Reagan administration. Behind the scenes, White House advisers argued that compensating veterans for Agent Orange–related illnesses would upset the "delicate balance between Reagan-era tax cuts and large-scale defense spending" and "might end up bankrupting the government as future toxic claims continued to pour in."[35]

After conducting its own study of Vietnam veteran readjustment problems and healthcare needs, the DAV became the old-line VSO most responsive to the needs of a new generation of veterans. Along with the Legion, it started to incorporate more Vietnam vets into its headquarters staff and leadership, realizing belatedly that they "were clearly the organization's future membership base."[36] Meanwhile, a Vietnam veteran didn't reach the top leadership of the VFW until the mid-1980s, more than two decades after that war began. The VFW preferred to innovate as an inside-the-Beltway player by becoming the first VSO to create a national political action committee (PAC). But, as Bonior observed, "old habits die hard." One of the first candidates the new PAC opposed was a California Democrat on the House Veterans Affairs Committee with a 100 percent voting record on veterans' issues but positions on foreign policy and defense spending that the VFW found objectionable. The VFW PAC also played a role in Carter's reelection defeat despite VA improvements made in the face of Republican opposition.[37]

MEMBERSHIP IN DECLINE

In recent decades the inside-the-Beltway clout of the old VSOs has—for better or worse, depending on your view of them—been eroded by shrinking membership. Their organizational decline parallels the erosion of labor union influence and infrastructure nationally and locally, with similar adverse consequences for their overlapping working-class membership. While the Legion still claims on its website to have more than 2 million members, the actual number is 1.8 million and dropping, down from a peak membership of 3.1 million in the 1990s. By 2019 more than 70 percent of Legionnaires were over the age of sixty. Similarly, the VFW has lost a third of its dues-payers in the last twenty years. The average age of the 1.3 million left is sixty-seven, and 400,000 are eighty or older. A thousand of its local posts have closed in the past decade. Half of all veterans—about 10 million—don't belong to any veterans' organization. Only 15 percent of those who've served in Iraq and Afghanistan have joined the Legion or VFW.[38] And the total number of post-9/11 vets is, of course, much smaller than the huge multigenerational, drafted cohort from World War II, Korea, and Vietnam, which is aging out of existence.

Some VSO members, particularly in the VFW, are not in denial about these trends. They have bravely tried to modernize the culture of local posts in order to make them more welcoming to veterans who are female, nonwhite, or trying to avoid addictive behavior. In Denver, for example, VFW Post 1 has relocated to a hipster neighborhood and now doubles as an art gallery while offering classes in acting, photography, yoga, and tai chi, with a resulting boost in membership. Post 1 takes particular pride in welcoming female and gay veterans. Its senior vice commander is thirty-two-year-old Brittany Bartges, a former intelligence officer who returned from Iraq in 2007 and initially felt out of place at VFW posts elsewhere because "people assumed you were there to pick up your dad or something."[39]

Lindsay Church is one young veteran who tried to reform the Legion before leaving it to cofound and direct Minority Veterans of America. She became commander of Legion Post 40 at a time when even the Legion's national headquarters was suggesting that local posts consider offering childcare, Wi-Fi, and video games to make them more family friendly. But in Post 40, too many members had a retrograde view of what constituted a "family." As one told Church, "It's okay that you're gay, but you don't need to talk about your wife." Some of the female veterans she recruited to the post were asked out on dates or otherwise made to feel uncomfortable. "I kept telling my friends, 'It's going to get better,'" Church said. "But I was harming my people, and it weighed on me. One day I realized that my work was perpetuating an old school mentality, so I left."[40]

Local resistance to racial integration was long part of that old-school mentality in the Legion, which is why there are some posts, like Cathay 384, whose members are almost exclusively veterans of color. As of 2020, no nonwhite person has ever been elected national commander of the Legion, and just one woman has served in that role—Denise Rohan, Brett Reistad's predecessor. The slate of candidates for vice commander positions in 2020 was entirely white; at Legion headquarters in Indianapolis, only one African American has ever served in a senior leadership role. Legion commission and committee leaders included only one person of color, Chanin Nunta-vong, an Asian American who serves as executive director of the Legion's Washington, DC, office.

One of the most prominent Black female veterans working there in recent years—Melissa Bryant, director of the Legion's national legislative division—left in dismay over the organization's response to Black Lives Matter protests. In a statement issued by Brett Reistad's successor, James Oxford, the Legion likened BLM to a "virus" capable of causing "more long-term destruction than COVID-19."[41] This reaction to the killing of George Floyd in 2020 was reminiscent of the Legion's claim four years earlier that NFL quarterback Colin Kaepernick was guilty of a "vicious attack on law enforcement" when he knelt during the national anthem.[42] The Kaepernick flap led some Legion posts around the country to inform members that the TVs mounted on the walls of their bars would not be showing any NFL games played by teams whose players engaged in similar peaceful protests.

Even on an issue once controversial but now far less so, the Legion managed to fumble the ball badly. As cannabis use was legalized to varying degrees around the country, younger veterans bridled at the federal ban on medical marijuana prescriptions from the VA, which forced them to pay out of pocket elsewhere. At the local level, Legion membership sentiment shifted in favor of expanded veteran access to medical marijuana. But according to several former Legion staffers, a group of headquarters insiders, known informally as the "God Squad," prevented this from becoming a national legislative priority. Fed up with this in-house opposition, one Legion legislative aide, Eric Goepel, left to found the Veterans Cannabis Coalition (VCC). The VCC has cultivated bipartisan support in Congress for VA clinical trials on the use of cannabis to treat chronic pain and PTSD. "There's a lot of ageism in the Legion," said Goepel, when asked about his job switch. "It felt like I was paddling a canoe upriver by myself."

CONSERVATIVE COMPETITION

While the Big Six were experiencing membership decline and varying degrees of organizational dysfunction, their traditional role as a friendly watchdog over the VA was being undercut inside the Beltway by a new veterans' group. Called the Concerned Veterans for America (CVA), it was backed by the billionaire Koch brothers and quickly developed its own competing relationships with Republicans in Congress who were definitely not VA friendly. The Kochs initially tried to influence policy affecting veterans and line up GOP support for their ideas via the conservative Cato Institute, which they also funded. Cato came up with a plan to replace VA-delivered care for veterans with vouchers that they could take to any private doctor or hospital, which would then be reimbursed in Medicare fashion. Leading Republicans like Senator John McCain, House Speaker John Boehner, and their party's 2012 presidential candidate, Mitt Romney, were all initially receptive to "voucherization" of the VA. But when the American Legion and other VSOs strongly objected to this concept, all of them backed away from it.

The Kochs had better luck promoting privatization via House Republicans they helped finance and elect. In 2010, for example, a Koch-backed oil industry executive named Bill Flores successfully challenged a pro-VA congressional Democrat in Texas. The defeated twenty-year incumbent, Chet Edwards, had secured new educational benefits for children of service members, created a public-private military family housing program, and helped boost funding for veterans' healthcare by 70 percent while serving on a Veterans Affairs subcommittee and other House bodies. Edwards was backed by the National Rifle Association, the Texas Farm Bureau, and many veterans' groups. His campaign accused Flores of favoring privatization of both Social Security and the VA. Flores argued that he only wanted to give "veterans the choice to use private doctors at government cost if they don't want to travel to a VA hospital."[43] Aided by a TV ad blitz featuring John McCain—a fellow proponent of "choice"—Flores beat Edwards by twenty-five points.

One year later, the Kochs and other right-wing funders launched CVA so their ideological challenge to public provision of healthcare would have more veteran cover. CVA was then, and is now, a case study in corporate-backed astroturfing. Unlike the old VSOs, it has no grassroots infrastructure in the form of veterans' posts or chapters. Its national leadership and staff have no accountability, via internal elections or conventions, to decisions made or resolutions passed by any dues-paying members—which the old VSOs, for all their flaws, still have. But with a big startup budget, CVA easily recruited a small cadre of conservative veterans who were personally ambitious, energetic, articulate, and, most of all, media savvy.

One of the most telegenic of these upstarts was Pete Hegseth, now a star pundit on Fox News. Hegseth became a commissioned Army officer via the ROTC program at Princeton University, where he wrote for a student publication called the *Princeton Tory*. He later served in Iraq and Afghanistan and with a National Guard unit in charge of detainees at Guantanamo Bay. After winning two Bronze Stars and leaving the military as a captain, Hegseth returned to his home state of Minnesota. There he attempted to enter politics as a Republican candidate for the US Senate; he later withdrew from a primary race because of Tea Party candidate competition. As CVA's newly hired CEO, Hegseth made his first media splashes conflating two very different federally funded healthcare programs—the VA and President Barack Obama's newly enacted Affordable Care Act (ACA). According to Hegseth, both were proof that "government healthcare doesn't work."[44] The same message was delivered by Arizona veteran and fellow CVA leader Dan Caldwell in opinion pieces that appeared in *USA Today*, *The Hill*, and the *Washington Examiner*. In 2015 the *Arizona Republic*, which, like *USA Today*, is owned by the Gannett Company, was lauding CVA's advocacy work and criticizing Obama for excluding it from a White House roundtable with other veterans' groups.[45]

As CVA honed its critique of the VA, Republican legislators and congressional candidates began parroting it. Among them was Congressman Jeff Miller, a tan, affable former TV weatherman and Florida Democrat who became a Tea Party Republican and, in 2011, new chair of the House Veterans Affairs Committee.[46] In that capacity, Miller welcomed testimony from the CVA on veterans' issues and began to coordinate closely with the group. Florida's new Republican senator, Marco Rubio—also a Tea Party and Koch brothers favorite—promoted CVA-inspired legislation to strip VA employees of workplace rights.

Their growing hostility toward the VA coincided with expansion of its medical coverage under the leadership of Eric Shinseki, a retired four-star general and Vietnam veteran who served as Obama's first VA secretary. In 2010, Shinseki added three new health conditions presumptively tied to Agent Orange exposure. Much applauded by the Big Six, this reform finally allowed hundreds of thousands of additional Vietnam-era veterans to access VA care. Unfortunately, this long-overdue change inundated a still-understaffed Veterans Benefits Administration (VBA) with new claims, creating a backlog, and simultaneously expanded the patient load of hospitals still struggling to cope with an influx of post-9/11 veterans.

The VBA, the official portal for accessing VA services, has long been "a broken door," according to benefits expert Paul Sullivan. While Congress, on a bipartisan basis, has traditionally backed ever-larger military budgets, federal spending on VBA claim processing rarely keeps up with any postwar surge in new claims from recently damaged veterans as well as additional patients. When veterans objected to VBA delays or longer wait times for mental health appointments, Chairman Miller wove these complaints into what one observer called "a broader narrative of government mismanagement and inefficiency under the Obama administration."[47] In response, VA Undersecretary for Health Robert A. Petzel made an ill-fated decision. VA medical centers were directed to schedule all appointments, whether for mental health issues or any other, within fourteen days of a patient's request. It was a goal that could not be met with available resources.

With the Senate still under Democratic control, the chair of the Veterans Affairs Committee, longtime VA supporter Bernie Sanders, tried to meet the agency's critical resource needs. By early 2014, Sanders knew that the VA had about thirty-four thousand vacancies due to retirements, transfers, or promotions but lacked sufficient funds to hire new employees to fill those slots. Roughly 40 percent of the VA's workforce was approaching retirement age, meaning there would be even more vacant positions in the near future.[48] At the same time, the number of veterans over age seventy-five—a population more dependent on VA services—was expected to increase by 46 percent over the next fifteen years. As committee chair, Sanders held hearings to highlight these issues and lay the groundwork for remedial legislation. In early 2014, he got top VA officials, the Legion, and other VSOs all lined up behind an ambitious proposal called the "Comprehensive Veterans Health and Benefits and Military Retirement Pay Restoration Act of 2014." If enacted, it would have authorized $24 billion for new VA hiring and infrastructure improvements. The bill would also have created an education and peer support program for military family members and caregivers with mental health disorders, expanded veteran dental care coverage, and expanded VA services for victims of military sexual assault.

Sanders's initiative was dead on arrival in the Republican-controlled House. In the Senate, Sanders had to contend with John McCain, whose past opposition to VA budgetary supplements had earned him poor ratings on the legislative report cards of some VSOs. True to form, McCain helped rally the Senate minority to block Sanders's bill as well. A few months after new VA funding was thwarted, CVA, along with its allies in Congress and the media, was able to weaponize the issue of VA "wait times" in a way that put Shinseki's job in jeopardy and Obama on the path toward a legislative compromise with lasting consequences.

MANUFACTURING A SCANDAL

In the House, Jeff Miller fired the first shot. During a Veterans Affairs Committee hearing, Miller announced a discovery made by his staff—namely, that top administrators at the VA's Phoenix Health Care System had falsified data about how long patients there were waiting for appointments.[49] This information came from Dr. Sam Foote, a whistleblowing VA doctor, who alleged that actual wait times were longer than fourteen days. Nevertheless, a few VA administrators in Phoenix were collecting performance bonuses based on their false reports that appointment-scheduling goals had been met. Reducing wait times was a bigger challenge in Phoenix than at other VA hospital locations for several reasons. In addition to an influx of newer patients from post-9/11 wars, Arizona already had a sizable year-round population of older veterans, plus a seasonal increase in patient loads during the winter due to visiting "snowbirds" from the Northeast and Midwest.

Despite the recommendations of a Bush administration commission, no new VA medical centers were added to handle an increase in patient demand in Sunbelt cities like Phoenix and Tampa. Miller and other Republican lawmakers turned a problem inherited by Obama into a sweeping indictment of the VA by claiming, falsely, that forty Phoenix-area veterans had died as a result of delayed care. CVA's media star, Pete Hegseth, cited additional cases of veterans dying while awaiting benefit approvals and demanded the immediate resignation of Secretary Shinseki, who had, in reality, managed to reduce the VA disability claim backlog by 84 percent.[50]

An extensive investigation by the VA's Office of Inspector General (IG) later uncovered no evidence to support Miller's widely reported accusation. According to one former VA official, Miller was too busy conducting Joe McCarthy–style press conferences to assist the official investigation of his own charges. "We asked him repeatedly for the names of the forty people who died in Phoenix," this official reported, "so that we could look at their medical files and investigate, but he never actually provided them. We never knew if he actually had a legitimate list or if it was all part of his circus show." The IG concluded that only six veterans had died during the period when wait time data was tampered with. But even in those cases, it was not possible to determine whether they died *while* waiting for a medical appointment or *because* they were waiting for a medical appointment.[51]

To capitalize on the controversy, CVA launched a ten-city "Defend Freedom Tour," replete with press briefings and dozens of interviews. CVA made costly ad buys and produced its own propaganda film, *The Care They've Earned,* which told the story of six veterans dissatisfied with the VA. According to Hegseth, the care they received was "socialized medicine at its worst."[52] Congressman Miller used his ample budget to mount a campaign-style press operation of his own. The Senate Veterans Affairs Committee, led by Sanders, was unable to counter the steady stream of negative publicity generated by the agency's right-wing detractors. Miller was thus able to turn a local VA wait time cover-up into a national "scandal" with the help of pack journalism at its worst.

New York Times reporters, including David Philipps, led the pack with their relentless depiction of the VA as a "demoralized and dysfunctional agency" that had lost the "trust" and "confidence" of its patients. Among those following that lead were CNN, the Washington Post, the Boston Globe, NPR, and other major media outlets. On talk radio, cable TV, and newspaper editorial pages, pressure grew for President Obama to take dramatic action in order to demonstrate his personal concern for veterans. Sanders continued to defend Secretary Shinseki as someone who'd made significant improvements in VA programs, but that support was soon undercut by the American Legion itself. For the first time since 1941, the organization demanded that a cabinet member be purged. The White House replaced Shinseki with Robert McDonald, the West Point graduate and recently retired Procter & Gamble CEO we met briefly in chapter 3.

The administration's hope was that McDonald's reputation for "taking over struggling business units" and turning them around would help restore public confidence in the VA. To assist this effort, Dr. David Shulkin, a longtime private hospital administrator, was made undersecretary for health. As secretary, McDonald got personally involved in trying to recruit more clinical staff for VA facilities. However, even with Shinseki gone, there was little change in Congressman Miller's behavior, which the Legion rewarded by giving him its 2014 Patriot Award for "providing needed oversight and attention to make [the VA] a system truly worth saving."[53] Miller was soon skirmishing with McDonald over issues like his handling of disciplinary action against Phoenix managers fired for misconduct.[54] Miller objected to VA caregivers being given modest bonuses, even though, as former VA official Kenneth Kizer pointed out, enhancing "the government's below-market-value-salaries" was absolutely necessary "to attract new medical specialists" and reduce "a shortage of primary-care physicians or psychiatrists." With much of the mainstream media acting as an echo chamber for Miller and the CVA, it was not long before public opinion was negatively impacted. A 2015 Pew survey of attitudes toward government revealed that the VA's favorability rating had dropped from 68 percent to 39 percent in just two years.[55]

VETERANS CHOICE

In the summer of 2014, the political fallout from Phoenix led Sanders and Mc-Cain back into negotiations over VA funding and patient access to care. The result was bipartisan legislation, approved by President Obama, that would have fateful and—as far as Sanders was concerned—unintended consequences. The VA Choice Act established new outsourcing guidelines that were supposed to last only three years. During that time, veterans could get private-sector care, at VA expense, if they faced wait times longer than thirty days or lived more than forty miles from the nearest VA facility. Of the $16.3 billion allocated by Congress by the Choice Act, just $6 billion was earmarked for VA facility upgrading and expansion and hiring of healthcare staff. This was just one-quarter of what Sanders had proposed six months earlier, and not nearly enough to address staff shortages exacerbated by a slow and overly complex hiring process that Secretary McDonald was trying to speed up.

More than $10 billion in the funding package was set aside for reimbursement of private doctors and hospitals, which became part of the Veterans Choice Program. Two private companies, TriWest Healthcare Alliance and Health Net, were hired to manage this outside network. Both were involved in recruiting private providers, scheduling approved patient appointments with them, sharing medical records, and paying provider-submitted bills. TriWest managed to secure its lucrative piece of the VA Choice contract despite a history of overbilling the federal government for its services.[56] It helped that the firm was based in McCain's home state of Arizona and that its president, David J. McIntyre, had previously served on his Senate staff. Within two years of Choice being launched, VA reimbursement payments to Tri-West and Health Net totaled $649 million.[57] An audit by the VA's IG found evidence of medical claims being paid more than once, payments made at incorrect rates, and overpayments to Health Net and TriWest totaling nearly $89 million during that period.[58] In addition, the IG faulted both contractors for their flawed transfer of medical records from the VA to private providers and poor performance scheduling outside appointments. Some veterans were left waiting between 31 and 389 days to see a private-sector doctor.[59] In January 2021 TriWest settled with the DOJ for $179 million to resolve allegations of overbilling. That news elicited no calls from lawmakers or VSOs to reassess the company's ongoing role in coordinating veteran healthcare.[60]

However problematic it might prove to be for veterans—or costly for taxpayers—VA outsourcing was a potential bonanza for private healthcare interests. Anthem, United Health Group, Emory Healthcare, and other firms began marketing care networks for veterans. This development coincided with a big uptick in healthcare industry spending on lobbying and electoral politics related to veterans affairs. Since 2014, more than four hundred businesses, trade groups, and other special interests have lobbied on veterans' issues—a level of activity about equal to all the reported efforts by the same groups during the entire decade before passage of the Choice Act.[61] By no coincidence, TriWest was among the listed campaign donors to both John McCain and Jeff Miller. It was similarly generous to VSOs old and new, making a $500,000 donation to the Legion to help cover its national convention costs.[62]

Thanks to appointments made by Congress or President Obama, the healthcare industry was heavily represented on the fifteen-member VA Commission on Care, a body created by the Choice Act. Its mission was to develop recommendations for the VA's future direction. Among the influential players involved in its deliberations were commission chair Nancy Schlichting, CEO of the Henry Ford Health System in Michigan, and Toby Cosgrove, CEO of the Cleveland Clinic, whom the White House briefly considered as a replacement for Shinseki until timely media exposure of the Cleveland Clinic's own patient safety problems upended that possible nomination.[63] Two other commissioners also represented "major medical centers that stood to gain from the outsourcing of veterans' care to private providers."[64] Thanks to Congressman Jeff Miller's continuing patronage, CVA was represented by Darin Selnick, a former Army captain and VA official during the Bush administration. AMVETS, a frequent ally of CVA, had one representative on the commission; the Legion and VFW had none. Fortunately, the VA did have two strong defenders in the form of Michael Blecker, a Vietnam veteran who directs Swords to Plowshares, a nonprofit group serving homeless veterans in San Francisco, and Phillip Longman, a Washington, DC, journalist, editor, and author of *Best Care Anywhere: Why VA Health Care Is Better Than Yours.*

The best thing the Care Commission did was hire the RAND Corporation to conduct an "independent assessment of the VA's health care capabilities." RAND researchers confirmed that the VA lacked sufficient caregivers and needed infrastructure improvements. Despite those handicaps, their study revealed that the VA's delivery of inpatient care was "the same or better than non-VA hospitals" and that its outpatient care "outperformed non-VA outpatient care on almost all quality measures."[65] To maintain that level of quality, the commission urged the VA to hire more staff and offer its clinicians more competitive salaries. After noting that veterans with other-than-honorable discharges are denied VA care, commission members even called for congressional reform of VA eligibility rules.

Despite these affirmative findings and constructive proposals, a majority of commissioners favored further expansion of VA outsourcing. In their preferred scenario, the care received by 40 to 60 percent of all veterans would be outsourced to the private sector—in effect, making Choice Act referrals permanent, much wider, and far more costly. In his dissenting opinion, Michael Blecker warned that incremental privatization would undermine the VA and lead to its eventual dismantling.[66] CVA's Darin Selnick dismissed the majority report as "a lost opportunity for the bold reform that the VA needs."[67] In a separate CVA report, called "Fixing Veterans Health Care," Selnick demanded that veterans be given "the same degree of choice that is available to other Americans."[68] Seven months later, CVA was well positioned to implement this "bold reform" when Selnick became an influential member of Donald Trump's Domestic Policy Council and top adviser to his first VA secretary.

MORE BARK THAN BITE?

As the bandwagon for VA privatization gathered momentum in the last years of the Obama administration, the agency's putative defenders reacted with more bark than bite inside the Beltway. In their initial monitoring of Choice Act implementation, the Legion and other VSOs received much negative feedback from their own members. In testimony before Congress, Legion legislative staffer Jeff Steele cited complaints over wait times in the private sector, how medical records were handled there, and the varying quality of outside care. Steele warned about the skyrocketing cost of the outsourcing and insisted that "choice is not the answer."[69] But none of the VSOs sounded the alarm among their hundreds of thousands of remaining members, whose grassroots rallying around an embattled VA might have stiffened the resolve of Democrats while they still controlled the White House.

In the meantime, Senators John McCain and Jerry Moran began drafting legislation that would further institutionalize VA outsourcing when the three-year sunset provision of the Choice Act expired. The Koch brothers were among Moran's top campaign contributors in multiple election cycles. As one critic later described the McCain-Moran bill, it would allow any eligible veteran "to visit a VA facility or a facility in the private sector whenever he or she wanted" and, in the process, "put the entire VA system at risk of harm by diluting its delivery capabilities and costing the U.S. Treasury billions more each year."[70]

As a courtesy to the Big Six, McCain and Moran circulated a draft of their bill among the VSO staffers, seeking their reactions before introducing it. The Legion's legislative director at the time was Lou Celli, a brash and colorful character who adorned his Washington, DC, office door with pictures of Al Pacino playing Tony Montana in *Scarface* and Marlon Brando in *The Godfather*. To his credit, Celli sometimes tried to buck Miller's agenda, at the risk of incurring his wrath. On one occasion the Republican chair of the Veterans Affairs Committee called Celli into his office to complain about a Legion op-ed piece that displeased him. Miller cursed Celli out and demanded an apology, which Celli did not provide, even after Dan Wheeler, the Legion's national commander, urged him to patch things up.

When Celli took his first close look at a hard copy of the McCain-Moran bill, he was working at home over the weekend. The draft legislation so angered him that he set it on fire in his backyard—then displayed its ashy remains in an iPhone image forwarded to VSO friends and colleagues. Unfortunately, when news of this stunt reached Moran, McCain, and their staff, all were much offended. Having ruffled feathers on Capitol Hill but not alerted or mobilized Legion members to bombard McCain or Moran with angry emails or phone calls, "the Legion had lost a lot of bargaining power," according to one of Celli's coworkers. By December 2017 the Legion was waving the white flag of surrender. Along with CVA and AMVETS, it decided to endorse the Veterans Community Care and Access Act of 2017, which McCain and Moran claimed "would transform the VA into a modern, efficient and easy-to-use system that will increase veterans' access to quality care."[71]

As one lobbyist for a dissenting VSO noted, "None of the major veterans' service organizations liked the McCain-Moran bill, but then suddenly the Legion came out in support of it. Instead of us having a united front, we had the largest veterans' group supporting the most conservative path forward." McCain-Moran was never enacted in its own form but did help build momentum for passage of the MISSION Act of 2018, which is described in chapter 6. For one Legion staffer in Washington, the whole disheartening episode was a reminder that the glory days of his veterans' organization were long gone. "We used to be a leader," he privately lamented. "Now we ride coattails."[72]

A NEW REVOLVING DOOR IN DC

In the past almost all the key players involved in veterans affairs worked within the same triangular set of institutions: the vsos, the va, and the Veterans Affairs Committees on Capitol Hill. As Stephen Trynosky notes in *Beyond the Iron Triangle: Implications for the Veterans Health Administration in an Uncertain Policy Environment*, there has long been a revolving door that led vso officials to later administrative positions at the va or staff roles at these two congressional committees. Now, Trynosky says, that traditional "iron triangle" has become a rectangle.[73] Its new fourth side is composed of actual or potential va vendors and outsourcers, who have started to hire vso alumni in the same way that Pentagon contractors have long employed and utilized the connections of former military officers.

Among those who left the Big Six for a new gig in the private sector was Lou Celli, of backyard bill barbecuing fame. The Legion's former legislative director was recruited by Zyter, a Rockville, Maryland, startup that offers it infrastructure improvements for paying customers in private and public healthcare organizations. One of Celli's former Legion colleagues, Matthew Shuman, took a job with Philips, the healthcare technology giant, which has a $100 million contract to help the va upgrade its telehealth system. Carlos Fuentes, former director of the vfw's National Legislative Service, became a senior government strategist for Cerner Government Services, winner of a $16 billion contract to overhaul medical record keeping at the va. Kayda Keleher, a former coworker of Fuentes at the vfw, went to work for Aptive Resources, a DC-area healthcare consulting firm. Adrian Atizado, a Gulf War veteran and former deputy legislative director for dav, was hired by TriWest, which employs a large stable of lobbyists, including former va secretary Anthony Principi.[74]

Even as amvets continued to partner with Humana, the nation's third-largest for-profit insurer, in return for an undisclosed annual donation, its own executive director, Joe Chenelly, was worried about so many former colleagues being wooed away by firms that "want to make their billions off the va." Chenelly explained, "They reach into the [vso] community and pick out folks for their connections. It can be tempting. You make a lot more for a corporate giant. . . . [But] anytime you lose one great advocate it hurts. To lose a whole slew of them can be very difficult to recover from." According to one Legion insider, "There is almost total turnover in staff who worked on the va and no expertise anymore." Making matters worse at Legion headquarters is the fact that several new department heads tend to view the VA as unfavorably as the CVA does. Kris Goldsmith, who was laid off by VVA after its national staff was reduced, agreed with Chenelly. "There's now just a handful of true veteran advocates shaping federal policy," he observed sadly. "Many more of the people influencing decisions and politicians are now just driven by a profit motive." The "corporatization" of veterans affairs is also a trend that extends well beyond the Big Six. As we'll see in the next chapter, new VSOs formed by post-9/11 veterans have their own problematic connections with corporate America, its wealthy political donors, and private foundations.

5. THE NEW VSOS

The young veterans are saying we need to do
things differently with a different emphasis.
—CHUCK HAGEL, Vietnam veteran,
former senator and defense secretary

Every year what one ex-Marine calls "the talented tenth" of post-9/11 veterans flocks to the national convention of Student Veterans of America (SVA). Founded in 2008, SVA is a campus-based support network for younger veterans and markets itself as the "guardian and steward" of the Post-9/11 GI Bill passed by Congress that same year. In 2017 SVA spearheaded efforts to enact the Forever GI Bill, which further expanded benefits for new student veterans. By 2020 it had 1,500 local chapters, representing about 700,000 of the 1 million veterans currently enrolled on campuses across the country. SVA officers, including its national president and CEO, Jared Lyon, see their role as helping "yesterday's warriors" become "today's scholars" and "tomorrow's leaders," particularly in sectors of the economy "ranging from investment banking and industrial manufacturing to technology and communications." To that end, SVA has positioned itself as the vets' organization best able to "help leading companies meet their staffing needs by attracting well-educated veterans who are uniquely qualified to fill their very specific high-growth, high-demand positions." Its impressive roster of business partners includes Google, Microsoft, AT&T, Morgan Stanley, Chevron, Dupont, General Dynamics, Walgreens, Walmart, Bank of America, Aetna, Citi, and Fidelity.[1]

While most participants in SVA's 2020 convention were in their twenties and thirties, a few older VSO members could be spotted among them at a swanky Marriott Hotel in downtown Los Angeles. For the most part, these Big Six officials weren't there to help SVA members find jobs or smooth their personal transitions to civilian life. Their mission was to replenish their own aging and dwindling ranks with younger vets already organizationally active in SVA. The Legion, VFW, AMVETS, DAV, PVA, and VVA made their joint recruitment pitch at a well-attended workshop chaired by thirty-five-year-old Kris Goldsmith, an SVA member studying at Columbia University. Goldsmith, the Army vet from Long Island we met in chapter 1, has tattooed arms, a shaved head, and a long beard that gives him the look of a stern Amish farmer; he stands next to the head table with his service dog, Frosting, resting at his feet.

Goldsmith recalled that his own first contact with older veterans' groups was in smoky bars with no windows and with drinkers old enough to be his father or grandfather. He attended his first SVA convention in 2014 and found it "super eye-opening" because "there were all these young folks." Two years later, he cofounded High Ground Veterans Advocacy, a small nonprofit. Its goal, Goldsmith explained, was "to develop leadership which could help breathe new life into the old-school VSOs." To do that, "you must have skin in the game," which is why Goldsmith encourages fellow post-9/11 veterans to join one or more of these groups.

Goldsmith's panelists included Ryan Gallucci, an Iraq War vet now employed by the VFW in Washington, who explained how his organization helps members file VA benefit claims. Shaun Castle, a former military police officer and staff member of the PVA, touted his group's advocacy on behalf of "everyone with a disability." Joe Chenelly, executive director of AMVETS, reported that his staff of seven hundred served a membership "open to all veterans," 40 percent of whom did not serve in wartime. VVA president John Rowan described how Vietnam vets waged a long struggle to win VA benefits for Agent Orange exposure, which "killed far more of us than the VC [Viet Cong] ever did." DAV legislative staffer Jeremy Villanueva spoke movingly about helping fellow veterans from blue-collar backgrounds like his own overcome the stigma of disability. Wearing his organization's traditional cap, John Kamin from the Legion played up its role in enacting the original GI Bill.

When Goldsmith opened up the session for audience participation, none of the panelists seemed prepared for the question fired at them by former Army sergeant Kayla Williams, author of *Love My Rifle More Than You* and a fellow conference speaker. Williams asked why all six groups—if they were serious about attracting a younger and more diverse membership—had sent a man to represent them on the panel. Her query produced a moment of awkward silence, followed by a series of defensive replies. John Rowan called the roll of past VVA board members or officers who were female. Joe Chenelly pointed out, more impressively, that AMVETS's current national commander, Jan Brown, was a woman. Chenelly also noted that AMVETS's female membership has doubled in recent years. The American Legion representative declined to answer.

Five months later, Williams was locked and loaded for more criticism of the same targets. In a *Task and Purpose* opinion piece coauthored with Lindsay Church, founder of Minority Veterans of America, Williams blasted the Big Six for "failing to address the issue of racism in America and in the veteran community" in the wake of nationwide protests over the killing of George Floyd by Minneapolis police. With the exception of the PVA, Williams and Church noted, "none of the largest and oldest organizations in the country serving veterans" had responded, as top military leaders quickly did, by "addressing the presence of racism and calling on their own organizations to do better." Instead, four Big Six members released statements that placed as much focus on "vandalized memorials, civil unrest, and property damage as on the existing systemic inequalities that led to the protests." Williams and Church urged fellow veterans to "fight for change both inside and outside" the VSOs, noting that "young veterans are more diverse than ever, and many are abandoning these organizations."[2]

During Williams's own presentation later at the same SVA conference, she described the decline of "legacy VSOs." As *New York Times* correspondent Dave Philipps has reported, they are now competing with hundreds of faster-growing "post-9/11 new economy organizations," which also purport to speak for veterans, locally or nationally. Few operate as membership-based groups, with elected leaders and actual dues-payers. Instead, they take the form of "nonprofit corporations," with a CEO, board of directors, and a business-minded "focus on data, scalable products, quarterly numbers and branding."[3] They actively recruit on the basis of the shared generational experience of post-9/11 military service, local social networks, personal identity (in addition to being a vet), progressive or libertarian views of US foreign policy, or—in the case of SVA—student veteran status. According to a Center for a New American Security (CNAS) study coauthored by Williams, about one-third of the $3.6 billion now raised annually by "veteran-serving non-profits" is going to newer groups with less "brick-and-mortar infrastructure, legislative knowledge, and membership role in electing leaders and setting policy."

CLIMBING THE CORPORATE LADDER?

What these new players in the field of veterans affairs do have is plenty of corporate partners, foundation grants, and donations from wealthy individuals. As noted in the previous chapter, the Koch brothers have been a key investor in Concerned Veterans for America. A much broader swath of corporate America was well represented at SVA's 2020 convention, where SVA staff and volunteers were dressed in red-and-gold shirts with Raytheon's name on them. Every registered convention guest got a swag bag courtesy of Rocket Mortgage, a product line of Quicken Loans. The convention theme was "Learn Today, Lead Tomorrow"—a message echoed throughout the corporate exhibit area. The Wells Fargo booth hailed each job-seeking SVA member as "a leader for our country" today, and, "tomorrow, a leader for our company." Nearby, at Procter & Gamble's table, glossy brochures assured new hires that they would "lead from Day One," thanks to the company's "veterans and reservist affinity network."

In the telecom and cable TV industry aisle, Charter Communications touted its broadband technician apprenticeship program and its hiring of twelve thousand veterans. Smiling young employees of Comcast/NBCUniversal dispensed advice under a banner that proclaimed, "Service Matters—to Country, Community, and Customer." Not to be outdone, T-Mobile staff buttonholed veterans with the pitch that their wireless company was the "best place to work for veterans." And a display sponsored by Disney announced, "Only Heroes Work Here." SVA members were also invited to join twenty thousand fellow veterans on the payroll of Boeing, where "veterans make us better" at "building the world of tomorrow." Amazon, a Seattle neighbor now fielding its own "military recruiting teams," highlighted its recent placement of "more than 18,500 veterans and spouses" in office and warehouse jobs, where a company-created "affinity group" called Warriors@Amazon provides a ready-made "professional network."

Two older white males on the Koch Industries payroll stood before a sign assuring SVA members, "Our Mission Is Your Success." Koch cleverly provided job application data on memory sticks made in the form of dog tags with the Koch corporate logo on them. BP, another energy firm with a controversial environmental record, encouraged veterans "to stand up for your planet" by joining its workforce. At Raytheon's booth one of its recruiters was a former SVA chapter president now employed as a cyberthreat operations technician. He offered information about the defense contractor's internship program, its national collegiate cyber defense competition, and the RayVets support network. Next to dramatic photos of Patriot missiles being launched, a big poster proclaimed that, at Raytheon, "we rely on the unique perspectives and skills of veterans" to "enable our customers to achieve their most challenging missions and make the world a safer place."

JOINING FORCES WITH LABOR

In a hotel corridor outside the ballroom filled with big corporate displays, SVA provided much smaller tables for the Legion, VFW, AMVETS, VVA, and other VSOs to peddle their wares. Yet GI bill beneficiary and Columbia University graduate Alex McCoy, then political director of Common Defense, was not allowed space to advertise his organization's work with veterans seeking social and economic justice. The miffed former Marine was not happy about Corporate America getting such an easy opportunity to "blow smoke up our ass, but, in the end, just hire enough veterans to issue a press release about it." McCoy came to Los Angeles loaded down with copies of a new brochure about a Common Defense project called the Veterans Organizing Institute (VOI), which he handed out to SVA members before and after convention sessions.

In New York, just a few months earlier, VOI participants from across the country spent a weekend together learning new skills useful in electoral campaigning and veterans' issue advocacy. VOI's goal for the presidential election year was to train a national network of younger veterans who could organize effectively in their own communities, counter the influence of big money in politics, and make politicians more accountable to poor and working-class people. While SVA has oriented itself toward corporate management, Common Defense hopes to become an ally of organized labor, particularly at companies like Amazon, T-Mobile, and Comcast. As noted in chapter 3, these firms brand themselves as "veteran friendly" while simultaneously engaging in unfair labor practices that violate the rights of veterans and non-veterans alike whenever they try to unionize. Among past VOI participants are members of a network called Veterans for Social Change, sponsored by the Communications Workers of America (CWA).[4] One CWA priority is passage of federal legislation that would bolster private-sector organizing and bargaining rights, a long-overdue reform fiercely opposed by most corporate funders of SVA.

Common Defense grew out of grassroots organizing against Donald Trump's first run for president. Cofounders of the group met during protests over Trump's failure to donate money to veterans' charities after promising to do so during a campaign event in Iowa. One of those protesters was McCoy, who joined the Marines because for him, like many others, it was "the family business," and he "didn't have a ton of good prospects other than the military." The son of a naval officer, McCoy became a Barack Obama admirer while still in boot camp and then served six years, primarily as an embassy guard. In 2016 he and a group of like-minded vets "felt really strongly about how Trump was constantly using veterans as props while running a campaign that was so founded in hate and division." During Trump's first term, Common Defense built up a network of twenty thousand supporters who called for his impeachment. In 2020, the group made a dual endorsement of Senators Bernie Sanders and Elizabeth Warren after both presidential candidates helped round up other congressional signers of a Common Defense pledge to end "forever wars" in the Middle East.

THE "RATINGS KING" OF IAVA

The largest advocacy group for post-9/11 veterans is Iraq and Afghanistan Veterans of America (IAVA), which has chosen a more establishment orientation than Common Defense. Like CVA and SVA, IAVA has been an impressive cultivator of media coverage and wealthy donors, including companies with a pecuniary interest in veterans affairs. While Common Defense got its start skirmishing with Donald Trump on the campaign trail in 2016, IAVA traces its roots as a nonprofit group to founder Paul Rieckhoff's role in the 2004 presidential race between George Bush and John Kerry. At its peak of influence since then, IAVA boasted of having 425,000 "members," although neither dues payment nor proof of veteran status was required.[5] It has raised millions of dollars for veterans' advocacy and services. And it became a platform for hundreds of media appearances by Rieckhoff, which made him, in the words of a former coworker, the "ratings king of the veteran space."

Rieckhoff decided to enlist in the military during his senior year at Amherst College. After graduation, he became an Army reservist, then found work in finance. He switched to the Florida National Guard, received officer training, and volunteered for active duty after serving as a civilian first responder at "the pit" in lower Manhattan created by the leveling of the World Trade Center in the 9/11 attacks.[6] In his 2006 memoir, *Chasing Ghosts*, Rieckhoff reports that he was "against the Iraq war from the beginning" because he "feared that President Bush's decision to invade was not in the best interests of our country." Nevertheless, what he calls his "hunger for combat" and fear of being "left on the sidelines during the biggest game of my generation" trumped any "distrust of the president." Rieckhoff's father, a Vietnam-era draftee and later Con Edison worker in New York City, was baffled by his son's decision "to turn down a great job on Wall Street, and all that money, to roll around in the mud with a bunch of rednecks."[7]

Rieckhoff's ten-month tour of duty as a first lieutenant and platoon leader confirmed his distaste for how the Bush administration was handling the war. When he got back home and saw TV coverage of the fighting, he didn't like hearing "policy wonks, retired generals, and Sean Hannity talk about something they knew nothing about." He contacted media outlets, offering his own services as a more informed commentator. Getting no response, he then reached out to John Kerry's presidential campaign. The candidate himself was sufficiently impressed with the brash young National Guard officer to arrange a life-changing opportunity for him. In May 2004 the Democrats needed someone to offer an official response to a weekly message from the White House. President Bush offered ABC radio listeners a reassuring update on "one of the swiftest, most successful, and humane campaigns in military history." Rieckhoff's rebuttal questioned whether the current "leadership in Washington" was worthy of the "extraordinary courage and incredible capability" of his fellow soldiers in Iraq. He woke up the next day widely hailed as "the next John Kerry." He made the rounds of CNN, ABC, NPR, the Associated Press, the *Los Angeles Times*, the *New York Times*, and *Fox News*, where Sean Hannity demanded, "What are you doing to my president?"[8]

After Bush beat Kerry, Rieckhoff resolved to take "the fight for American hearts and minds to where it could be waged most effectively: the media." In 2005 he launched Operation Truth as a "nonpartisan forum for the troops to tell their stories so the American people could make informed decisions . . . and hold leaders from both parties accountable."[9] Later rebranded as IAVA, Operation Truth brought together a "new generation of activists, criticizing a new kind of war." Right from the start, Rieckhoff kept his distance from the antiwar movement, because "we weren't tree-hugging peaceniks and we weren't throwing our medals at the White House."[10]

At the time, other Bush critics, like Iraq Veterans Against the War (IVAW), Military Families Speak Out (MFSO), and Veterans for Peace (VFP), were rallying active-duty service members, their relatives, and post-9/11 veterans around the demand for immediate withdrawal from Iraq. As war correspondent Dahr Jamail reports, some soldiers being deployed went AWOL, others sought conscientious objector status, and a few endured court-martials and imprisonment because of their antiwar views.[11] Rieckhoff dismissed "Bring Them Home Now" as a goal that was "unrealistic for Americans and irresponsible for Iraqis." Plus, he believed that groups like IVAW and MFSO were "stuck in an outmoded model of protest that had been superseded by online organizing and appearances on talk shows."[12] As one former colleague explains: "Paul knew if he criticized the purpose of the war or the Bush administration too heavily, there was going to be a backlash. It was better to rant and rave about lack of armor for Humvees or to lambast the VA, because those are easy targets."

A BLUE-CHIP BOARD

Taking aim at the VA as an "easy target" is a topic we'll return to below and in chapter 6. But figuring out how to balance the work of assisting individual veterans while amplifying their collective voice was not easy for IAVA. Early on, the organization set up an interactive website to help veterans better access VA benefits and a Rapid Response Referral Program that connected them with direct service providers, including at the VA, who could help with problems like homelessness and depression. But media outreach—lining up interviews for Rieckhoff and other IAVA spokespeople—always took top priority during its formative years, according to one ex–staff member.

To its credit, IAVA tackled a number of high-profile legislative issues, from repeal of "Don't Ask, Don't Tell" to MST and veteran suicide prevention. It launched an advertising blitz criticizing predatory for-profit schools like those described in chapter 3, and in 2017 it worked with SVA and other vet groups on passage of the Forever GI Bill.[13] This important work was backed by a blue-chip advisory board, which included bankers, corporate lawyers, real estate developers, and tech industry entrepreneurs recruited by Rieckhoff, a former J. P. Morgan trader. To maintain its growing base of wealthy, well-connected donors, IAVA threw fancy fundraisers where star attractions like Meghan McCain, Stephen Colbert, and Henry Kissinger walked down camo-patterned carpets, rather than red ones. At MSNBC, both Brian Williams and Rachel Maddow became big fans of the organization. Rieckhoff, in turn, became Maddow's favorite go-to guy for the "veterans' perspective" on her show. In 2011–12, Maddow and her partner, Susan Mikula, personally donated more than $50,000 to IAVA.[14] Its corporate media patrons included NBC News and MSNBC itself.

In 2011 Rieckhoff and four IAVA members landed on the cover of *Time*, which hailed them as leading members of "the new greatest generation."[15] Hollywood connections helped the IAVA founder land a small speaking role in *Green Zone*, a 2010 film about the Iraq War that starred Matt Damon. To beef up IAVA's inside-the-Beltway presence, Rieckhoff recruited and promoted Allison Jaslow, a former Army captain, Iraq War veteran, and Bronze Star winner. She became IAVA's political director, then chief of staff, and finally executive director, in charge of the $6.5 million budget and fifty staff members it had in 2016. During that year's presidential campaign, Jaslow worked with NBC on an IAVA-hosted "Commander in Chief Forum" that drew an audience of 15 million and was addressed by both Donald Trump and Hillary Clinton.

A SCIENTIFIC APPROACH?

Unfortunately, IAVA's impressive media reach rarely helped members of the press or public better understand veterans' healthcare issues. Instead, Rieckhoff used his frequent guest appearances on *The Rachel Maddow Show* to laud Republican Jeff Miller when the House Veterans Affairs Committee chair was trying to turn the Phoenix wait time cover-up into a rationale for VA privatization. Meanwhile, he accused Senator Bernie Sanders of "basically being an apologist for the VA as the scandal erupted around him."[16] In the pages of the *New York Times*, Rieckhoff declared that there was now "a total loss of confidence in the VA" among veterans. Like the American Legion, he demanded that President Obama fire his VA secretary immediately.[17]

As always, Rieckhoff purported to speak on behalf of a nonpartisan group, which, according to its website, takes a "scientific approach" to veterans' issues, using "data as well as stories from our community" when staking out policy positions.[18] However, any quick scan of IAVA financial reports reveals a steady income stream from corporate interests that are not part of the veteran "community" but eager to curry favor within it. IAVA's big business donors over the years have included TriWest Healthcare Alliance and Cerner, two recipients of multi-billion-dollar VA contracts during the Trump administration. Two years after TriWest gave more than half a million dollars to IAVA, it was a major beneficiary of legislation, backed by IAVA, that required the VA to outsource more care to the private sector.[19] As a result, TriWest was hired as one of two outside administrators of the VA's new Veterans Choice Program, both of which performed poorly, as reported in the previous chapter. Cerner received a huge contract to revamp the VA's health-care information technology.[20] Another IAVA benefactor is Cigna, a giant private insurer whose foundation received one of IAVA's annual Corporate Leadership Awards.[21] Other donors include the Pharmaceutical Research and Manufacturers of America and several of its affiliated biotechnology firms.[22]

When IAVA was criticized in *Washington Monthly* for its TriWest ties, Rieckhoff wrote an indignant letter to the editor calling the piece "over-simplistic and misinformed."[23] He sidestepped the question of who was donating to IAVA or why—and denied that the group was "peddling a message of VA privatization." Rieckhoff acknowledged that his own members "want to see a better VA, not a dismantled one." Nevertheless, he insisted that "many veterans, regardless of political background, are rightfully critical of the VA" because "there's no shortage of new scandals and failures to criticize."[24] Allison Jaslow was particularly fixated on one largely symbolic "failure." Her signature campaign at IAVA was called "She Who Has Borne the Battle." Its goal was to get VA leaders to adopt a new, gender-neutral motto, modifying the original quotation from Abraham Lincoln's Second Inaugural Address, which appears on veterans' hospital signage everywhere.

Despite motto change resistance from Trump-appointed VA secretaries, the department itself was making substantive changes beneficial to the 7 percent of its patients who are female. In 2015 the VA did a major internal study on reducing institutional barriers to better care for women veterans.[25] Based on the results, all VA major medical centers, which deliver primary and mental health care, created places in their facilities specially designated for their treatment. Staff members received additional training on MST and other relevant service-related conditions.[26] In 2016 Kayla Williams, author of two memoirs about her military service—one of which deals with the challenges of being the spouse and caregiver of a badly disabled fellow Iraq veteran—took the lead in this area. Working in the VA's Washington, DC, headquarters as director of its Center for Women Veterans, Williams launched national initiatives designed to educate staff and patients about the needs of female veterans and make them feel more welcome. Under her leadership the center had a digital communications outreach program that sent out newsletters, news roundups, and health research reports to female veterans already enrolled in the VA and those seeking coverage.

A VA patient herself, along with her husband, Williams explained how the VA provided "high quality, culturally competent care," including "the highest rates of breast and cervical cancer screenings of any healthcare system in the country." She also helped publicize the fact that the VA "understands women's specific military experiences and risks and is able to give women veterans the support and services they need—at lower cost," while "most providers in the private sector don't even know what military sexual trauma is." Williams even helped coordinate the first-ever VA "baby shower," an event that provided essential items to 2,500 VA patients who had just become mothers.[27]

To the IAVA, however, not much had changed at all. In an op-ed for the *Philadelphia Inquirer*, Jaslow reported still hearing "from women who are 'welcomed' at their local VA hospital by staff addressing their husbands first."[28] In her view, "the very agency meant to acknowledge and serve veterans falls short." IAVA's singular focus on a gender-neutral motto put Williams in the cross fire. She did her best to placate Jaslow in a letter explaining that "for many years I—along with other senior VA leaders—have honored the population we serve today by using a modernized version" of the VA motto, which replaced the word *him* with *those*. Williams's assurance that "this symbolic update" was being "gradually incorporated alongside the original in digital and print materials, as well as spoken remarks" outraged political appointees like VA press secretary Curt Cashour, a former campaign staffer for Republican governor Scott Walker of Wisconsin. Cashour publicly chastised Williams for expressing her own "personal view . . . not the VA's position."[29] At this point, Williams felt she had no choice but to resign. "If you have the press secretary of the organization you are working for lying to the media about you, it is not a good sign," she said.[30]

A TERRIBLE MANAGER

In his memoir Paul Rieckhoff rates himself as having been a popular platoon leader. But near the end of his thirteen years as commander in chief of IAVA, he was getting bad reviews from current and former subordinates. On the job website Glassdoor, the IAVA founder was variously rated as a "self-obsessed megalomaniac who drives good people and ideas into the ground," a "horrible boss," and a "terrible manager" who lacked "integrity, transparency, and human decency." One Glassdoor source wrote that IAVA should be renamed AIVA—"An Iraq Veteran of America, because only one veteran matters at this organization, the CEO and Founder."[31]

In early 2018 Rieckhoff left IAVA for greener pastures, amid a flurry of self-congratulation. "When IAVA started in 2004 the veterans' landscape was a desert," he declared. "Now it's a metropolis. We are very proud of the fact that a lot of people who come through the IAVA team have gone on to do really cool stuff."[32] Among those alumni he hailed were former IAVA lobbyist Tom Tarantino, who went to work for Twitter; Todd Bowers, who landed on the payroll of Uber; and Matt Miller, who became a Trump campaign staffer. According to Rieckhoff, it was better to have "Taratino [sic] at Twitter changing the culture there than have him at the House VA Committee talking to a bunch of other veterans for the ninetieth time." In ten years, he predicted, a growing and disproportionate number of "CEOs are going to be veterans . . . and that's going to be exciting to watch."[33]

Rieckhoff handed his CEO reins to Jeremy Butler, an African American Naval Reserve officer with twenty years of experience in the military. The IAVA founder left to create a media and podcasting company—more on that below—while remaining on the IAVA board and, according to one source, collecting an extra year's salary on his way out the door. In March 2018 testimony on Capitol Hill, Butler told the Senate and House Veterans Affairs Committees that VA outsourcing, which had begun under President Obama and continued under his successor, "will require strong Congressional oversight to ensure that it does not turn into an expansion of privatization."[34] This timely warning notwithstanding, IAVA—like the American Legion and other VSOs—was still maintaining its own wait-and-see attitude toward a major policy experiment of questionable value to veterans.

Kris Goldsmith is one of many former IAVA staffers still disappointed by its unfulfilled potential. In his view, the group too often sacrificed substance for flash, favoring quick media hits over the hard slog of real membership recruitment, leadership development, and long-term campaigning. It spent money carelessly and pursued organizational self-promotion over effective partnering with other veterans' advocates. According to Goldsmith, IAVA became overly "focused on symbolic things, like changing Abraham Lincoln's words in the VA motto to be gender neutral rather than getting obstetricians in VA hospitals."

A "MONEY FUNNEL" FOR WEALTHY DEMS?

Paul Rieckhoff was not the only post-9/11 veteran with a Kerry campaign connection who later became a full-time advocate for other veterans. After volunteering for Kerry, former Army captain Jon Soltz became a cofounder of VoteVets. Based in Portland, Oregon, VoteVets brands itself as the largest "progressive organization of veterans" in the country while simultaneously proclaiming its muscular commitment "to the destruction of terror networks around the world." Like CVA on the right, VoteVets has little formal membership in any traditional VSO sense—no local chapters or posts and no elected leadership. Its frequent email blasts publicize online protest petitions about military, foreign policy, and veterans' issues—and seek donations for itself in the process. By 2020 VoteVets had collected enough email addresses, names on online petitions, and contributors to claim "over 700,000 supporters," counting among them "troops, veterans, military families, and their supporters." The group also boasts 420,000 followers on Facebook and Twitter.[35]

VoteVets's work is carried out through multiple legal entities. The first is VoteVets Political Action, a federal PAC that does voter education about "veterans and military issues" and backs Kerry-style "service candidates" (profiled in chapter 7)—usually veterans who have served in Iraq and Afghanistan.[36] VoteVets Action Fund is a 501(c)(4) that "primarily focuses on non-partisan education and advocacy on behalf of veterans and their families" and operates as a "dark money" group: in other words, it does not have to reveal the identity of its donors. And then there is the Vet Voice Foundation (VVF), a 501(c)(3) organization committed to "building a national network of 21st century veterans, using a combination of new technologies and social media tools—as well as traditional organizing methods."[37] Under the banner of a campaign called "The Land We Love," VVF tries to protect public land from mineral exploitation and get veterans involved in green energy projects.

Since its founding, VoteVets has raised and spent an impressive $120 million on politics. About $50 million of that bought TV and radio ads urging the reelection of "veterans' allies and defeat of those who do not support troops and veterans."[38] In 2014, one candidate that VoteVets failed to defeat was Tom Cotton, a conservative vet from Arkansas. That year Cotton was trying to move up from the House of Representatives to the Senate; unfortunately, he succeeded and now sees himself as a future GOP presidential candidate. On issues, if not candidates, Soltz, an Iraq War veteran, and his CVA counterpart, Dan Caldwell, have found common ground on a policy objective that both progressive and libertarian vets favor but that the traditionally hawkish Tom Cotton does not: revoking the open-ended congressional authorization for using US military force anywhere in the world since the 9/11 attacks. This blank check for the Pentagon's Global War on Terror proved hard to cancel on Capitol Hill even two decades later, as reported in chapters 7 and 8.[39]

Only a handful of veterans' groups have tackled the seemingly intractable problem of "forever wars." They include VFP, Common Defense, VoteVets, Win Without War, About Face, and, on the libertarian right, CVA and a new group called Bring Our Troops Home.[40] Most, like VFP and Common Defense, don't have much money for advertising. Thanks to the deep-pocketed patronage of the anti-interventionist Koch brothers, CVA does have such resources. In 2020 alone, it was able to spend "over $3 million on advertisements in support of an Afghanistan withdrawal."[41] Soltz's collaboration with Caldwell does not extend to the latter's former CVA colleague, who became a *Fox News* commentator. "I have been debating Pete Hegseth for 12 years," Soltz says, "and I can't tell you what he stands for other than himself and his own ambition."[42]

During election years, VoteVets activates a network of "state captains organizing in all 50 states," like holding candidates' forums and "get out the vote" (GOTV) drives. It boasts of having made "50 million voter contacts since 2006" via millions spent on direct mail, phone banking, and canvassing.[43] Because of its close ties to the Democratic Party, VoteVets Action Fund also attracts PAC donations from unions; in one election cycle, the AFL-CIO-affiliated Plumbers and Pipefitters Union reported giving it $500,000. AFGE, the embattled bargaining representative of VA employees, has also been a donor.

But one leader of another progressive veterans' group, also pro labor, believes that VoteVets has become part of the "big money in politics" problem. This critic questions the validity of its opaque candidate endorsement process—mainly online polling to help determine which candidates to back and then help finance. He describes VoteVets as a "money funnel" for wealthy individuals and business interests that have "maxed out" on their direct donations to candidates, which are limited by federal election law. By its own account, during the 2018 election cycle VoteVets was "one of the largest outside spending organizations" on either the Republican or Democratic side when control of the House shifted to the latter. According to Federal Election Commission (FEC) filings, one of its biggest benefactors that year was billionaire Michael Bloomberg, a nonveteran who donated $1.5 million (but became far less generous in 2020 when VoteVets didn't back his own Democratic presidential candidacy). Various Wall Street money managers, private equity firms, and the pollution-prone Duke Energy contributed hundreds of thousands of dollars as well. This pattern of private industry generosity persisted in the 2020 election cycle, when VoteVets PAC donors also included the defense contractor General Dynamics, Pfizer, and Cigna.[44]

When the authors of this book sought more information than what's available in FEC filings about the exact mix of veteran versus nonveteran funding of VoteVets in 2020, we ran into the same stone wall that Carrie Levine, from the Center for Public Integrity, did a few years earlier.[45] When Levine sought the names of the fifty-two donors who raised $5.5 million for VoteVets Action Fund in 2016, her request was denied by VoteVets PR person Eric Schmeltzer "because the law does not require disclosure of people's identities" and "we maintain that privacy for individuals." When we tried to arrange a phone interview with Jon Soltz to find out whether its 2020 election-year ads were funded by actual veterans or by corporations and wealthy individuals, Schmeltzer proposed that any questions be submitted via email instead. Explaining that he was personally "walled off" from "the IE [independent expenditure] side of VoteVets," Schmeltzer then handed us off to Doug Gordon, cofounder of UpShift Strategies, a Washington, DC, consulting firm. Via email Gordon told us that VoteVets "follows all FEC guidelines when it comes to fundraising and reporting," but beyond that, "we don't comment too much on VoteVets PAC spending."

WOMEN IN COMMAND

Among the post-9/11 veterans' advocacy groups—from CVA on the right to VoteVets and Common Defense on the liberal and left side of the spectrum—different political orientations are not the only source of division. Most modern-day rifts between younger advocates are related to race, gender, ethnicity, or class differences. But even among women of color from immigrant backgrounds in the same generational cohort, divergent voices have emerged.

Consider, for example, the activist careers of Anuradha Bhagwati, who penned a scathing critique of military culture called *Unbecoming: A Memoir of Disobedience*, and Brittany DeBarros, an Afghan War veteran now employed by About Face—formerly Iraq Veterans Against the War.[46] Both women have been critical of the leadership style of men in VSOs, old and new. They share a strong antipathy toward what DeBarros calls "the white male veteran hero narrative." But Bhagwati's reform project was making the military into an equal-opportunity employer with less workplace harassment and sexual assault. DeBarros became a radical critic of the Pentagon, particularly its deployment of troops at the Mexican border to deter asylum seekers and, in 2020, to help suppress protests against police brutality.

As revealed in *Unbecoming*, Bhagwati's personal story is a case study in how military service can make preexisting mental health issues worse among young people trying to escape troubled civilian lives.[47] A bisexual graduate of Yale, she was estranged from her high-powered and overly controlling parents, both Ivy League professors. The Marine Corps beckoned as a "culture in which degradation and humiliation were entwined with belonging." Even as an officer, Bhagwati's prior experience of sexual harassment as a teenager and psychological abuse at home made her particularly vulnerable to hazing, harassment, and "fierce misogyny" within the Corps. After she left the Marines, Bhagwati waged a four-year fight with the VBA to get a 40 percent disability rating as a result of MST. She later appealed and won a higher rating for her service-related condition. Meanwhile, she became a high-profile advocate for other enlisted women as the cofounder and first director of the Service Women's Action Network (SWAN), which lobbies for full integration of women into combat roles and an end to sexual harassment and discrimination within all branches of the Armed Forces. With funding from corporate law firms and foundations, SWAN won much-needed improvements in the treatment of women on active duty and female veterans who suffer from MST—a problem so widespread, as noted in chapter 1, that even Senator Martha McSally, the first woman to fly in combat, was scarred by it.[48]

Before she joined the Marines, Bhagwati was a youthful supporter of Ralph Nader and once made a trip to Mexico to visit the Zapatistas, an insurgent group in Chiapas. However, as director of SWAN, Bhagwati steered clear of fellow veterans like DeBarros who had been radicalized by their military service. In her memoir she criticizes those who approached SWAN "with mixed agendas that started with opposition to the wars in Iraq and Afghanistan." Bhagwati accuses them of "writing off the military in broad brushstrokes" and trying to impose "an antimilitary ideology on a relatively conservative group of women . . . who needed a safe place to heal."[49] Under her leadership, SWAN "avoided antiwar partnerships" because it wanted "to win over mainstream flag-waving Americans, whom we needed on our side in order to reduce sexual violence in the ranks."[50]

Far more than Bhagwati, who grew up in a wealthy liberal suburb of Boston, DeBarros was raised among those "flag-waving Americans." But that hasn't deterred her from becoming a fierce critic of militarism and coordinator of a national campaign called "Drop the Military Industrial Complex." The focus of that work for About Face—which has a membership of about five thousand, plus another twelve thousand "followers"—is repealing congressional authorization for open-ended warfare in the Middle East and exposing the political influence of big military contractors. Later, as organizer-director of About Face, she helped enlist hundreds of other veterans to sign an open letter urging members of the National Guard and other military units to refuse riot duty in the wake of nationwide protests over the killing of George Floyd. Why would she be involved in such a call for high-risk, active-duty disobedience? As she explained to the press, "I can say from experience that the moral cost, the cost to your soul, of following an order that you wish that you hadn't, is far greater and far more sustained than whatever the military can do to you in the short run."[51]

DeBarros grew up in a mixed-race family, but being raised in a "very Republican, libertarian-leaning" part of Texas initially made her an "evangelical neo-con crazy person." Lacking sufficient money to attend college, she enlisted in the Army right after high school. When first deployed to Afghanistan as a platoon leader and strategic communications officer, she believed that America was trying to make the country more secure and help Afghan women. But, she recalls, "it soon became apparent that the U.S. military was the wrong vehicle for achieving that mission." After returning to the United States, and while still a captain in the Army Reserves, DeBarros attended a meeting of VFP in New York City. She was introduced to the organization by former Navy nurse Susan Schnall, a leading activist in the GI antiwar movement of the 1960s. DeBarros didn't find VFP's local chapter very welcoming to women or younger vets—although she told a VFP national convention audience several years later that "the fact so many of you have been in this struggle for decades gives me hope." In that 2019 speech, she raised questions that have long vexed VFP and now its newer competitors: "How do we move from fighting each war, one by one, and begin dismantling the system that allows these wars to keep popping up? How do we get at the roots of the system?"

As DeBarros became more involved in veterans affairs, she noticed that newer groups, and the political candidates they backed, had their shortcomings too. A Staten Island resident, she was not a fan of Congressman Max Rose, despite his service in Afghanistan, where he won a Bronze Star and a Purple Heart as an infantry officer. In 2018, with backing from VoteVets, Rose ran against a conservative Republican to become the first post-9/11 combat veteran elected to the House from New York City. VoteVets chair Jon Soltz hailed Rose as "one of the most energetic and exciting candidates in the country." But DeBarros was "turned off by his gross nationalism" and later by his aggressive House floor criticism of a newly elected colleague, Ilhan

Omar from Minnesota. In DeBarros's view, VoteVets was just a corporate Democratic front group, overly focused on veterans' issues as opposed to broader social justice concerns, in addition to being "another organization controlled by a bunch of white dudes." Common Defense, she believes, also has too many "white bro staff members making all the decisions," which results in a lot of "toxic bullshit" and "tokenism." Such accusations were made in a letter of protest signed by DeBarros and eighteen other female vets over the sudden departure of Common Defense executive director Pam Campos-Palma in 2019.[52] Campos-Palma had served in the Air Force for over a decade as an operations and antiterrorism intelligence analyst working in Germany, Kyrgyzstan, Iraq, and Afghanistan.

BRO CULTURE CRITICS

In their "Open Letter on the Systemic Mistreatment of Womxn of Color Leaders in Social Justice Spaces," Common Defense critics accused the group of "silencing Pam's voice and leadership" and "valuing the time, energy, resources and contributions of white and/or male staff members over minority members."[53] As one structural remedy for this, the signers demanded that the group's board of directors be replaced by one "that includes a supermajority of traditionally marginalized voices." The change was not adopted, and Campos-Palma moved to form a new group, Vets for the People, launched in conjunction with the labor-backed Working Families Party. In *Unbecoming*, Bhagwati is equally scathing about "conservative dudes and good old boy veterans" in the Big Six in DC. One exception, she reports, was VVA, "one of the few VSOs that regularly had our backs, signing onto our litigation to change the VA's PTSD regulations for sexual trauma and supporting sweeping sexual assault reforms." But for her, the inside-the-Beltway veteran community—new and old—was "mostly male and white and fiercely uninviting to women."[54]

Bhagwati directs particular scorn at the "bros"—like IAVA's Paul Rieckhoff—who were overly preoccupied "with branding their own images and increasing their followers on social media." Despite Allison Jaslow's prominent role in IAVA and high media profile, Bhagwati believes that Rieckhoff's frequent appearances on shows like Rachel Maddow's "did not help create space for a diverse array of veteran voices." According to Bhagwati, "most veterans grumbled privately about Paul's infamous ego and tendency to hang out with Hollywood celebrities, but few challenged him on anything because of his far-reaching influence with politicians, news networks, and funders."[55] That changed somewhat when the IAVA negotiated a sponsorship deal with Miller Brewing Company that "got a lot of pushback from outraged veterans who had struggled with substance abuse," Bhagwati contends. Then IAVA aroused Bhagwati's ire when it decided "to host a NYC outreach event at Hooters, the big-boobs, beer-and-wings, chain restaurant that entertained its customers with 'female sex appeal.'"[56] Rieckhoff initially defended this choice of venue on the grounds that the chain had a long history of supporting veterans. Bhagwati reminded him that "lots of extremely sexist people and organizations support veterans' charities," but that doesn't mean they should receive reciprocal backing. Because "women make up 15% of the military" and "our PTSD disproportionately stems from sexual harassment and sexual assault while serving," Bhagwati insisted that Hooters was no place for IAVA membership recruitment.[57] Threatened with an embarrassing social media blitz by SWAN, Rieckhoff finally called the event off.

As noted earlier in this chapter, newer VSOs have an organizational culture far more entrepreneurial than that of their older counterparts. Former headquarters staffers of the old VSOs may have gravitated toward lucrative employment with private firms in more traditional inside-the-Beltway, revolving-door fashion, as chronicled in chapter 4. But several former leaders of new VSOs have, in more modern fashion, become social entrepreneurs. They've capitalized on their past political, media, and donor connections to build a more personal brand as writers or podcast hosts, consultants and commentators, visiting professors, or motivational speakers. True to form, Paul Rieckhoff remains the most self-promotional of this cohort, which also includes Bhagwati, Jaslow, and Campos-Palma.

On the website for his *Angry Americans* podcast, the IAVA founder now hails himself, with typical modesty, as "a fighter, a patriot, an independent political and media force to be reckoned with . . . one of the most dynamic political and social leaders in America." After being "at the forefront of American history for the last 15 years . . . fearlessly leading America during some of our most important times, and creating multi-million dollar advertising campaigns and impactful partnerships with companies ranging from Google to Uber . . . while forging creative partnerships with Lady Gaga, Linkin Park, and NASCAR driver Cale Conley," Rieckhoff has become a "voice for the voiceless." On his new interview show, he "takes on Republicans, Democrats—and everyone in between. If you're in the angry middle, Angry Americans reminds you that you're not alone. We're all in this together." He invites listeners to "join the Angry Americans movement" by subscribing to his podcast and wearing an "Angry American" T-shirt—ordered from a veteran-owned business that advertises on his site.[58]

After leaving SWAN, Bhagwati first reinvented herself in a more quiet and meditative way as a teacher of yoga in Brooklyn. However, to promote her newly published book in 2019, she came out swinging in the pages of the *New York Times*—on behalf of President Donald Trump. She penned an op-ed directing her anger at the VA and applauding Trump's partial privatization of veterans' healthcare at a time when most VSOs, other than the CVA, were still very wary of it.[59] She dismissed outsourcing foes as being "out of touch with the needs of a younger and more diverse veterans' population." In her view these VSOs were only concerned about "older men whose cultural norms are becoming increasingly obsolete," a rather broad-brushed tarring of the VA's far more diverse patient population of 9 million. Meanwhile, Bhagwati was able to sell her book rights to Hollywood. The buyer was *Slumdog Millionaire* star Freida Pinto, who plans to play Bhagwati in a cable TV series for Entertainment One based on her military career. The author of *Unbecoming* views this project as a way of "advancing the voices and stories of women of color, immigrant families, and queer women" and says she "cannot wait to see Freida become a #Marine."[60] In a way, Anuradha Bhagwati had come full circle, since her own decision to enlist was due in part to seeing a buff and buzz-cut Demi Moore "pushing feminist boundaries" in the 1997 Hollywood action film *G.I. Jane*.[61]

Like Bhagwati, Allison Jaslow also developed Hollywood connections. According to her personal website, she forged "leading impact partnerships" with the producers of *Dunkirk*, *War Machine*, and *Blood Stripe*, an independent film that depicts a woman Marine's transition from combat to civilian life. But her first post-IAVA gig, as executive director of the Democratic Congressional Campaign Committee, was short-lived; in July 2019 she resigned amid a controversy about "the lack of diversity in its senior management."[62] She then became an adjunct professor at Duke University's Hart Leadership Program, where she offers "coaching from someone who's been tested in nearly every aspect of our political system, from campaigns to Capitol Hill to the White House."[63] Jaslow has also been a member of the elite Council on Foreign Relations and an Aspen Security Forum scholar.

Drawing on her own military service and following Common Defense work, Pam Campos-Palma now brands herself as a "partner with national-level leaders in policy, politics and movements, peace and security organizations and think tanks, political campaigns and electoral organizations."

Her areas of expertise as a consultant include "strategic coalition-building, organizational management and culture, institutional diversity, equity, and inclusion." In coalition with the Working Families Party, a ten-state network of progressive labor and community groups, Campos-Palma now coordinates Vets for the People (VFP). Not to be confused with the other, much older Veterans for Peace, her new project hopes to "create an organizing community of bold, progressive veterans that will work for all our people to create a more just, inclusive, and reimagined world."[64] In the summer of 2020, she was taking up the cause of Vanessa Guillen and questioning why VSOS, old and new, weren't putting more pressure on Congress to investigate the Army's handling of her case. "You don't see the Guillen family flanked by officer associations or political organizations that claim to be doing great by veterans," she said in one interview. "The family is mostly surrounded by other Latinos and people of color."

Embracing so many good progressive causes and, of course, greater diversity certainly sets younger veteran advocates apart from their older counterparts in the ever-so-last-century American Legion. But one worrisome result of declining old VSO influence—and related organizational dysfunction, as described in the previous chapter—is less effective lobbying for the VA. The new VSOS that have upstaged the old ones—albeit in fragmented, far less membership-based form—have generally not been vigorous defenders of the nation's largest public healthcare system. Instead, past leaders of IAVA and SWAN—like Rieckhoff, Jaslow, and Bhagwati—chose to snipe at the VA in the same shortsighted fashion as old VSO officials, but in op-ed page commentaries or MSNBC sound bites with much broader reach.

The VA does, after all, serve 9 million predominantly poor and working-class patients, many of whom are people of color. It represents a good working model for "socialized medicine" that's quite popular among blue-collar veterans who are not college-educated former officers—like Rieckhoff, Jaslow, or Bhagwati—and don't have similar access to higher-paying civilian jobs with good private insurance coverage. About a third of the VA healthcare workforce served in the military before helping other veterans. Having worked for VSOS old and new, Army veteran Kris Goldsmith now worries that "younger advocates often don't see the damage done by their negative messaging." Goldsmith believes that veterans from all generations need to come together "to protect the VA because the VA saves lives every day. It saved my life." But how many other lives the VA will save in decades to come depends on the outcome of the political struggle described in the next chapter.

6. A VA HEALTHCARE STRUGGLE

The Choice program has been a wreck.
Every veteran up here will tell you that.
—SENATOR JON TESTER (D-MT)

On a wet and dreary afternoon in February 2020, seventy-two-year-old Mick Cole marched up the steps of the Capitol Building in Washington, DC. He was part of a delegation of more than a dozen veterans who belong to Veterans for Peace. As a member of its "Save Our VA" working group, Cole was visiting members of Congress and their staff involved in veterans affairs.

From 1965 to 1969, Cole flew bombing missions over Vietnam as an airborne voice intercept operator. After learning Vietnamese, Cole's job was to monitor the communication of the North Vietnamese Air Force and provide real-time intelligence to American pilots. Because of his Air Force assignments, Cole eventually lost hearing in one ear. He has also been operated on several times for prostate problems, which he believes are related to Agent Orange exposure.

Cole's most debilitating problem is PTSD, a condition he attributes to experiencing the battlefield trauma of both sides in the conflict. "When I was monitoring the Vietnamese pilots and one of them got shot down, I could hear the anguish in their voices," he told us. "They were just like us." After he left the Air Force, Cole spent years self-medicating with alcohol. Finally, someone convinced him to seek treatment at the VHA. "If it weren't for my weekly therapy groups," he said, "I wouldn't be here today." Nevertheless, Cole's emotional state is still fragile enough that telling his story over and over again during a long day of lobbying can be difficult. In one meeting with a young congressional aide, he choked up, broke down, and began to weep quietly.

His most critical appointment of the day was a face-to-face meeting with Representative Mark Takano (D-CA), who was chair of the House Veterans Affairs Committee. This was an opportunity for Cole to remind a key player on Capitol Hill how he and 9 million other VHA patients have been impacted by the Trump administration strategy of shrinking the VHA and outsourcing veterans' care to private-sector doctors and hospitals. Understaffing at the VHA facilities in upstate New York that Cole has used for years has led to caregiver burnout, higher turnover, and—he believes—compromised care. The VHA psychologist who runs Cole's weekly group therapy session is now so overburdened that scheduling individual appointments with veterans in crisis takes longer than it should. "My psychiatrist left to go into private practice and hasn't been permanently replaced," he told Takano. "So every time I have to go get checked up on, I have to tell my story to someone new; it is very painful to relive that trauma over and over again."

Takano, who became chair of the Veterans Affairs Committee after Democrats regained control of the House in 2018, was a sympathetic listener. Sitting in a crammed conference room with Cole and other VFP members, he assured his visitors that he strongly supported the VHA. As evidence of this, he cited his recent opposition to a bill backed by the Trump administration that would have outsourced more mental health services. When Cole and his delegation asked to take a photo with Takano, the California Democrat stood with them and proudly displayed a "Save Our VA" bumper sticker. Eight months later, however, Takano pushed through yet another bill that took money out of the VHA's budget and allocated it to outside providers of unproven ability to treat the complex mental health problems of VHA patients.[1]

By 2020, when Cole and his fellow veterans made their rounds on Capitol Hill, there was already much alarming data on the impact of incremental privatization. The Choice Act had diverted nearly $10 billion from the VHA to private-sector hospitals, doctors, and administrators while letting in-house services suffer.[2] According to several studies, the VHA's budget for private-sector care grew almost fourfold between 2014 and 2018.[3] In 2016 alone, the VHA made nearly 25.5 million outside appointments. Meanwhile, its own hospitals and clinics had more than fifty thousand vacancies, up from thirty-four thousand in 2014.[4] And even this vacancy rate failed to capture the extent of the VHA's actual staffing problem because it only reflected attrition, which often occurred in facilities that were understaffed to begin with.

While lawmakers like Takano were debating solutions to the problem of veteran suicide, many positions for VHA psychiatrists went unfilled. In New Mexico, a chronic shortage of VHA mental health providers led to four-month wait times for new patients.[5] In response to similar delays in Rhode Island, mental health counselors were ordered to double their number of weekly visits to meet demand.[6] PTSD support groups at the West Los Angeles VA Medical Center were shut down.[7] In Kokomo, Indiana, a new VHA clinic—much praised by veterans for increasing their access to care—was shuttered less than a year after it opened.[8] In New York, the VA closed its ear, nose, and throat clinic in Brooklyn, along with an outpatient clinic in Buffalo.[9] In New Jersey, even a small woodshop program for veterans was shelved.

If local administrators argued for facility expansion, based on projected increases in their patient loads, VA headquarters was not responsive. An effort to boost capacity at the North Texas VA Health Care System, the second-largest in the country, was blocked despite an expected 12 percent increase in the patient population within ten years. In this demoralizing environment, dozens of top VA officials resigned or retired, resulting in a serious talent drain.[10] In 2019, the VA's inspector general found that 14 percent of the agency's local medical center directors were serving in an acting or interim role. When one left, it took an average of eight months to find a permanent replacement.

MAKING THE VA GREAT AGAIN

This grim picture was not part of the rosy scenario painted by Donald Trump at presidential campaign rallies like one near a Navy battleship in Norfolk, Virginia. "We are going to make the VA great again," he promised his supporters there.[11] First, however, the new president had to find a new VA secretary, willing to do his bidding. Among the initial contenders for that job was Jeff Miller, whom we met in chapter 4 in his role as Republican chairman of the House Committee on Veterans Affairs. Miller was an early

Trump endorser but did not run for reelection to Congress himself in 2016 and would soon become a well-compensated lobbyist for private health-care interests seeking VA contracts.[12] Senate Democrats, who were not fans of Miller, breathed a sigh of relief when Trump instead picked Dr. David Shulkin, a former private hospital administrator. Shulkin was the only cabinet undersecretary under Obama who secured his agency's top job in the new administration. His nomination won unanimous Senate approval, which earned him the presidential nickname "Mr. 100 Percent."

Shulkin had the personal backing of Ike Perlmutter, a Trump megadonor, fellow billionaire, and CEO of Marvel Entertainment. After Trump's surprise electoral college victory in November 2016, Perlmutter was one of three Mar-a-Lago club members who became key White House advisers on VA issues, even though none had ever served in the US military or worked at the VA. In his first "State of the VA" address, Shulkin pledged to tackle pressing issues like veteran suicide and a backlog of ninety thousand disability claims.[13] He compared the VHA to a patient who, while improving, was "still in critical condition and requires intensive care." That analogy was a striking departure from the message of a 440-page book about the VHA that Shulkin had just coedited while serving as deputy undersecretary for health. Titled *Best Care Everywhere,* this collection of clinical case studies by 120 VA doctors, nurses, social workers, and psychologists described how their research and innovative treatments were "changing veterans' lives" and "leading American health care."[14] (Published by the Government Publishing Office, Shulkin's book oddly went "out of print" soon after publication.)[15]

During his fifteen months in office, Shulkin had to contend with a cadre of new VA political appointees, who were either alumni of Concerned Veterans for America (CVA) or former Trump campaign workers. Their goal, he reported later, was "unfettered VA patient access to private care" that would pave the way for "the dismantling of the government-run system set up to serve veterans." Shulkin feared that VA patients would end up with "fewer options, a severely weakened VA, and a private healthcare system not designed to meet the complex requirements of high-need veterans."[16] Nevertheless, on his watch, the percentage of patients referred outside the VA increased from 19 to 36 percent.[17] That was not good enough for Darin Selnick, CVA's inside man at the White House, or Trump's informal adviser Pete Hegseth, who "never worked at the VA, knew nothing about managing a healthcare system and had little understanding of the clinical and financial impact of the policies he was advocating."[18]

When Trump named Shulkin to his cabinet, he publicly assured him that he would never hear the words "You're fired!" like so many failed contestants on *The Apprentice*. Shulkin's perceived foot-dragging on privatization, and negative publicity over a VA-funded trip to Europe with his wife and personal security team, made Trump's promise one of many he did not keep.[19] In March 2018, the White House sacked Shulkin via a presidential tweet.[20]

LEADERSHIP ACCOUNTABILITY?

One irony of Shulkin's own summary dismissal was his prior embrace of legislation that made it easier to fire VA staff not serving at the pleasure of the president. The VA Accountability and Whistleblower Protection Act of 2017 was championed by Senator Marco Rubio, whose 2016 reelection campaign benefited from $90,000 worth of CVA spending on his behalf. CVA then made a six-figure investment in getting this legislation passed, via media buys and creation of a digital tool that enabled constituents to contact their members of Congress. Strong bipartisan majorities in both the House and Senate voted to weaken due process protections for VA employees and limit their right to appeal job-related discipline.

In a sign of things to come for the American Federation of Government Employees (AFGE), Trump's VA refused to bargain over the act's implementation and impact. Six months after it was enacted, only five senior leaders had been removed for alleged misconduct. The other 1,264 discharge cases all involved low-level employees who worked in claims processing, food service, and housekeeping jobs. Among them, of course, were some of the veterans who comprise a third of the VA's overall workforce, either in regular jobs or the agency's compensated work-therapy programs, which offer economic stability to veterans with a history of homelessness or mental illness.

The 2017 law established an Office of Accountability and Whistleblower Protection, with dozens of investigators. Its first director was Peter O'Rourke, a Republican Party operative later forced to resign from the VA for "collecting pay, but doing little work," as the *Washington Post* reported.[21] O'Rourke was also accused of protecting political allies who were under investigation and failing to provide timely reports to Congress. As of late 2019, several thousand whistleblower complaints had been received, but only one resulted in any recommended discipline of a senior official, according to the Project on Government Oversight.[22] In some cases investigations were undertaken that appeared to single out VA union activists for minor infractions. Complaints about misbehavior by some VA police officers, a well-documented internal problem, led to few operational improvements.[23]

In 2018, the White House used a series of executive orders to further modify disciplinary procedures, weaken seniority rights, and limit the long-established practice of allowing union stewards to spend compensated time representing their coworkers during working hours. The VA also sought to remove union offices from VA property, where they had long provided easier access for workers seeking job-related assistance.[24] An AFGE lawsuit temporarily blocked these changes, but they were finally implemented in February 2020. In contract bargaining with AFGE, VA management sought major concessions, including weakening workers' rights related to job safety and health.

Whether VA workers belonged to a union or held a higher-level career job, the Trump administration succeeded in creating a toxic work environment for many of them. In the view of Steve Robertson, former legislative director for the American Legion, the VA's new personnel policies did far-reaching and intentional damage. "It no longer made sense for people to prioritize VA when seeking government work," he points out. "Why would someone come to work at the VA when they could work at the DOD or NIH or other agencies where there are more protections?"

FROM CHOICE TO MISSION

With David Shulkin out of the way, the Trump administration focused on passing successor legislation to the Choice Act, which had a 2018 sunset provision. This effort was overseen by new VA secretary Robert Wilkie, a veteran of both the Air Force and Navy Reserves, whose father was wounded in Vietnam. As a Republican political operative, Wilkie had served as an aide or adviser to southern Republicans in Congress, including Jesse Helms, Trent Lott, and Thom Tillis.[25] He came to the VA from the DOD, where he had helped codify and defend Trump's discriminatory ban on transgendered troops. In an earlier tour of duty at the Pentagon, during the Bush administration, he helped restrict congressional access to hearing testimony by military officers about the status of the Iraq War. Wilkie was a North Carolina native, and his longtime admiration for Confederate heroes like Jefferson Davis and Robert E. Lee triggered a few questions at his own confirmation, but not many. The Senate confirmed him by a vote of 86 to 9.[26]

A good starting point for any congressional debate about further VHA outsourcing would have been a candid assessment of actual patient experience with it since 2014. Another smart move would have been determining private-sector capacity to handle a large influx of VHA patients versus the small number, referred outside on the basis of medical need, prior to the Choice Act.[27] In 2018, RAND published one such study, titled "Ready or Not?," that assessed healthcare capacity for veterans in New York state in the context of possible Choice Act expansion. The authors created a rigorous set of standards to evaluate whether doctors, nurses, mental health clinicians, and even physical therapists were "ready to serve" VHA patients but found that only 2 percent met the criteria.[28]

Even Senator Jon Tester, cosponsor of what became the MISSION Act of 2018, acknowledged that "the Choice program has been a wreck. Every veteran up here will tell you that."[29] Representing a rural state, Tester was familiar with the difficulty that even nonveterans face accessing certain kinds of healthcare. According to one government study, 77 percent of all US counties face a severe shortage of practicing psychiatrists, psychologists, or social workers. Fifty-five percent—all of them rural counties—have no mental health professionals at all.[30] Even when private-sector psychiatrists are available, some are unwilling to accept either private insurance or federal reimbursement.[31] Under such "market conditions," not only do patients wait too long for appointments, according to the National Institute of Mental Health, 40 percent of Americans with schizophrenia and 51 percent suffering from bipolar disorder go untreated in any given year.[32] By contrast, data available on Capitol Hill in May 2018 showed that the waiting time to see a VHA mental health professional averaged four days. One in five VHA patients was seen on the same day that they made an appointment.[33] Even though roughly 16 percent of VHA primary care facilities were then operating at over 100 percent of capacity, for the system as a whole, the average wait time to see a VHA primary care doctor was five days—nine days for specialist appointments.[34]

Nonetheless, Tester and Georgia Republican Johnny Isakson, then chair of the Senate Veterans Affairs Committee, moved ahead with replacement legislation authorizing the VA to establish new standards for outside referrals that might be looser than Choice Act metrics of wait times, mileage from the nearest VA facility, or both. Private providers reimbursed under Choice would become part of a reorganized and expanded Community Care Network (CCN) assembled by a third-party administrator of the TriWest type. Private-sector providers would not have to demonstrate that their own wait times were comparable to or better than the VA's. Sponsors of the bill also balked at requiring them to meet the rigorous in-house quality standards met by VA clinicians.

Industry lobbyists, like the American Health Care Association, and individual companies, like Ascension, wanted so few obstacles to increasing their "market share" among veterans that even Joe Manchin was concerned. In a Senate hearing, the West Virginia senator questioned Dr. Baligh Yehia, then VA deputy undersecretary for health, about whether outside providers had the necessary skill sets to care for patients with complex service-related conditions. The VA official informed Manchin that free continuing medical education (CME) credits would be offered to all approved network physicians, but only on a voluntary basis, until private doctors and hospitals had a larger volume of veteran patients. "If you put a lot of burdens on the community providers and they're seeing a handful of veterans, they won't sign up," Yehia explained.[35] Joanne Frederick, vice president of WellPoint Military Care, a division of Anthem, gave similar testimony, arguing that if the VA instituted quality criteria for private providers, "people that don't want to meet those standards won't deliver the service."[36] (Doctor Yehia later left the VA to become a senior vice president at Ascension, one of the firms with a growing interest in veterans' healthcare; after Joe Biden's election, Yehia served on the new president's VA transition team.)[37]

A SYSTEM WORTH SAVING?

During this crucial debate about the future of VA healthcare, VSO officials—some of whom are VA patients—had plenty of ammunition to defend the VA. But not much was ever used, nor were rank-and-file members encouraged to use their own organizations' critique of privatization in any sustained grassroots lobbying effort. In 2015, the Veterans of Foreign Wars summarized the views of its membership in a report titled "Veterans Prefer VA Care."[38] Two years later, the Legion commissioned a forty-thousand-word report titled "VA Healthcare: A System Worth Saving," written by Phillip Longman and a coauthor of this book. The report documented how the VA performed "as well as, and often better than, the rest of the U.S. health-care system on key quality measures," while providing "highly integrated care specific to the needs of veterans that is typically not available at any price to patients outside the VA system."[39]

A link to what the Legion called the "Longman-Gordon Report" appeared on its national website, in the "Publications" section. Thousands of hard copies were apparently printed up as well, but not widely distributed. At the Legion's 2017 national convention, neither the report nor its subject matter were ever mentioned. There wasn't even a small-group workshop to share information on saving the VA so some of the several thousand Legionnaires attending would return home better equipped to lobby their members of Congress.

The DAV produced an excellent series of videos called *Setting the Record Straight*.[40] These creative animations showed why turning the VA into just another federal government payer of big bills from private doctors and hospitals would lead to its eventual extinction as a direct care provider. Unfortunately, YouTube has a lot of competing social media content. Even within the DAV's own claimed membership of 1 million, the videos never attracted more than a couple thousand views.

In an interview with one of the co-authors on the VA in 2017, Sherman Gillums Jr., then executive director of PVA, was consistently "on message" about his positive experience as a VHA patient with a spinal cord injury. "When I go to the private-sector emergency room, it's dreadful for me," Gillums confessed. "It's a dismal experience." Yet in his official capacity at PVA, Gillums focused on protecting the VHA's spinal cord injury program from privatization, not fighting outsourcing in general. "If we stand pat, we look like we're intransigent, pro-status-quo supporters, and we don't want to be labeled that," he told us. "To be honest, I can't expend that kind of energy to fight every aspect of privatization."

The Big Six and more than thirty other advocacy organizations, like IAVA, signaled their acceptance of the MISSION Act in a May 7, 2018, open letter to the Republican chairs of the Veterans Affairs Committees and their ranking members from the minority party in both chambers. What swayed them was the act's inclusion of long-sought financial assistance for family members caring for aging and disabled veterans at home. The VA's previous Caregiver Support Program, which provided case support services and stipends to caregivers of severely disabled veterans, was restricted to post-9/11 veterans. Expanding "comprehensive caregiver assistance" to veterans of all eras was a major gain for VSOs with an older membership, but it came with a price. That took the form of what the letter signers called a "carefully crafted compromise" that "would develop integrated networks of VA and community providers to supplement, not supplant VA healthcare, so that all enrolled veterans have timely access to quality medical care."[41]

As one well-informed congressional staffer told us, this VSO intervention pulled the rug out from under House Minority Leader Nancy Pelosi and others in the Democratic party still trying to mitigate MISSION's likely impact on future VA budgets and functioning. Congressman Raúl Grijalva (D-AZ), then chairman of the House Progressive Caucus and another VA defender, believed that many more Democrats were prepared to vote against MISSION before this letter arrived and provided necessary political cover to buck their House leader. The House passed the MISSION Act by 347 to 70; Pelosi and Grijalva were among the dissenters. According to Pelosi, "Handing Trump Administration ideologues and the Koch Brothers the keys to an underfunded VA" was only going to further "their campaign to dismantle veterans' healthcare."[42] In the Senate, only Bernie Sanders and four others stood against MISSION. Sanders said, "My fear is that this bill will open the door to the draining, year after year, of much-needed resources from the v.a."[43]

Not surprisingly, CVA director Dan Caldwell celebrated the outcome as "a big win for those who want to see the VA better integrate with the private sector."[44] It also enabled President Trump, just a few months away from losing Republican control of the House, to claim a major bipartisan victory. "This is a very big day," Trump declared at a White House signing ceremony. "All during the campaign, I'd say, 'Why can't they just go out and see a doctor instead of standing on line?'" Now, he proudly announced, "we're allowing our veterans to get access to the best medical care available, whether it's at the VA or at a private provider."[45]

WILKIE'S RULES

From the moment the MISSION Act became law, the Trump administration tried to implement it with minimal congressional oversight.[46] Fears that the VHA budget would be cannibalized to pay for a much greater volume of private care than expected were soon confirmed. Instead of basing outside referrals on the clinical needs of patients or the quality of private providers, Wilkie proposed new access standards tied to wait and drive times. Under his proposed rules, any patient who had to drive more than thirty minutes for a primary care or mental health appointment or sixty minutes for a specialty appointment could automatically choose private doctors and hospitals instead. (If a veteran had to wait more than twenty days for mental health or primary care or twenty-eight days for specialty care, they could also seek care outside the VHA.) In many heavily trafficked urban centers, as well as scantily populated rural areas, drive times to the nearest VA medical center or clinic can easily exceed thirty to sixty minutes. According to internal VA estimates, this change alone would direct more than 60 percent of all patients toward the private sector.

Wilkie's access standards were drafted, as the VFW noted, without "proper stakeholder input." Yet proponents of VHA privatization made sure that public comments on Wilkie's draft access standards would be overwhelmingly favorable. Both CVA and the Independence Fund (TIF) helped orchestrate a comment filing blitz. As the VA's IG found later, a "substantial portion" of the twenty-three thousand comments received contained wording identical to a form letter created and distributed by TIF. This spamming operation was protested by Senator Tammy Duckworth and others, but to no avail.[47]

By January 2019 even Senate Democrats, like Duckworth, who voted for the MISSION Act were displaying some degree of buyer's remorse. Twenty-nine of them, including Jon Tester, expressed concern that the projected cost of expanded outsourcing—ranging from $1 billion to $21.4 billion over five years—was not being "adequately assessed" or properly funded. President Trump's refusal to support additional funding, combined with escalating costs for that private-sector care, "would likely come at the expense of VA's direct system of care . . . something we cannot support," the signers declared.[48]

One VA medical center chief who chose to remain anonymous confirmed the accuracy of this prediction. At the physician's large VA medical center in the South, $32 million was spent on private-sector care in the year before MISSION was passed. In just the first quarter after the new access standards went into effect, the cost of outsourcing at the facility ballooned to $54 million. A senior VA administrator reported that fourteen out of eighteen VA integrated service networks (VISNs) were being starved of funds for staff retention and recruitment. In 2019, another source, at VA headquarters in Washington, expressed concern that the agency's 2019 budget lacked sufficient funding for increases in pension contributions or cost-of-living adjustments.

The threat to the VA's direct-care capabilities was more than just financial. One reason many caregivers choose to spend their career at the VHA is the absence of private health insurance paperwork and related "network" restrictions, which require clinicians to spend countless hours dealing with outside "managers" of care. The MISSION Act saddled VHA caregivers with a burdensome new responsibility—monitoring the care of outside providers, many of whom are employed by private healthcare systems with scant internal care coordination. As outlined in March 2019, these new MISSION Act duties included everything from helping veterans choose a network provider to conducting root-cause analyses of hospital infections acquired in the private sector. Instead of spending more time with their patients, VA doctors and nurses had to be on the phone tracking down outside providers, who were slow to return their calls or provide necessary documentation of their treatment of veterans.[49] In one Nevada VA medical center where RNs were needed for in-house care, management tried, unsuccessfully, to dispatch some, like temp agency staff, to local for-profit private hospitals to help with discharge planning for veterans referred there.[50]

While reducing in-house wait times was the rationale for the Choice Act and then MISSION, VA staff members had no ability to speed up the outside appointments of patients they referred to "community care." In Vermont, for example, a patient sent out to the private sector for a first-time dermatology appointment might face a delay of seven months or more. But, as one VA doctor there pointed out, if a veteran couldn't get a dermatology appointment at the VA medical center in White River Junction within thirty days, or had to drive too far for it, MISSION Act access standards dictated an outside referral, even when the comparative local, private-sector wait times led to even greater delays in getting an appointment.[51]

The MISSION Act may have spawned a new community care network, but one major contractor involved with it was not new. Along with Optum, a subsidiary of UnitedHealth Group, the long-troubled TriWest was hired again as third-party administrator.[52] According to an IG report, "The VA was paying the contractors at least $295 every time it authorized private care for a veteran. The fee was so high because the VA hurriedly launched the Choice Program as a short-term response to a crisis. Four years later, the fee never subsided—it went up to as much as $318 per referral."[53] In 2019, TriWest won a lucrative VA contract from the Trump administration to facilitate outsourcing in thirteen western states. Once again, the firm was tasked with "getting authorizations from the VA to the providers, coordinating patient care, scheduling appointments for veterans, and serving as their primary customer service contact."[54]

When that process does not go smoothly, the VA often gets blamed, unless a patient is aware of the contracting-out arrangement. In New Mexico, one of the states assigned to TriWest, Vietnam veteran Robert Anderson spent three months trying to arrange a second opinion outside the VA about problems with his back. "The outsourcing to TriWest is a joke," he told us. "They called me no less than four times to ask the same questions about preparing an appointment time with the University of New Mexico health center." Meanwhile, staffing cuts left Anderson's own VA medical center "like a ghost town." He noted that a dental lab with rooms for twenty hygienists had just three left "to serve thousands of vets needing dental care." In Anderson's view, "vets are suffering and paying the price of privatization right now."

At a February 2019 Veterans Affairs Committee hearing, Representative Conor Lamb, a veteran elected to the House just a year before, confronted

Wilkie about such understaffing and resulting workload increases for VA doctors and nurses. At a time when the VA had an estimated forty-nine thousand vacancies overall—forty-six thousand in healthcare delivery—Wilkie did admit to being "concerned." But, he informed Lamb, "I would not be honest with you if I told you that my focus would be filling 49,000 vacancies."[55]

A COORDINATED PANDEMIC RESPONSE

A year later, the coronavirus pandemic created threats to VA patients and their caregivers that would have been serious even if VA privatizers had not been on a collision course with reality before half a million Americans became fatally infected. As deadly as it was, COVID-19 provided two important lessons for veterans and their advocates. First, it demonstrated the practical impossibility of outsourcing their care to a private healthcare system quickly overwhelmed by its existing patients. Second, the pandemic provided a timely reminder of the VHA's little-known "fourth mission"—acting as a backup system during a national public health crisis or smaller-scale emergency.[56]

As the pandemic spread, getting a quick appointment with a primary care provider, dentist, or eye doctor was not easy for any patient in the private sector, much less for new patients from the VA. By May 2020, "a survey of primary care doctors found that nearly a fifth had temporarily closed their practices, owing to the pandemic, and two in five had laid off or furloughed staff."[57] Veterans are generally older and less healthy than the overall US patient population. Their common chronic conditions put many at increased risk of contracting COVID-19, being hospitalized, or dying from a severe case. As private hospitals throughout the country became more crowded and hazardous for non-COVID patients, Wilkie was forced to announce a "temporary strategic pause in the MISSION Act access standards for 90 days, or until the soonest possible time that routine care resumes."[58]

This seemingly reasonable decision triggered howls of protest from CVA and privatization hard-liners in Congress. Eager to avoid his predecessor's fate, Wilkie quickly clarified that referrals were still being made but "on a case-by-case basis for immediate clinical need and with regard to the safety of the veteran." The White House offered additional assurance that President Trump was "not stopping or pausing" MISSION Act implementation, only "ensuring that the best medical interests of America's veterans are met."[59] As part of its first coronavirus stimulus package, Congress authorized—and President Trump approved—an emergency infusion of $20 billion for VA hospital expansion, equipment purchases, and new hiring. This enabled the VA to fill twenty-four thousand staff positions by the end of 2020.

The VA quickly emerged as the only national healthcare system able to mount a coordinated response to the pandemic. Its emergency response was not hobbled by a fee-for-service model or the need to generate revenue sufficient to meet shareholder dividend demands. As one VA hospital chief of staff told us, she had no problem canceling knee replacements or other elective surgeries for patient safety reasons. "When I talk to colleagues in the for-profit sector," she reported, "they are much more reluctant to do this because they will lose money." Because all VHA healthcare professionals are on salary, they could also be switched more easily from their normal duties to COVID-19 testing or any other assigned task. In contrast, as University of Washington medical school faculty member Hugh Foy explained, "50 percent of private-sector doctors are on contract—you can't tell them where to work or what to do."

In lieu of face-to-face visits, VA caregivers could utilize their agency's world-renowned telehealth capacity to see more patients that way. As the *New England Journal of Medicine* noted, this federal response offered "a blueprint for rapid expansion of telehealth services during the COVID-19 pandemic."[60] In early 2021, when vaccination became possible, the *Minneapolis Star-Tribune* found that "at VA clinics and hospitals across the region, distribution of the shots was swift, efficient, and highly coordinated—a sharp contrast to the chaos and dysfunction that have marred the rollout in the fragmented private health system." Veterans enrolled with the VA were "able to secure vaccine appointments within minutes, often for the next day." Vaccination acceptance rates "have stayed persistently high," and by March the VA had fully vaccinated nearly 1.6 million people, more than many states or some of them combined.[61] In July 2021, the VA became the first federal agency to mandate that its own employees be vaccinated, when 115,000 frontline caregivers were ordered to get shots.[62]

The VA's system of coordinated and integrated care led to far fewer healthcare disparities during the COVID-19 crisis. Initial reports suggested that fewer African American veterans died or suffered devastating health consequences from COVID-19 than men and women of color outside of the VA. Experts believe this is because the VHA manages chronic health problems more effectively than our fragmented, private-sector healthcare system.[63] Using data from millions of VA patients, VA researchers began tracking "long COVID," the chronic ailments afflicting many survivors, whether or not they were ever hospitalized. In April 2021, they published a study "believed to be the largest yet to evaluate such a comprehensive array of health conditions."[64]

Most impressively, the VA acted swiftly to protect residents of its own nursing homes, known as community living centers. These facilities have better-paid, unionized staff and more of them, as well as rigorous infection control training and procedures. As a result, none experienced the deadly outbreaks that plagued for-profit nursing homes or mismanaged state veterans' homes like a now-infamous charnel house in Holyoke, Massachusetts.[65] As *Politico* reported, these state-run homes serve "a little more than twice as many people as the federally-run community centers, but their pandemic-related deaths were almost five times higher."[66] When COVID-19 cases exploded in state veterans' homes in Louisiana, North Carolina, and Hawaii, VA staff were dispatched to help patients there and in some private long-term care facilities as well. VA clinicians also assisted more than 122 private hospitals.[67]

The VA's available resources for civilian pandemic victims included more than 16,500 acute care beds, 1,000 isolation rooms, 3,000 ventilators, six mobile nutrition units capable of churning out 1,200 meals a day, twelve mobile command units, and a network of nearly 4,000 deployable volunteers known as disaster emergency medical personnel. They also distributed nearly 1 million pieces of personal protective equipment. Staff were embedded with the Centers for Disease Control and helped run the CDC's sixty-five emergency coordinating centers. The VA also deployed nurses to screen returning soldiers for COVID-19 and built a website to keep VA patients updated throughout the crisis.

Unfortunately, even a belated hiring spree and impressive displays of fourth-mission capacity could not undo three years of workplace damage inflicted by the Trump administration. "In the early days of the pandemic, VA nurses went to work facing dangerous shortages of personal protective equipment and caring for more patients than we could handle," recalls RN Linda Ward-Smith, an AFGE local union leader in Las Vegas. "When we were exposed to COVID and got sick, we were initially denied paid leave, and often denied leave altogether depending on the manager."[68]

The Federal Emergency Management Agency (FEMA) contributed to this personal protective equipment (PPE) shortage by directing "vendors with VA orders to instead send equipment to FEMA for the federal stockpile of such supplies," according to Dr. Richard Stone at VA headquarters.[69] At the VA's Hampton Medical Center in Virginia, workers faced "a scarcity of everything from masks to hand sanitizer to test kits," according to AFGE chapter president Sheila Elliott.[70] In press interviews, Elliott also criticized the lack of training and safety protections in her hospital's COVID-19 unit, which she attributed to local management freezing out the union.[71]

Frozen out as well to varying degrees were the VSOs, although some did rouse themselves to challenge Wilkie's risky homage to President Trump's favorite COVID-19 remedy—hydroxychloroquine. This antimalarial drug proved to be not only ineffective but actually hazardous for COVID-19 patients and others. In mid-June 2020, the Food and Drug Administration (FDA) revoked its earlier emergency authorization for off-label use, citing side effects like cardiac arrest. In various media appearances, Wilkie continued to make unsubstantiated, Trump-like claims about the drug's effectiveness.[72] Two days after the FDA revoked its emergency use authorization, he informed Congress that $2 million worth of VA-purchased hydroxychloroquine would still be available to treat COVID-19 "along with current information on potential risks."[73] A later study of 1,300 infected veterans who received the drug experimentally found that they received "no benefit" and experienced even "higher rates of death."[74]

THE VA DEFENDERS

If frontline workers like Sheila Elliott or Linda Ward-Smith had always been the face of AFGE during its many struggles with the Trump administration, the union would have been better off. Unfortunately, its workplace mobilization and political action were hampered by an embarrassing scandal, which Republican foes were quick to exploit. Investigative reporting by Bloomberg News in the fall of 2019 revealed AFGE president J. David Cox's sordid history as a sexual harasser—misbehavior that had "driven away talented employees, violated labor's values, and undermined the union's mission."[75] Sixty-eight-year-old Cox, a former VA nurse, was forced to take an administrative leave from his $300,000-a-year job. Four months later, in February 2020, he finally resigned as national union president, while dismissing any accusations against him as "lies and scurrilous, politically-motivated attacks."[76]

In the midst of evicting AFGE local unions from long-occupied office space on VA property, Wilkie found time to exploit Cox's misconduct for maximum PR advantage. In a November 21, 2019, letter to AFGE Secretary-Treasurer Everett Kelley, who became Cox's successor, Wilkie noted that the union had "allowed a culture of sexual harassment to develop and thrive at the highest levels."[77] Wilkie demanded that Kelley take steps to "protect VA employees who are members of your union from any form of harassment by union officials."[78]

National Nurses United (NNU), which represents about twenty thousand VA nurses, came to the anti-privatization struggle with no similar political baggage. In fact, it enjoyed a national reputation for being a progressive union, a longtime advocate for patient safety, and the labor movement's leading proponent of Medicare for All. In 2016 and 2020, the NNU backed Bernie Sanders for president and poured substantial resources into his campaigns. However, the union's VA membership was much smaller than AFGE's and was located only in some facilities. The NNU also lacked an exclusive focus on federal employee labor relations issues, since most of its members work in other public or private healthcare systems. Working together and apart, NNU and AFGE organized press conferences, protest picket lines, and a series of town hall meetings with congressional opponents of VA outsourcing.

These anti-privatization events in San Francisco, Portland, Phoenix, Reno, Milwaukee, New York, Washington, and other cities featured both liberal Democrats like House Speaker Nancy Pelosi and Capitol Hill progressives like Raúl Grijalva and Alexandria Ocasio-Cortez. When COVID-19 put healthcare workers of all kinds at risk, AFGE, NNU, and three other unions representing VA employees took some promising steps toward more coordinated action. As Betsy Zucker, a longtime VA nurse practitioner and union activist in Portland, reported, this pandemic-related pushback included "filing OSHA complaints, local and national grievances, and class action suits; lobbying and activating members of Congress; and raising union demands for adequate PPE through social media, press statements, TV appearances, online petitions and social-distancing rallies."

No veterans' group provided more grassroots support for unionized VA staff than Veterans for Peace (VFP). VFP activists like Mick Cole had firsthand experience with VA care and a strong personal commitment to rallying their fellow veterans against privatization. Some VFP members, like Paul Cox, who also belonged to local posts of the VFW or Legion tried to get membership resolutions passed on this issue that would encourage the big VSOs to weigh in more effectively. Unfortunately, VFP's own membership base of four thousand was far smaller. Most of its volunteer energy flowed into campaigns against nuclear weapons, ongoing US military operations in the Middle East, attempts to destabilize governments in South America, fossil fuel industry threats to Native American land, and deportation of undocumented veterans, to name just a few of VFP's many worthwhile causes. Where VFP local chapters or individual members engaged in "Save Our VA" campaigning and lobbying, their low-budget efforts showed what kind of resistance to privatization could have been mounted, with far more impact, if the organizational resources and ground troops of the Big Six had been similarly deployed.

ANOTHER BIPARTISAN WIN?

Instead, in mid-2020, under the banner of suicide prevention, VSOS old and new embraced another misguided bipartisan effort on Capitol Hill. This time the budgetary impact on the VHA was less significant than that of the MISSION Act, but too many Democrats once again displayed their inability to learn from past legislative mistakes. Prominent among them was MISSION Act cosponsor Jon Tester, the home-state senator of John Scott Hannon, a much-decorated Navy SEAL team leader. After Commander Hannon's twenty-three-year career in the military ended, he moved back to Montana. There he was diagnosed with PTSD, a TBI, severe depression, and bipolar disorder. He received help from the VA locally and also sought solace in nature. A gun owner like many other vets, Hannon had easy access to what the VA calls "lethal means." On February 25, 2018, he ended his life, leaving his wife and family behind. A year later, with Republican Senator Jerry Moran cosponsoring, Tester introduced S. 785: the Commander John Scott Hannon Veterans' Mental Health Care Improvement Act.

This memorial legislation could have boosted the VHA's own suicide prevention services—while expanding veteran eligibility for them. The agency employs thousands of well-trained clinicians, peer support specialists, researchers, dedicated support staff, and compassionate volunteers. Collectively they have unparalleled institutional experience treating PTSD, MST, depression, suicidality, and other mental health conditions. There are now two VA national centers exclusively focused on developing pioneering treatments for PTSD and TBIS. But under the Trump administration, job vacancies for psychiatrists were among the many not filled. As Mick Cole reported to Congressman Takano, VA mental health staff shortages were leading to four-month wait times for new patient appointments in some states. Plus, more than half of all veterans who die by suicide are not VA patients. Expanding their access to VHA care would require that Congress end its legislative exclusion of veterans with no provable service-related condition, too high an annual income, or other-than-honorable discharges.

The Hannon Act, in its Senate form, did none of that. To expand access to treatment and reduce the veteran suicide rate, it directed the VA to dispense $200 million in grant money to private-sector providers.[79] Under this pilot program, grant recipients would be free to treat VA patients and veterans not eligible for VA coverage, but only for mental health issues. As drafted by Tester and Moran, the bill had several major flaws. The VA itself was given little role in coordinating or supervising this outsourced care. There was no requirement that grant recipient staff members undergo competency training for treatment of PTSD or depression to ensure that their caregiving met VA standards. As noted in chapter 3, among those angling for Hannon Act grants were the Independence Fund and other politically connected proponents of nontraditional therapies of unproven value to veterans.

The most important subject of training not mandated by the Hannon Act was the lethal means used by Hannon himself. Seventy percent of veterans who die by suicide use guns—almost always with fatal results. Because many suicide attempts are impulsive acts that may not be repeated if thwarted, VA suicide prevention experts now stress the importance of veterans voluntarily reducing their firearm access, with the help of family and friends, where possible. "If you really want to make a dent in preventing suicide, this would have the most impact," says Russell Lemle, former chief psychologist at the San Francisco VA Healthcare System and senior policy analyst at the Veterans Healthcare Policy Institute. Despite lobbying by Lemle and other experts in the field, backers of the bill in the Senate ignored this "safe storage" approach to suicide prevention.

After the Hannon Act was passed unanimously there, Republicans in the House opposed a parallel effort by Congresswoman Lauren Underwood to require that VA-funded outside caregivers receive lethal-means training to inform their work with suicidal veterans. The success of Underwood's amendment was dependent on House Veterans Affairs Committee Chair Mark Takano. His own staff wanted to improve the Senate version of the legislation. But for months, Takano had faced mounting VSO pressure to respond to the much-publicized veteran suicide toll of nearly twenty a day. Sherman Gillums Jr., who had left PVA and become an adviser to AMVETS, led the charge against any legislative inclusion of firearm safety, claiming that it "misses the point."[80] Just six weeks before an election that promised to replace the Trump administration, Takano moved an identical version of the Hannon Act to a floor vote in the House, with no amendments.

Once again, Democrats on Capitol Hill facilitated VA outsourcing that Republicans would, in the future, try to convert from a "pilot program" into a permanent diversion of VA resources. For the VSOs, "it's all a win, even if veterans lose," says Steve Robertson, former legislative director for the Legion. "When veterans can go to private-sector care, or Minute Clinics, or get mental health care, no matter the quality of the services they receive, the

VSOS can claim, 'We've worked diligently to win you great new benefits.'"
Too many lawmakers, whether they have lots of veterans in their district or
only a few, pay no price for backing legislation that may have a detrimental
effect on vets, if it's packaged as "pro-veteran." And what better way to do
that than name a bill after a fallen hero like Scott Hannon or pass privatization measures under the guise of giving veterans more "choice" or access to
"community care"?

NO SOLDIER LEFT BEHIND?

The VSOS justified their support for the Hannon Act as an expansion of mental
healthcare access that would benefit all veterans, not just the 50 percent who
were VA patients. At the same time, most were unwilling to reconsider their
own past opposition to any broader extension of VA health coverage to hundreds of thousands of former military personnel with other-than-honorable
discharges. As one official claimed, "Our members don't support that." This
stance has left the uphill fight for bad paper reform in the hands of smaller
advocacy groups like San Francisco–based Swords to Plowshares and the
National Veterans Legal Services Program (NVLSP).

In 2015, Swords and NVLSP began a five-year process of trying to change
how the VA handles appeals from veterans denied healthcare because of
discharge status. Their rule-making petition, which languished under both
the Obama and Trump administrations, argues that the intent of Congress
when it passed the Servicemen's Readjustment Act in 1944 was only to exclude veterans "discharged under dishonorable conditions," not those with
other-than-honorable discharges. The petitioners urged the VA to conduct
discharge reviews that more carefully weighed the many extenuating circumstances, including multiple combat deployments, that might have produced behavioral changes and then military discipline leading to VA benefit
disqualification under existing rules.[81]

On July 10, 2020, Trump's VA rejected almost all of the changes sought in
the petition.[82] The VA invited further public comment on its own proposed
modification of discharge review procedures from individual veterans, their
organizations, and other advocacy groups, so Swords and the NVLSP solic-
ited additional filings supportive of their original legal position. No VSOS
wrote in support of the petition. That was not surprising to Swords director
Michael Blecker, who told us that even "the general public is way in advance
of the VSO community when it comes to veterans with bad papers. The VSOS
are really behind the eight ball on this issue."

In another VA-related initiative, affecting the processing of benefit claims filed by veterans without a disabling discharge status, the Trump administration expanded the role of outside contractors doing compensation and pension (C&P) exams.[83] During these appointments, non-VA staff examine a claimant's military health records and conduct tests to understand whether certain injuries, physical or mental, might be service-related and to what degree. Roughly 1.4 million C&P exams are conducted every year, and the result is a disability rating that either provides VA access or denies it, which can lead to further appeals either way. Over the years, lawmakers, veterans, and their organizations have questioned both the cost and the quality of these outside examinations. A 2018 report from the GAO, for instance, found that the major C&P contractors routinely subjected veterans to long wait times and made significant errors in their reports.[84] One of the companies cited by the GAO was Veterans Evaluation Services (VES), which has been faulted for its pursuit of C&P exam volume at the expense of accuracy and quality.[85] In 2015 the *Tampa Bay Times* reported that the company sent dozens of veterans to a Tampa doctor who was under federal investigation.[86] Margaret Rajnic, a registered nurse, says she was fired after questioning VA practices that were "failing veterans," in her view. "Their operational efficiency is poor," she told us. "It's a money-making machine, and the VA is not evaluating the true outcomes."

If there's anyone in Congress who should be taking a closer look at VA outsourcing costs and risks, large and small, it's politicians who served in the military and their colleagues on the House and Senate Veterans Affairs Committees. Not surprisingly, healthcare industry donations to those committee members more than doubled from their 2012 level to nearly $10 million in 2018, as profit-making opportunities created by the Choice and MISSION Acts have proliferated.[87] As we demonstrate in the next chapter, big money in politics has also become a major force behind "service candidates" fielded by both major parties. As struggles over the VA's future reveal, some of those "playing the veteran card" to get elected—like the late Senator John McCain—are not even great allies of their fellow veterans. Nor have post-9/11 veterans distinguished themselves in Congress yet by using their military experience to support much-needed changes in the foreign and military policies that led to our "forever wars."

7. PLAYING THE VETERAN CARD

> Veterans are people you can talk to who will cut
> through the (bull) because we come from a common
> background of non-partisan service.
>
> People talk to me, and they're like, "So are you lefty,
> or are you ultra-conservative and a hawk?" I'm like,
> "I'm just about the strength of America."
> —SENATOR TAMMY DUCKWORTH

In Paul Rieckhoff's memoir about his military service, the IAVA founder denounced the entire "generation of politicians currently in power" who have "failed America's veterans—and the American people." Criticizing the shortcomings of both major parties, he argued that "only veterans have the credibility to reach across party lines and represent all Americans." That's because veterans, far more than civilians, "have been trained and hardened in the most extreme conditions and possess a unique set of skills that make them exceptional political candidates." They will "not shy away from difficult decisions," because "they've seen first-hand the need for strong leadership in difficult times." They "can heal our divided country, strengthen our tattered reputation and remind us what is important." Writing in 2005, Rieckhoff predicted that a future president would emerge from the "new generation of leaders . . . forged on the battlefields of Fallujah and Ramadi." On Capitol Hill, other men and women who served in the military would "lay the groundwork for a populist political movement that challenges the status quo in America and propels veterans into Congress for decades to come."[1]

Since Rieckhoff made this optimistic prediction, both major parties have recruited, trained, and funded more "service candidates" with past experience in the Armed Forces, foreign service, or national security agencies. Along with allied groups, the Democrats and Republicans are trying to reverse or slow a half-century decline in veteran representation on Capitol Hill. As the percentage of veterans in the overall US population has gotten smaller, their presence in Congress has shrunk to historic lows. In the early 1970s, about 390 members—more than 70 percent of the total—had military backgrounds. By 2001 that number was below 200, and in recent years it has fallen under 100.[2]

One of the groups now investing in service candidates is a Super PAC called the With Honor Fund. Its wealthy founders believe that veterans have historically been more bipartisan than nonveterans. As their federal government role has declined, "extreme partisanship has corroded our national legislature," and "public confidence in Congress has plummeted over the last fifty years." Describing itself as "a cross partisan movement," With Honor seeks to end legislative "gridlock and partisan bickering" by funding "principled veterans" willing to take what it calls "The Pledge." This commits them, if elected, to joining "a cross partisan veterans caucus," conferring regularly with members of the opposing party, and cosponsoring "at least one piece of substantial legislation each year."[3]

Thirty-three congressional hopefuls got a big funding boost during the 2018 election cycle when Amazon founder Jeff Bezos gave $10 million to With Honor. This donation was announced the same week that Super PAC critic Bernie Sanders introduced a bill in the Senate called the Stop Bezos Act. Its goal was to force Amazon to reimburse the federal government for the cost of public benefits, like Medicaid or food stamps, that thousands of its workers were eligible to collect because their pay was so low. Nineteen candidates backed by Bezos, via With Honor, ended up winning House seats. Sanders's legislation to hold his company accountable was not successful.

In January 2019 these newly elected representatives comprised the largest cohort of veterans among freshman lawmakers on Capitol Hill in a decade. Ten among them were Democrats who helped their party retake control of the House as part of a wider midterm election backlash against Donald Trump. "There's no question those veterans and service members were central to our work to build a Democratic majority," a spokesman for the Democratic Congressional Campaign Committee (DCCC) confirmed.[4]

VoteVets, which spent $18 million on these and other candidates without military backgrounds, was exultant about their showing. "Veterans have more power than ever," declared its director, Jon Soltz. "We're raising more money. And we're having our voices heard in the halls of Congress like never before."[5] The editorial page of the *New York Times* was duly impressed by how much veterans would contribute "to a body whose practical skills and knowledge about war, peace, foreign aid, diplomacy and geostrategic thinking are in short supply."[6]

The new Congress seated in January 2019 included six female veterans, the most in US history. The Democrats among them quickly made plans to expand their numbers by creating a Service First Women's Victory Fund to raise money for future candidates with national security backgrounds.[7]

Along with Republican colleagues, they also created a bipartisan caucus to support women in the military, whose numbers are expected to double in the next twenty-five years, eventually making one out of five living veterans a woman. Senator Martha McSally (R-AZ), appointed to replace John McCain when he died in office, helped draw attention to the problem of MST by speaking publicly about her own sexual assault by a superior officer in the Air Force. Joni Ernst, an Army combat veteran and the highest-ranking woman in the GOP's Senate leadership, cosponsored legislation to deal with MST after revealing past physical abuse by her ex-husband.

Regardless of their gender or race, almost all successful service candidates are college-educated former officers with good political connections and affluent donors. Contrary to Paul Rieckhoff's prediction, few have demonstrated much interest in building a progressive "populist movement that challenges the status quo" in the United States. If that was their announced goal, they would not benefit from big spending on their behalf by billionaire Super PAC donors like Jeff Bezos or Michael Bloomberg. Instead, just like other centrist Democrats or conservative Republicans, most military veterans on Capitol Hill have dutifully embraced "bipartisanship" in the form of rubber-stamping Pentagon budgets, backing US military intervention abroad, or favoring privatization, which threatens poor and working-class VA patients. In their personal behavior, some veterans in Congress have been less ethical than their colleagues or political rivals who lack military laurels.

In January 2021, almost all the Republicans among them voted against accepting the results of the previous year's presidential election.

WHITE HOUSE HOPEFULS

During the 2020 election cycle, four veterans of post-9/11 wars did seek the Democratic nomination for the presidency, as Rieckhoff foresaw. But none succeeded. Since 2000 only four veterans from either party have made it onto the presidential election ballot—and the only winner among them was George W. Bush, a former Texas Air National Guard member with a famously spotty attendance record. Thanks to the electoral college and a Bush-friendly Supreme Court, Democrat Al Gore, the only vet in the race who actually set foot in Vietnam, ended up losing in 2000 (though he received more popular votes).

Two Vietnam veterans with actual combat experience—John Kerry and John McCain—both failed in their later bids for the White House. Their presidential campaigns demonstrated that running for office with military laurels does not always bulletproof a candidate, particularly against flak from fellow veterans. As noted in chapters 4 and 5, Kerry built his political career on the controversial antiwar activism that made him a household name in the early 1970s. After becoming a US senator, he initially backed the invasion of Iraq in 2003 and, like many others in Congress, only started questioning the conduct of the war later on. When Kerry ran for president in 2004 against George Bush, the latter's status as an incumbent and wartime commander in chief made him difficult to beat. The senator from Massachusetts tried to counter those advantages by playing up his own stronger credentials as a military veteran.

However, during his campaign, Kerry failed to offer convincing policy alternatives to open-ended occupation of Iraq and Afghanistan. To make matters worse, Kerry became the first target of what is now known in the campaign trade as "swift-boating." Backed by big Republican money and led by a retired admiral, a small group of conservative veterans, known as the "Swift Boat Veterans for Truth," used press conferences, negative ads, and a factually challenged book titled *Unfit for Command* to discredit Kerry's war record. His critics falsely accused him of misrepresenting the events that won him a Purple Heart and Bronze Star as a Swift Boat commander, throwing his campaign on the defensive. By the fall of 2004, the airwaves and cable TV were, according to Kerry, "full of lies about my military record. . . . At the Republican national convention, crowds thought it was clever to wear purple camouflage Band-Aids on their cheeks to mock the severity of the wounds I received in Vietnam. . . . I had volunteered to go to Vietnam. Bush didn't. Politics had clearly entered a dark, new chapter."[8]

Kerry's friend and Senate colleague John McCain, a former Navy pilot and Vietnam prisoner of war, was swift-boated four years before that term entered the political lexicon by political operatives within his own party. During his first bid for the presidency, McCain won the New Hampshire primary in February 2000, an upset that left his opponent, then–Texas governor George W. Bush, running scared. During their next contest, in South Carolina, "literature began to pepper the windshields of cars at political events suggesting that McCain had committed treason while a prisoner of war in North Vietnam" and "that he was mentally unstable after years in a P.O.W. camp."[9]

Bush also appeared on stage with an angry South Carolina veteran who claimed that McCain "came home from Vietnam and forgot us" on issues like Agent Orange. But such accusations—and McCain's greater willingness to question the Confederate flags flying in the state—helped Bush defeat him, 53 percent to 42 percent, and force his withdrawal from the race three weeks later.[10] During his second run for the presidency eight years later, McCain faced a primary challenge from fellow veteran Ron Paul, a libertarian critic of US military intervention and Pentagon spending. After not getting the 2008 Republican nomination, Paul refused to back McCain in the general election because of his continuing hawkishness. Back in the Senate after his defeat by Barack Obama, McCain never stopped rattling the saber on foreign and military policy issues. When McCain died in 2018, he was nevertheless widely eulogized as "the ultimate public servant" who "personified everything that is good . . . about modern politics."[11]

FIGHTING DEMOCRATS

In 2006, as more Americans turned against the Iraq War that John McCain always championed, the DCCC plotted a strategy to regain control of the House during the last two years of George Bush's presidency. Chaired at that time by Congressman Rahm Emanuel of Illinois, the DCCC searched for younger veterans who could run as moderate Democrats but tap into emerging antiwar sentiment. It was, after all, John Murtha, a conservative House member from Pennsylvania and former Marine, who made waves a year after Kerry's defeat when he renounced his own past support for the

Iraq War and demanded a timetable for a US withdrawal within six months. "The war in Iraq is not going as advertised," Murtha declared. "Our military is suffering. The future of our country is at risk." This announcement lent credence to progressive criticism of the war and created, for the Bush administration, what was dubbed a political "Murthquake."[12]

With Emanuel's recruitment and fundraising help, forty-nine veterans ran as Democratic candidates in congressional races across the country in 2006. Their efforts were backed by a Veterans and Military Families Council, newly created by the Democratic National Committee. Overall the party won thirty seats and regained control of the House. But only six of the Democratic service candidates succeeded. Military veterans running as Republicans that year—both as challengers and incumbents—did much better than Emanuel's heavily promoted "Fighting Democrats."[13] One who lost narrowly was Tammy Duckworth, a retired Army lieutenant colonel who nearly died in Iraq when a rocket-propelled grenade tore through the cockpit of her Black Hawk helicopter, leaving her a double amputee.

During Duckworth's initial run for Congress, she presented herself as a fiscal conservative and foe of "illegal immigrants." Yet she remained a mentee of leading Democrats like Illinois senator Dick Durbin, who arranged for her to speak at the 2008 Democratic National Convention in Denver. Duckworth served as the state director of veterans affairs in Illinois and, later, at VA headquarters in Washington during the Obama administration. In 2012 she made another run for the House, this time defeating Joe Walsh, an incumbent Republican. According to Walsh, she was the "perfect biographical candidate," who wore "that biography on her sleeve," making it "really, really difficult to attack her because of it." As Walsh recalled their campaign debates, "Every other word out of her mouth was about her service."[14] Four years after this victory, Duckworth moved up to become her state's junior senator. By November 2018, when the Democrats won control of the House by winning forty seats, one-quarter of their winners had personal biographies like Duckworth's.

One of those campaign stars was Conor Lamb, a western Pennsylvania lawyer and Marine Corps Reserve major. Lamb ran against a Republican incumbent in a congressional district carried by Trump, by a large margin, in 2016. Lamb's opponent touted his votes for twelve major pieces of veteran-oriented legislation backed by the White House and passed with bipartisan support thereafter. Lamb highlighted his record of service in the military and as a former federal prosecutor. In 2018, he won upset victories in both the special and regular elections held in his district.

According to retired four-star Army general Wesley Clark, a past candidate for the Democratic nomination for the presidency, the key to Lamb's success was his refusal "to make the race about the [Trump] White House or ideology." Instead, Lamb "focused on local issues and the solutions which best fit for his district," a reflection of the fact that post-9/11 veterans, in general, have "little patience for petty partisanship or rigid ideology." Clark predicted that candidates like Lamb would be an "antidote to Washington's toxicity" because of the "qualities that distinguish them" from other office-holders there. "Want a politician you can trust?" he asked readers of the *Baltimore Sun.* "Elect a veteran."

A POLITICIAN YOU CAN TRUST?

Clark's claim that veterans, by virtue of their military service, are more trustworthy than ordinary politicians was called into question by the career of Duncan Hunter. Unlike Tammy Duckworth, a total newcomer to Illinois politics when she first ran for office, Hunter laid claim to a Southern California congressional seat held by his Republican father for nearly thirty years. As a first-time candidate in 2008, the Iraq and Afghanistan War veteran highlighted his three tours of combat duty, including participation in the battle for Fallujah. "The U.S. Congress needs more military veterans, people who have walked the walk," Hunter declared. After his election he served on the House Armed Services Committee and boasted that he was bringing the best of "warrior culture" to Capitol Hill. In 2016 Hunter became one of the first House Republicans to back Donald Trump, who later considered him for several national security posts in his administration.[15]

Hunter's career began to unravel when he was accused of converting $250,000 in campaign funds to support his lavish personal spending. Donor money he embezzled helped finance a series of extramarital affairs, including one with a Capitol Hill lobbyist that began soon after he first took office in 2009. He even listed some improper purchases for himself as gifts to "wounded warriors." After being charged with fraud and campaign finance violations in a sixty-count federal indictment, Hunter gallantly tried to shift the blame to his codefendant and wife, Margaret, a mother of three who handled the couple's finances. "Whatever she did, that will be looked at, too, I'm sure," he told *Fox News.* "I didn't do it. I didn't spend any money illegally."[16]

While under indictment, the former Marine devoted himself to a veterans' cause of questionable merit—winning presidential pardons for military personnel convicted or accused of war crimes, including Navy SEAL Eddie Gallagher. According to Hunter, Gallagher "is the kind of guy we want out there killing for us, killing bad guys. He shouldn't be going to court at all for doing his job."[17] In November 2018, Hunter managed to hold on to his House seat by running a vicious smear campaign against his twenty-nine-year-old opponent, Ammar Campa-Najjar.

Long an immigrant basher, Hunter depicted this Latino Arab American Democrat, who had worked for the US Department of Labor and the Hispanic Chamber of Commerce, as an Islamic terrorist sympathizer and national security risk. Campa-Najjar took the more compassionate and exculpatory view that Hunter was a soldier who "never made it back from the battlefield" and then "lost his way" in Washington, which "chewed him up and spat him out." In December 2019 Hunter finally copped a plea and resigned from Congress. A federal judge sentenced him to eleven months in prison and ordered his soon-to-be ex-wife to serve a shorter period of home confinement. (Both Hunters were later pardoned by President Trump, who also intervened on Gallagher's behalf to nullify Navy discipline against him.)[18]

In Jason Kander's race for a US Senate seat in Missouri, it was impossible for his opponent, Republican Roy Blunt, to depict a former military intelligence officer who served in Afghanistan as a terrorist sympathizer. Yet Kander was, by his own description, "a thirty-three-year-old progressive Democrat who was pro–single payer, a vocal supporter of Planned Parenthood, and had an F rating from the National Rifle Association" while in the state legislature.[19] So Senator Blunt's negative ad blitz in 2016 focused on his opponent's support for background checks on gun purchasers. To fend off this propaganda assault and showcase his military experience, Kander produced a viral video of himself reassembling the parts of a fieldstripped assault rifle while blindfolded. This performance drew 1.6 million views but not enough in-state votes to oust Blunt, who got three draft deferments during the Vietnam War and never served in the military. After losing this Senate race—in which $75 million was spent by all sides—Kander continued to be a rising star in the state Democratic Party. In 2018, he decided to run for mayor of Kansas City, planning once again to use his background in the military as an additional selling point for his candidacy. As his campaign manager explained, "A politician doesn't start with the benefit of a doubt, but someone who served in the military does. People know you have sacrificed something. They may not agree with you, but they are willing to listen to you."[20]

That observation rang true with Alex McCoy, based on his personal experience as a Common Defense canvasser in electoral campaigns in other states. "When I knock on a door and the person I'm talking to identifies as a conservative or a Republican, when I tell them I was in the Marines, they'll often give me a second look," McCoy says. "They'll actually listen to what I have to say. If the voter who answers the door also served in the military, the connection is much stronger than with any civilian who never wore a uniform or served abroad." The extent of Kander's "sacrifice" for his service abroad soon became apparent when he abruptly withdrew from the Kansas City mayoral race, despite strong momentum and record-breaking fundraising. "Instead of celebrating that accomplishment," he explained, "I found myself on the phone with the VA's Veterans Crisis Line, tearfully conceding that, yes, I have had suicidal thoughts. And it wasn't the first time."[21]

Kander's public admission that he was suffering from service-related PTSD and depression—and needed treatment—was widely applauded and contrasted with service candidate behavior in an earlier era. As Max Cleland, the disabled Vietnam vet who later became a US senator for Georgia and secretary of veterans affairs, told the *New York Times*: "We never talked about it because you couldn't—you couldn't say you had problems and still be elected. . . . And we didn't have a name for the issues from combat. We just called it alcoholism." After Kander ended his campaign and before he launched the Veterans Community Project, which provides housing and support services for homeless veterans, he went to regular therapy sessions at the VA Medical Center in Kansas City. "I'm not cured, but I'm so much better," he later reported. "PTSD is like an old knee injury. It's always going to be there. If you treat it and manage it, it doesn't have to restrict what you do."[22]

TALKING ABOUT PATRIOTISM

Kander's public testimonial to the importance of VA care stands in sharp contrast to Massachusetts Democrat Seth Moulton's persistent sniping at the VA. Moulton is a model, mentor, and frequent fundraiser for other ex-military men and women seeking congressional seats, as Democrats, around the country. In 2019 he tried, unsuccessfully, to make that network a base of support for his long-shot bid for the Democratic presidential nomination. The winner of a Bronze Star during four tours of duty in Iraq, Moulton attributes his own prior electoral success to his willingness "to talk about patriotism, about security, about service . . . issues that for too long Democrats have ceded to Republicans."[23] This personal branding won over Democratic primary voters in his own district—north of Boston—in 2014, when he ran against a nine-term incumbent favored by organized labor and the national Democratic Party.

But Moulton's primary campaign against John Tierney was not an Alexandria Ocasio-Cortez–style challenge from the left. Moulton ran against Tierney from the right, with backing from fellow veterans like General Stanley McChrystal, former commander of US forces in Afghanistan, and General David Petraeus, who supervised Moulton's work on a special counterinsurgency team in Iraq. Once in Congress, Moulton became such a champion of bipartisanship that, according to *Politico*, he made sure guests at his own wedding included "an even number of Republicans and Democrats from Congress." As a presidential candidate, Moulton touted his work with Republicans on the Faster Care for Veterans Act of 2016. Signed into law by President Obama, this bipartisan measure required the VA to experiment with an online self-scheduling app for VA patients. According to Moulton, a VA patient himself, this allows them to make medical appointments "from their smart phones or computers with the click of a button."[24]

However, as Rick Weidman from Vietnam Veterans of America notes, scheduling convenience for some is not the same as better access to care for all. "Scheduling apps just mean that one veteran gets ahead of someone else in line," Weidman points out. The real challenge is properly funding VA hospitals and clinics so they have enough caregivers to assist all the new patients coming through the door. "You don't do that with a scheduling app," Weidman says. "You do that by filling the almost 49,000 vacancies at the VA." In 2018 Moulton joined forces with conservative Republicans and other Democrats flouting the leadership of Nancy Pelosi when he voted for the MISSION Act. As noted in the previous chapter, this legislation diverted billions of dollars from the VA to private-sector providers. Among the other Democrats who cast a "yes" vote over Pelosi's objections was newly elected Conor Lamb, who, once seated in the House, rarely "voted against the party's leadership on any significant issues."[25]

When Moulton then tried to replace Pelosi herself, in the interest of "generational change," his failed attempt was not supported by influential advocates for veterans in Washington, DC. Three of them—who had served as past national legislative directors of the DAV, Legion, and VFW—penned an opinion piece for *The Hill* praising what they called Pelosi's "incredible legacy of leadership on behalf of our nation's veterans and their families."[26]

When Common Defense lobbied Congress to bring ongoing US global military conflicts to a "responsible and expedient" conclusion, neither Moulton nor Lamb signed its "End the Forever War" pledge. After his election to Congress from Staten Island in 2018, Afghanistan War veteran Max Rose, a fellow moderate Democrat, did agree to cosponsor a measure introduced by Representative Barbara Lee from California that would have rescinded congressional authorization for US military activity in Iraq.[27] In July 2020 Rose became one of the few veterans in Congress to support an accelerated time-table for withdrawal of US forces from Afghanistan, a measure defeated in the House. As noted in the next chapter, he also became one of the first House members from a military background to support removing the names of Confederate Army generals from US military bases.[28]

One of the best-known critics of military intervention in the Middle East was Rose's more left-leaning colleague Tulsi Gabbard from Hawaii. In 2019 and 2020, Gabbard took her political career to a new level when she ran for president in a field that initially included three other veterans. On a political stage where many candidates shy away from foreign policy issues, Gabbard bravely made ending "regime change wars" the centerpiece of her campaign. She also opposed any renewed arms race with Russia and called for the United States to rejoin the nuclear pact with Iran that the Trump administration had repudiated. But even such a staunch anti-interventionist as Gabbard was "not nearly as dovish as non-veteran Bernie Sanders," according to a Code Pink analysis of the 2020 Democratic presidential primary field. In the six years prior to her run, Gabbard voted for nineteen of twenty-nine military spending bills and thus earned only a 51 percent Peace Action voting record.

Many of the votes counted against her were to fund controversial new weapons systems, including nuclear-tipped cruise missiles, an eleventh US aircraft carrier, and various parts of Obama's anti-ballistic-missile program—which helped fuel the new arms race with Russia she later criticized on the presidential campaign trail. Gabbard voted at least twice against repealing the much-abused 2001 Authorization for the Use of Military Force, and she voted three times against curbing the use of Pentagon slush funds. In 2016 she even voted against an amendment to cut the military budget by just 1 percent.

Code Pink questioned what kind of commander in chief Gabbard would prove to be if she made it to the White House in her long-shot 2020 campaign. "Would it be the Army Reserve major with a self-described 'military mindset' who cannot bring herself to deprive her military colleagues of new weapons systems or even a 1% cut from the trillions of dollars in military spending she has voted for? Or would it be the veteran who has seen the horrors of war and is determined to bring the troops home and never again send them off to kill and be killed in endless regime change wars?"[29]

Not many officers—whether successful in politics or not—shift from a traditional "military mindset" that embraces "regime change wars" as being just and necessary to a stance more critical of US foreign policy. Andrew J. Bacevich Jr. is one well-known veteran who did, but not as a politician. Bacevich retired as an Army colonel after twenty years of service in Vietnam, the first Gulf War, and Germany; his son became an Army officer as well and a combat casualty of the war in Iraq. Bacevich's own account of his personal transition from tank commander to think tank critic of foreign intervention illustrates the hold that groupthink can have on most career officers.

"I myself have certainly changed my views on war," Bacevich told us during an interview in which his clipped answers and ramrod-straight demeanor reflected his many years in uniform. "Why did they change? Getting out of the Army was key to me. The military is an all-encompassing institution. It demands a certain level of intellectual conformity. It does not encourage free thinking. I went to West Point. Its purpose was to socialize and shape the individual to subscribe to a certain set of priorities. It's very difficult to resist that socialization process because they've been doing it for 150 years, and it was very powerful. They knew how to produce the product they wanted to produce." When he became a history professor and distinguished author after leaving the service, Bacevich began "to rethink some of the things I'd simply taken for being self-evident," a process that "was advanced by the recklessness with which we began using military power after the end of the Cold War, especially in the events that followed 9/11. I mean, my god, what the hell are we doing?"

In 2019, Bacevich became cofounder and president of the Quincy Institute for Responsible Statecraft, which promotes new approaches to US foreign and military policy. But few veterans who become service candidates—other than the brave but idiosyncratic Tulsi Gabbard—do much similar questioning of the status quo. Those who make it to Capitol Hill become part of an institution, like the military, in which intellectual conformity is rewarded and too much free thinking can be hazardous to your career.

THE CLASS OF 2018

The veterans elected in the class of 2018 soon proved this point—and made Gabbard look good in comparison. A mere six months after they were sworn in, the House was considering a Pentagon appropriation bill that offered the new Democratic majority an opportunity to begin reining in military spending. In the House Democratic caucus, among those carrying the ball for the DOD was VoteVets-backed Mikie Sherrill, a former Navy pilot and Annapolis graduate just elected from New Jersey. She criticized her liberal colleagues, who sought to reduce the proposed $733 billion allocation, for not believing "in a muscular foreign policy and muscular national defense like I do." As reported by the *New York Times*, moderate Democrats like Sherrill were "reluctant to cut that number" because it was less than the $750 billion annual budget previously approved by the Republican-controlled Senate—an amount greater than even the DOD itself had requested.[30]

In May 2020, in anticipation of House Armed Services Committee action on the National Defense Authorization Act (NDAA) for the next fiscal year, twenty-seven Democrats called for "a reduction in defense spending during the coronavirus pandemic." Among those House progressives championing this seemingly reasonable suggestion were nonveterans first elected to Congress in 2018 like Ilhan Omar, Ayanna Pressley, Rashida Tlaib, and Alexandria Ocasio-Cortez, whose Bronx-Queens district was decimated by COVID-19. The signers noted that "in the last three years alone—during a time of relative peace—we have increased annual defense spending by more than $100 billion, almost 20 percent." Because the coronavirus was now "our greatest adversary," the signers argued that resources should be devoted to that fight instead of "increasing military spending that already outpaces the next 10 closest nations combined."[31]

One veteran in Congress, Ruben Gallego—and two other Democrats who had signed the Common Defense "End the Forever War" pledge just a few months earlier—would not sign this appeal for "more testing, not more bombs." Tulsi Gabbard was also MIA. Ironically, the only veteran in the House who did sign was Peter DeFazio from Oregon, who had just crushed a Democratic primary challenger named Doyle Canning who was backed by Common Defense and tried to make a campaign issue out of DeFazio's acceptance of defense industry donations. As one Common Defense organizer sadly observed, there "really isn't any veteran in Congress yet who is part of the progressive wing of the Democratic caucus. Ruben Gallego is the closest."

In early July 2020, most Democrats on the House Armed Services Committee joined forces with conservative Republican Liz Cheney from Wyoming to win approval of an amendment to the NDAA that would restrict President Trump's ability to reduce US troop levels in Afghanistan below eight thousand. Cheney's bipartisan initiative was cosponsored by Colorado Democrat and former Army Ranger Jason Crow, who served three tours of duty in Iraq and Afghanistan and won the Bronze Star. Only Tulsi Gabbard and two other Democrats balked at the Crow-Cheney restrictions, but then the entire committee—including veterans like Crow, Gabbard, Gallego, Seth Moulton, and Anthony Brown—voted 56 to 0 to spend $740.5 billion on the Pentagon during the next fiscal year, an allocation later approved by the full House and Senate.

In September 2013, when Army Major Danny Sjursen was still on active duty, he had higher hopes for fellow veterans of post-9/11 wars then serving in Congress. Sixteen strong in the House at the time, they were asked to approve Obama administration air strikes in Syria. In *Ghost Riders of Baghdad*, Sjursen noted that only two Iraq War veterans favored this action. "At a time when the two parties can't agree on much of anything, *nine Republican* veterans joined their Democratic colleagues in strident opposition to intervention. Four others were undecided but leaning toward an anti-war stance." One new House member involved in that debate was Tammy Duckworth. If US forces were to get more involved in Syria, she reminded her colleagues, "families like mine . . . are the first to bleed." Duckworth declared that she would not support "pre-emptive intervention" until she felt it was "imperative for our national security."[32]

Seven years after applauding this healthy display of bipartisan skepticism, Sjursen was mainly disappointed by the performance of veterans in Congress because "we have a $750- to $800-billion-a-year military budget and nobody votes against it." Noting that it "takes less political courage to oppose intervention than the military budget itself, which takes an extraordinary amount of courage," Sjursen believes that veterans on Capitol Hill could take more political risks than their colleagues who didn't serve, but few are willing to do so. He expressed particular disdain for Jason Crow, who became "the king of Congressional combat veteran quislings" when he and other post-9/11 veterans in the House tried to "[block] the end of a long-lost war that some 73 percent of their fellow Afghan-alumni now oppose."[33]

Alex McCoy, then political director at Common Defense, agreed with Sjursen. "It's notable that—with the exception of Max Rose on Afghanistan withdrawal—100 percent of the swing district 'service candidate' veterans have been reliably pro hawkishness, pro–military-industrial complex votes." To McCoy, "Jason Crow partnering with Dick Cheney's daughter to prevent the end of a 'forever war,' in order to stick it to Trump, is a perfect example of what Common Defense tries to prevent and inoculate against."[34]

Like Sjursen and McCoy, Nan Levinson, a chronicler of post-9/11 veteran activism, also wishes that more ex-military personnel used "their capacity for leadership" to help Congress exercise its "constitutional responsibility as the custodian of war and peace." Levinson attributes "much of the reluctance of veteran-politicians to buck their parties on war-making" to their "loyalties to military contractors who support their campaigns or do business in their districts."[35] A Center for Responsive Politics analysis of how Democrats in the House voted on a proposed 10 percent Pentagon budget cut in July 2020 confirmed the extent of that campaign donor influence. On average, the Democrats who voted against that measure had received $29,731 in contributions from the defense industry since January 2019, while those in favor of the amendment received, on average, $8,800 from the industry during that same period.[36]

FAST TRACK TO THE OFFICER CLASS

Campaign contributions are not the only currency employed inside the Beltway when various components of the military-industrial complex are winning hearts and minds in policy-making circles. The Department of Defense has its own big stake in maintaining a status quo arrangement in which Congress defers to the president on the use of military force, while the White House, regardless of who occupies it, remains overly deferential to the DOD on its every budget request. So what better way to ensure such deference than helping well-connected civilians burnish their résumés so that, if they do become future members of the legislative or executive branch, they will remain military friendly? The US Navy has been particularly strategic in its use of a direct commission officer (DCO) program for such purposes. As former State Department staffer and Marine Corps company commander Matthew Hoh points out, this program was originally designed to quickly enlist certain kinds of specialists—doctors, lawyers, chaplains—during wartime crises or emergencies.

Now, Hoh argues, it has become a way of manufacturing "political actors in military costumes." Those "who are directly commissioned into the military do not attend the service academies, do not complete ROTC training while at college, and do not attend Officer Candidate School. Rather, they attend a ten-day direct commission officer indoctrination course where they learn how to wear the uniform, are taught the rank structure, practice saluting, etc. . . . Direct commissioning is a way for the politically well-connected to become military officers without enduring the selection and hardship involved in normal officer training."[37]

One of the best-known graduates of the DCO program is Pete Buttigieg, who served as an intelligence analyst in Afghanistan for six months, a military credential much brandished during his 2020 campaign for the Democratic presidential nomination. Before Buttigieg, forty-three-year-old Hunter Biden also used the DCO as a fast-track route to an officer commission. Hunter's father, vice president at the time, swore him in at the White House in May 2013, after he got special waivers because of his age and a past drug-related incident. A month later, the younger Biden tested positive for cocaine during a routine drug test and was drummed out of the program, a decision he questioned but did not formally appeal. At age forty-seven, former Republican National Committee chair and White House chief of staff Reince Priebus was even older than Biden when he got a DCO-assisted commission as a Navy Reserve human resources officer. In June 2019 Priebus was sworn in by Mike Pence, Joe Biden's successor as vice president.[38]

During the 2020 Democratic presidential primary race, Buttigieg was far more adept at playing the veteran card than Seth Moulton was. This apparently made the Bay State congressman rather touchy about who was an actual combat leader, as opposed to a DCO briefly deployed in a war zone. In an interview with the *New York Times*, Moulton pointed out that Buttigieg was just an "analyst and analysts don't make decisions" whereas he had made "life and death decisions involving American lives."[39]

WORKING-CLASS CANDIDATES?

What Harvard graduates like Buttigieg and Moulton both lack is the experience of serving in the ranks and then trying to run for public office. "Who ends up getting elected to Congress?" asks Andrew Bacevich. "It's not the sergeants. Ninety percent of veterans are former enlisted people. It's only about 10 percent—or maybe just 8 percent—who served as officers. . . . I don't think there are any former enlisted people in Congress or in the political conversation. And yet that's the veteran population. The typical vet is still politically powerless." As Harvard professor Michael Sandel points out, "About half of the U.S. labor force is employed in working class jobs, defined as manual labor, service industry and clerical jobs. But fewer than 2 percent of the members of Congress worked in such jobs before their election."[40]

When veterans from working-class backgrounds enter politics, their handicaps include not having elite connections necessary to raise money or even the ability to take time off from work to campaign. If they're running as genuine progressive populists, they must find a way to develop a base of Bernie Sanders–style small donors, as Alexandria Ocasio-Cortez (AOC) did during her 2018 campaign for Congress. The Democratic Party establishment and its big-donor class were no more welcoming to military veterans like Lee Carter, Richard Ojeda, or Kerri Evelyn Harris than they were to the Manhattan bartender now widely known as AOC.

A thirty-year-old former Marine, Lee Carter was, like AOC, inspired to run for office by Bernie Sanders's 2016 presidential campaign. Carter was also motivated by his personal difficulty, as a blue-collar worker, qualifying for state workers' comp benefits after being injured on the job. In 2017, Carter won his first race for Virginia House of Delegates when he challenged a six-term incumbent who was part of the Republican leadership in Richmond. Because the young red-haired veteran was a member of the Democratic Socialists of America, the state Democratic Party regarded his campaign as a joke; his opponent likened him to Lenin, Stalin, and Mao. Carter's detractors in both parties continued to fire away at him throughout his first term. During a House of Delegates debate in early 2019, a fellow Democrat stood behind Carter while he was speaking on behalf of tax reform and displayed a laptop image of a red hammer and sickle.

In 2019, Carter defeated a centrist Democrat opponent in the primary, winning 58 percent of the vote, and then won reelection by beating a Republican challenger 53.3 percent to 46.5 percent. Serving in the House of Delegates is a part-time job that pays only $17,640 a year. As one Carter admirer reports, "While many of his legislative colleagues had cushy jobs with corporations that influenced their votes, Carter worked as a Lyft driver in order to give him the flexibility to attend legislative sessions and meet with constituents."[41] In 2020, with Democrats in control, the Virginia legislature finally passed one of Carter's bills, extending the state minimum wage to workers at Dulles and Reagan Airports. Fearful of offending the business community, Carter's moderate Democrat colleagues squelched his attempt to repeal Virginia's right-to-work law, which has weakened its private-sector unions for seventy-five years.[42] In 2021, Carter waged a long-shot campaign for the Democratic nomination for governor of Virginia; he placed fifth in a field of five, and then lost a primary race to return to the House of Delegates, after which he announced his retirement from electoral politics.

Richard Ojeda, a fiery former Army paratrooper, became a tribune of the working class in neighboring West Virginia after he was elected state senator from Logan County. Ojeda began his twenty-seven-year Army career as an enlisted man and then went through officer training after completing college; he retired with the rank of major. In 2018 he became a leading public supporter of the twenty-five thousand public school teachers who staged a militant statewide walkout. Later that year, he ran for Congress against an incumbent Republican, despite voting for Trump two years before based on the billionaire's promise to "drain the swamp" in Washington, DC.

During his campaign, Ojeda expressed regret for that decision because Trump "hasn't done shit" and is just "taking care of the daggone people he's supposed to be getting rid of." In a district the GOP won by 49 percentage points in 2016, Ojeda lost by only 12 percent two years later due to the largest swing of voters away from Trump anywhere in the nation. Nevertheless, according to Ojeda's campaign manager Dennis White, a fellow veteran, his candidate faced primary opposition from a well-funded and better-connected "Hillary Clinton–type Democrat" backed by the state party leadership. Even after Ojeda won the primary, he struggled to raise money, and the Democratic National Committee (DNC) offered little help, apparently because Ojeda didn't fit the party's preferred service candidate profile. As White recalls with disgust, "They provided no fundraising, no insights on organizing, nor any help on basic things, even like how to file an FEC report."[43]

In 2018, Kerri Evelyn Harris, an Air Force vet and African American community organizer, had the audacity to challenge an incumbent US senator from Delaware, gaining 35 percent of the Democratic primary vote. Harris looked much like the insurgent congressional candidates in New York, Michigan, Massachusetts, and Minnesota who ran with greater success that year and then became known as "the Squad." As a kindred soul, she was definitely not a favorite of the party establishment nationally, or in Delaware, which had no need for a service candidate of her type, even though she was a woman of color. Harris criticized Senator Tom Carper for his coziness with the banking industry and his vote in favor of the Iraq War. "Democrats need to say, 'This war was our mistake, and we need to fix it,'" she declared. "We need to say 'We are going to pull back.' We need to say . . . we will not go blindly into another conflict that risks our working-class children."[44]

TWO, THREE, MANY VETS

By the 2020 election cycle, the fifteen-year-old romance between the DNC and its favored service candidates had even inspired a Hollywood movie. Called *Irresistible*, it was directed by comedian and former talk show host Jon Stewart, who has become an advocate for veterans seeking compensation for burn pit exposure. Stewart's film deftly satirized how veterans—in this case a retired Marine colonel named Jack Hastings, played by Chris Cooper—are recruited, funded, and deployed to regain red-state political turf. Carefully branded by his campaign consultant as a candidate "tempered by war, shaped by his faith," Colonel Jack woos the electorate with Jason Kander–style ads highlighting his weapons-handling skill; in one video, he fires long bursts from a heavy machine gun to convince voters that he's "Not Your Daddy's Democrat."

Two years after Democrats regained control of the House—with the help of two, three, many Colonel Jacks—the party viewed service candidates as a cornerstone of its 2020 strategy for retaining a House majority and retaking the Senate while ousting Donald Trump in the process. Not to be outdone— or outspent—the GOP doubled down on veteran candidacies. Before primary election contests reduced their numbers, about 250 Republican veterans sought seats in Congress. Some of them, like Mike Garcia, reflected the party's emphasis on greater racial, ethnic, and gender diversity. The GOP's branding of Garcia as a "Veteran, Businessman, Family Man . . . and definition of the American dream" helped the former fighter pilot and second-generation Mexican American win a vacant Southern California congressional seat during a special election in May 2020.[45]

In 2020 primary battles, competition between veterans in the same party was not uncommon; in some districts this morphed into veteran-only contests in the general election. In Texas, two Latino Republican vets vied with each other to become the potential successor to the party's only Black House member, Will Hurd, who was retiring. Tony Gonzales, a Navy cryptologist and combat veteran, faced off against Raul Reyes Jr., a retired Air Force lieutenant colonel. The Democrat seeking that same congressional seat was also a vet—Gina Ortiz Jones, a former Air Force intelligence officer who had lost a tight contest to Hurd in 2018.

In a Michigan Senate race against a Democratic incumbent, the GOP fielded John James, an African American West Point graduate who flew helicopter missions in Iraq. James styled himself as a nonpartisan Republican who didn't "have a problem with Democrats because I don't have a blue message or a red message. I don't have a Black message or a white message. I have a red, white and blue message."[46] Taking a more typically partisan stance was Dr. Ronny Jackson, Donald Trump's former White House physician and failed nominee for VA secretary following David Shulkin's firing. After retiring as a rear admiral, Jackson won his Republican primary race in Texas by denouncing another former patient, Barack Obama, as a "Deep State traitor" who "weaponized the highest levels of our government to spy on President Trump" and deserved to be prosecuted for it.[47]

In Oregon, Peter DeFazio, the seventeen-term Democrat who was the only veteran in Congress to call for Pentagon budget cuts during the pandemic, was opposed by a fellow vet who played himself in a Hollywood movie made by Clint Eastwood. Republican Alek Skarlatos served in the Oregon National Guard and was deployed to Afghanistan. On his way home in 2014, Skarlatos helped thwart a terrorist attack on a train in France, as depicted later in Eastwood's *The 15:17 to Paris*. For his off-duty heroism, Skarlatos was inducted into the French Legion of Honor.

In Virginia's fifth congressional district, the Democrats' encouragement of service candidates led former Marine Claire Russo to challenge first-term Republican Denver Riggleman, a former Air Force intelligence officer. Unfortunately for Russo, her competition in the four-candidate Democratic primary field included two other ex-Marines. To break out of that otherwise male pack, Russo highlighted not just her battlefield service "mapping out Al Qaeda networks in Iraq" but also her role in "taking on the military bureaucracy on issues like sexual assault." A month before the primary, she released a powerful TV ad revealing that she had been drugged and raped by a superior officer after attending a Marine Corps ball in San Diego. Despite Russo's compelling personal story, Democratic primary voters in her district opted for the one non-Marine in the race—Cameron Webb, a thirty-seven-year-old African American doctor and former Obama administration official, who was later defeated in the general election.

A SENATE "SQUAD" IN THE MAKING?

In 2020 Democratic primaries in three other southern states, candidates like Webb—African American, nonveteran, and more liberal leaning—couldn't overcome service candidates who got strong early backing from the Democratic Senatorial Campaign Committee (DSCC). In Kentucky and Texas, these would-be senators lacked the local legislative experience of their rivals but raised far more out-of-state campaign cash. Only in Tennessee—a state considered far less likely to help flip the Senate—was a young, Black environmental justice activist able to overcome the huge fundraising advantage of attorney James Mackler, an Iraq War veteran still serving in the National Guard. During the early stages of her primary race, Marquita Bradshaw—the eventual Democratic nominee—raised only $8,400, compared to Mackler's campaign war chest, which totaled $2 million thanks to the fundraising help he received from the DSCC.

In neighboring Kentucky, former fighter pilot Amy McGrath was considered a primary election shoo-in because of her service candidate credentials and similar fundraising edge. McGrath graduated from Annapolis and later taught there; during her twenty-year military career, she became the first female Marine to fly a combat mission in an F/A-18. By June 2020, with help from the DSCC, VoteVets, and other groups, McGrath had already raised $41 million, more than any other Senate candidate in the country. But McGrath's centrist politics and party establishment support proved to be a turnoff for enough Democratic primary voters to make thirty-five-year-old state representative Charles Booker an unexpectedly strong competitor.

Backed by Bernie Sanders and groups like Our Revolution, the charismatic Booker championed Medicare for All, the Green New Deal, and the protest demands of Black Lives Matter activists. Despite being outspent by 10 to 1, Booker lost to McGrath by only fifteen thousand votes. In the primary Booker also benefited from in-state liberal unease over McGrath's criticism of Mitch McConnell for not being helpful enough in turning Trump's "good ideas" into policy. When asked whether she considered herself a "pro-Trump Democrat," she defaulted to standard service candidate rhetoric: "You can't put me in some partisan box. . . . If it's a good idea, I'm for it. It doesn't matter if you wear a red jersey or a blue jersey."[48]

McGrath's 2020 general election appeal remained very much rooted in her personal story of growing up in Edgewood, Kentucky, in the 1980s and dreaming of becoming a fighter jet pilot. At the time, women were still barred from such combat roles, so thirteen-year-old Amy sat down and wrote to her US senator seeking his support for lifting that ban. In a letter to potential donors three decades later, McGrath accused Mitch McConnell—still in office after all those years—of never replying to her letter. Striking a populist note, McGrath claimed that her voice was ignored because McConnell was too busy helping "coal barons" and Big Pharma. If elected to replace him, McGrath pledged to put "people first and get things done," not be dependent on "millions of dollars in dark money."[49]

In Texas the military credentials of Mary Jennings ("M. J.") Hegar, a helicopter pilot injured in Afghanistan, tracked those of McGrath in Kentucky. As a teenager, Hegar also dreamed of becoming a pilot and proving herself in a combat role previously denied to women. Yet she, like Claire Russo in the Marines, became a victim of sexual assault, which the military was reluctant to punish. As Hegar recounts in her 2017 memoir, *Shoot like a Girl*, she "felt powerless to stop" the Air Force flight surgeon who conducted an unnecessary pelvic exam to violate and humiliate her. Even after he confessed, her assailant received no military discipline, she reports, because the "chain of command protected him."[50]

Once out of the military, after three tours of duty in Afghanistan, Hegar joined other female veterans lobbying against the Pentagon's Ground Combat Exclusion Policy. That fight left Hegar "with a lot of concerns about the dysfunctional mess" she found in the nation's capital. To take on conservative US senator John Cornyn in 2020, Hegar first defeated Texas state senator Royce West in two rounds of primary voting. An African American, West was a longtime advocate of criminal justice reform who touted himself as the "true Democrat" in the race. He made much of the fact that Hegar had been a past Texas Republican primary voter and even a one-time donor to Cornyn. "With the sparks flying—and the runoff fast approaching—Hegar's outside allies stepped into the fray. The DSCC was already heavily funding Hegar but, with only a few days left before the runoff, EMILY's List spent over $1 million on TV and digital ads boosting her. . . . Hegar's campaign and its allies outspent West $102 to $1 on TV and radio advertising."[51]

As Hegar quickly pivoted toward her general election showdown with Cornyn, she, like McGrath, became more populist. On the campaign trail, she pulled up her sleeve to compare her tattoos with those of a female admirer. Her body art, she explained, was a way of turning scars left by shrapnel wounds in Afghanistan, when she was "facing down 150 Taliban fighters," into "something beautiful." If sent to Washington, she pledged to "take on Big Pharma, the gun lobby, and corporate PACs that have a stranglehold on the Senate—and clean up the influence of big money in our politics." In another email blast, she aligned herself with fellow "servant leaders" like McGrath in Kentucky, Cal Cunningham in North Carolina, and Mark Kelly in Arizona. Since all "swore oaths to support and defend our Constitution, we won't be pushed around by the special interests or DC bosses," Hegar wrote.

Like McGrath and Hegar, Cunningham was the beneficiary of millions of dollars in preprimary spending by party leaders—not to be confused with any "DC bosses"—who viewed him as a stronger candidate against Republican senator Thom Tillis than African American state senator Erica Smith.[52] A lawyer and former state legislator himself, Cunningham was commissioned in the Army Reserve, Judge Advocate General's Corps, after the 9/11 attacks. He then served on active duty in Iraq and Afghanistan, reaching the rank of lieutenant colonel and earning a Bronze Star. Unlike his challenger, Tillis never served in the military. But, like other Republican incumbents who did—including Martha McSally and Joni Ernst—Tillis directed much campaign fire at China. To counter "national security threats posed by

China," Tillis favored more Pentagon spending and a "strengthened American military presence" in the Pacific.

To overcome a Democratic challenger in Iowa, Ernst rattled her saber in similar fashion against "so many bad actions out of China." In Arizona, McSally was running so far behind Democrat Mark Kelly in the polls that she also tried to make their election "about who can stand up to China, the world's communist bully." Playing the veteran card against a fellow veteran, McSally cited her own Air Force experience as the reason for her hawkish stance. "I learned the day I entered the military, never trust a communist," she explained. "China is to blame for this pandemic and the death of thousands of Americans." Put on the defensive, Kelly—a naval aviator who flew combat missions in the first Gulf War and later became a NASA space shuttle pilot—cited his own military experience as proof that he, no less than McSally, perceived China as a "threat."[53]

Among Democrats in the fall of 2020, there was rising poll-driven optimism that red-state voter turnout against Donald Trump would sweep McConnell, Cornyn, Tillis, and McSally from office along with their president. If that occurred, there would be a squad of veterans joining the Senate in January 2021 as part of a new Democratic majority. This group of potential newcomers—from Kentucky, North Carolina, Texas, and Arizona—would be very different from the four progressive House members who gained such celebrity in 2018 for their successful primary challenges to Democrats backed by the party establishment. Given their campaign dependence on wealthy donors and Democratic Party Super PACs, none of these DSCC-backed fighting Dems were likely to emerge, individually or collectively, as strong allies of any populist movement challenging big money in politics or the status quo in military and foreign affairs. Instead, they all campaigned very much like the nonveteran at the top of the Democrats' 2020 ticket, who marketed himself as a "pragmatic and nonideological" presidential candidate, eager to collaborate with Republicans and "uniquely capable of doing so effectively."[54]

8. VETERANS AND THE 2020 ELECTION

No one has done more for veterans than me.
—PRESIDENT DONALD TRUMP

As military historian Andrew Bacevich has observed, the quadrennial contest to choose a new president of the United States should be "an opportunity for stock taking." Instead, "candidates in every election since 1980 have assiduously avoided anything like a serious debate on U.S. military policy."[1] In 2016 there was, per usual, little substantive disagreement about the Global War on Terror (GWOT), a now $8 trillion project that Hillary Clinton heartily endorsed.[2] A more agile Donald Trump managed to distinguish himself from his Democratic opponent by criticizing forever wars in a way that resonated among veterans who were, by then, questioning the value of occupying Iraq and Afghanistan at such great cost.

Trump's campaign rhetoric about Obama- and Bush-administration failures abroad may have been accurate. But, predictably, it was followed by little or no actual change in US foreign and military policy. In his first cabinet and his White House staff, Trump proudly surrounded himself with four-star generals who were all part of those failed GWOT efforts. As this A-team wore out its welcome, the president promoted veterans of lower rank within his administration. They included his second secretary of state, Mike Pompeo—"a captain trained to follow orders, not a general used to giving them"—and two equally loyal colonels: Robert Wilkie, whose wrecking-ball reign at the VA was described in chapter 6, and Defense Secretary Mark Esper, whose White House nickname—"Yesper"—explains why he was picked.[3]

With either team of former military officers on board, the Trump administration posed no threat to the military-industrial complex or any other Washington, DC, swamp in need of draining. As Bacevich summed up the situation three years after Trump took office: "Our endless wars persist (and in some cases have even intensified); the nation's various alliances and its empire of overseas bases remain intact; U.S. troops are still present in something like 140 countries; Pentagon and national security state spending continues to increase astronomically."[4]

With such a far-flung military presence still in place, photo ops with the troops were a regular Trump temptation as he geared up, almost immediately, for his 2020 reelection campaign. Halfway through his first term, the president made a holiday trip to visit US troops in Iraq. On the way he stopped at Ramstein Air Base in Germany, where one woman in uniform welcomed him with a "Make America Great Again" flag. At Al Asad Air Base near Baghdad, after getting a standing ovation from the soldiers assembled there, the president autographed a "Trump 2020" patch and the red MAGA hats brandished by his fans in the crowd.

He boasted about boosting military pay and criticized congressional Democrats—who had voted for that increase—for their refusal to fund his Mexican border wall. In response to this legislative impasse back home, an Iraq War veteran named Brian Kolfage kicked off an online campaign called "We the People Will Fund the Wall" to secure private funding for Trump's favorite infrastructure project. Among Kolfage's key advisers was immigration critic Steve Bannon, a former naval officer, Trump campaign consultant in 2016, and recently departed White House staffer.[5]

During his formal reelection campaign kickoff in 2019, Trump highlighted his outsourcing of VA services via the MISSION Act as a great bipartisan achievement of his administration. Citing nearly a dozen other veteran-related bills that Trump had signed into law, VA Secretary Robert Wilkie told *Fox News* that "you can't find another president in American history who, first as a candidate and then as a president, put veterans at front and center."[6]

Events yet to unfold in the 2020 presidential election cycle would make Trump's cultivation of the vet vote more difficult than he and his Republican backers anticipated. One challenge on that terrain was already emerging from the very large field of potential Democratic presidential candidates, which included, by Veterans Day 2019, four men and women with military experience of their own. As noted in the previous chapter, former Marine Seth Moulton's bid for the presidency—which, when first announced, made him the twentieth contestant to join the race—failed to gain traction. The candidacy of retired three-star admiral Joe Sestak, a former congressman from Pennsylvania, was equally quixotic and short-lived. Two other veterans of service in the Middle East—Pete Buttigieg and Tulsi Gabbard—gained far more national visibility when both reached the early debate stage of the competition and used that platform to showcase their respective service candidate credentials.

For Gabbard, an Army Reserve major and Iraq War veteran, that provided an opportunity to sharply criticize "regime change wars" in stronger terms than anyone else in the race except Senator Bernie Sanders, whom she supported in 2016. But, as one admirer sadly observed, Gabbard's "unshakeable anti-war stance" drew much "vitriol and slander" from "social media trolls, mainstream media pundits, serious national newspapers, and leading Democrats like Hillary Clinton who labeled her a 'Russian asset,' a 'Vladimir Putin apologist,' and even un-American."[7] When her polling numbers stayed low and her fundraising efforts lagged, the Hawaii congresswoman was first dropped from the debate lineup for top-tier candidates and then, a few months later, formally quit the race.

VYING FOR THE VET VOTE

Pete Buttigieg, a former military intelligence officer who served two terms as mayor of South Bend, Indiana, demonstrated far more fundraising muscle and staying power in the race. He proved adept at playing the veteran card when contrasting his credentials with those of the current commander in chief, "who was working on Season 7 of *Celebrity Apprentice* when I was packing my bags for Afghanistan."[8] Buttigieg criticized Trump's frequent use of the military as "a prop" for his "fragile ego" and was particularly incensed about the president's rationale for pardoning several veterans either convicted of war crimes or still facing discipline related to such accusations. "The idea that being sent to war turns you into a murderer is exactly the kind of thing that those of us who have served have been trying to beat back for more than a generation," he said. "Frankly, [Trump's] idea that being sent to fight makes you automatically into some sort of war criminal is a slander against veterans that could only come from someone who never served."[9]

As a pioneering gay presidential candidate and voice of youthful moderation in the Democratic primary field, Buttigieg proved very popular with wealthy nonveterans—including nearly sixty billionaires. He was backed by VoteVets, whose cofounder and chairman Jon Soltz argued that "there's nobody better to end the Afghanistan War than a person who fought in it."[10] Ironically, before Buttigieg's poor Super Tuesday performance led to his presidential race withdrawal in March 2020, a nonveteran was polling much better than Buttigieg among voters in uniform surveyed by *Military Times*. By early 2020, soldiers, sailors, Marines, and Air Force personnel had donated $185,000 to Bernie Sanders's presidential campaign, an amount greater than their combined contributions to Buttigieg, Biden, and Warren. At that point Sanders had also raised $70,000 more than Donald Trump from donors on active duty.[11] His policy-oriented appeals to veterans stressed his record as a longtime ally of Vermonters who've served in the military, which he himself did not.

After the first Gulf War, Sanders championed the cause of veterans who returned with the service-related condition known as Gulf War Syndrome. As noted in chapter 6, when Sanders was chair of the Senate Veterans Affairs Committee, he worked closely with VSOs to come up with a plan for expanded VA funding, which Senate Republicans blocked in early 2014. Although often accused of ideological inflexibility that prevented him from securing bipartisan support for bills he favored, in 2014 Sanders negotiated the political compromise with Senator John McCain that secured passage of the Choice Act. Contrary to Sanders's intentions, Choice opened the door for VA outsourcing on a much larger and more permanent scale, as authorized by the MISSION Act of 2018.

Along with Nancy Pelosi in the House, Sanders was a lonely foe of MISSION Act passage. He defended the VA as a federal agency in need of better funding and staffing, not piecemeal dismantling. Instead of welcoming such support, Secretary Wilkie sounded the alarm about Sanders during a Breitbart News interview on the eve of Super Tuesday primary voting. If Sanders-style "socialism became the coin of the realm," Wilkie warned, "the care that was promised for warriors would disappear"—a claim not supported by the actual language of Sanders's Medicare for All bill, which preserved VA coverage for 9 million veterans while creating a single-payer system for other Americans.[12]

Throughout his second unsuccessful bid for the presidency, Sanders also repeatedly stressed the interconnectedness of US foreign and domestic policy. He called for congressional limits on military intervention abroad and cuts in Pentagon spending so that billions of dollars could instead fund Medicare for All, free public higher education, and a Green New Deal to avert climate disaster. After his own string of primary defeats and the onset of COVID-19 restricted further campaigning, Sanders bowed out of the 2020 race. He endorsed Joe Biden, whose commitment to any of these goals was seriously doubted by Sanders supporters, many of whom reluctantly backed Biden in the general election as the only viable alternative to Trump. On the question of national priorities, for example, Biden did not foresee the need for any Pentagon budget reductions during his presidency. In fact, as he told *Stars and Stripes*, some of his campaign advisers were already suggesting areas where that budget "is going to have to be increased" in order to address potential threats from "near-peer" powers like China and Russia.[13]

OUR SACRED OBLIGATION

On Biden's campaign website, voters could also find his "Plan to Keep Our Sacred Obligation to Our Veterans."[14] This document stressed Joe and Jill Biden's personal connection to military families as "the parents of a son who deployed to Iraq." The former vice president highlighted his past role as a champion of "up-armored Mine-Resistant Ambush Protected vehicles, which saved thousands of lives and limbs of U.S. service members in Iraq and Afghanistan." He criticized Republicans for taking steps "designed to privatize and dismantle the VA." Unlike Trump, he promised to achieve "the right balance" between "VA care and purchased care"; the latter term is a euphemism for outsourcing to the private sector (aka privatization). Biden displayed little appreciation for the VA's well-documented ability to outperform private hospitals on quality measures like wait times, coordination of care, and accountability to patients. Instead, he promised to "leverage the commercial best practices and modern technologies" of the private sector "to meet the demands of the VA's public sector mission" and chided the agency for its "poor organizational performance, staff shortfalls, leadership gaps, and IT systems failures"—as if these shortcomings were unrelated to Trump administration mismanagement.

Military Times arranged for both candidates to respond in writing or via video message to a series of questions submitted by VSOs old and new. In this campaign exchange, plus a *Stars and Stripes* interview, Biden promised pay increases for VA caregivers and greater efforts to fill thousands of job vacancies. He insisted again that he did not "under any circumstances support moving to total privatization," nor would he ever "defund the VA," because there patients get treatment that is "specialized, supportive, and second to none."[15] President Trump touted his administration's expedited hiring of twenty thousand additional VA employees during the pandemic. In Trump's view, "veteran trust in the VA reached an all-time high" in the spring of 2020, up nineteen points since he took office.

Neither candidate had much to say in response to a VFW question about the Pentagon's need to shield soldiers from future exposure to hazards like contaminated drinking water, Agent Orange, depleted uranium, or open-air burn pits. Instead, they debated whether and how future VA benefit claimants should get the benefit of presumptions about the cause of their service-related conditions. Referencing his son Beau's service on bases with burn pits and his death, six years later, of brain cancer, Biden promised "an epidemiological study of post 9/11 veterans" with such toxic exposures while expanding access to care in the meantime. Trump bizarrely claimed that "presumptions are not required to gain benefits" but then went on to boast about his administration's "historic expansions of Agent Orange benefits through the Blue Water Navy [Act]," which had resulted in 66,853 new claims and completed VA processing of 31,774 of them, with a 71 percent approval rate and payout, so far, of $629 million "in retroactive compensation and survivor benefits."[16]

Despite widespread military sexual assault—which Biden called "a crisis in the ranks"—neither he nor Trump endorsed the Military Justice Improvement Act, a bill backed by the IAVA that would take sexual assault cases out of the hands of commanders and assign them to independent investigator-prosecutors. Both candidates favored further study of the problem—in Trump's case by a task force already created by his DOD and, in Biden's case, by a special commission "of military leaders, survivors, advocates and experts" to be named by him after his election. In Biden's platform there was not much discussion of the VA's critical role as a backup healthcare system during pandemics and other national emergencies. As noted in chapter 6, the VA's fourth mission soon gained far more attention as COVID-19 cases multiplied by the hundreds of thousands, quickly overwhelming private hospital systems—even those with "commercial best practices and modern technologies." Despite the private sector's demonstrated lack of capacity, under pandemic conditions, to absorb new MISSION Act–authorized patients from the VA, Biden criticized Trump for not rolling out a bigger "community care network" fast enough![17]

MONEY FOR B-21S OR N95S?

As the coronavirus spread, Americans increasingly preoccupied with their own exposure risk got an offshore reminder of what a "toxic workplace" looks like in the military. Anchored off Guam, the USS *Theodore Roosevelt* provided a dramatic illustration of how military service, even under "peacetime" conditions, can be hazardous to your health. Densely packed on board, the aircraft carrier's five thousand sailors risked a COVID-19 infection on a scale larger than any of the private cruise liners that had already become giant floating sick bays. This led their brave captain, Brett Crozier, to accuse the Navy of failing to provide proper resources to combat the virus by quickly moving *Roosevelt* crew members ashore. "We are not at war," Crozier reminded his superiors in a letter leaked to the press. "Sailors do not need to die. If we do not act now, we are failing to properly take care of our most trusted asset—our sailors."

Crozier's commander in chief was not happy with this initiative. Trump's secretary of the Navy removed Crozier from his command—amid a chorus of criticism from Crozier's appreciative crew, his Naval Academy classmates, and former colleagues.[18] Crozier ended up in quarantine on shore after testing positive for the virus, along with more than 1,200 other sailors, one of whom died. After Crozier recovered, his removal from command of the *Roosevelt* was upheld, effectively ending his career as a well-respected officer on track to become an admiral. Crozier's superior officer, who approved the questionable port of call in Vietnam that brought the virus on board, was absolved of any responsibility.[19]

In the middle of this controversy involving a nuclear-powered aircraft carrier idling in the Pacific—along with three other carriers with infected sailors aboard—the Pentagon demanded more money for nuclear arms modernization, a new class of ballistic-missile-carrying submarine, and accelerated development of the B-21, a new stealth bomber. Its planners in the Indo-Pacific Command informed Congress that an additional $20 billion was needed just for naval deployments "to bolster deterrence against China after the coronavirus ebbs."[20] The feminist antiwar group Code Pink issued a timely reminder that no branch of the military should be seeking more funding when President Trump and Congress had just showered the DOD with nearly $738 billion—a sum bigger than the combined annual military budgets of the next ten largest defense spenders in the world.

In that same FY 2020 budget, a mere $11 billion was set aside for the now truly urgent mission of the Centers for Disease Control and Prevention (CDC). As the Costs of War project at Brown University pointed out, total spending on the FDA, the CDC, and the National Institutes of Health for 2020 amounted to less than 1 percent of the cost of the Iraq and Afghanistan Wars since 9/11. According to Code Pink, whose leaders include retired Army colonel Ann Wright, this reflected a long-standing misallocation of resources earmarked for national security. As a result, the United States had 1.3 million active-duty troops and another 865,000 in reserve, but not enough doctors, nurses, or medical equipment to confront an enemy that would cause more civilian deaths in 2020 than the total number of US soldiers killed during World War II.

Common Defense, Veterans for Peace, and sixty other groups joined Code Pink in calling for a coronavirus-related freeze on military spending. Nevertheless, Congress authorized an additional $10.4 billion for the Pentagon, bringing its total FY 2020 funding to over $756 billion. In late June, before Congress voted on military spending again, Bernie Sanders responded by introducing an amendment to the NDAA. "At this pivotal moment in American history," Sanders declared, "we have to make a fundamental decision. Do we want to spend billions more on endless wars in the Middle East, or do we want to provide decent jobs to millions of unemployed Americans here at home? Do we want to spend more money on nuclear weapons, or do we want to invest in decent jobs and childcare and healthcare for the American people most in need?"[21] Under Sanders's proposal, the Pentagon budget would be reduced $74 billion—or 10 percent—during the coming fiscal year, exempting military salaries and healthcare from any cuts. The money saved would be redirected into grant programs for healthcare, housing, childcare, and educational opportunities in cities and towns experiencing a poverty rate of 25 percent or more. In the House, with similar intent, Representative Barbara Lee proposed $350 billion in cuts.[22]

In late July, 139 House Democrats joined forces with the Republican minority to reject any 10 percent Pentagon budget cut of the sort proposed by Sanders in the Senate. Only two veterans, Ted Lieu and Peter DeFazio, voted in favor of it.[23] Just twenty-three of Sanders's Senate colleagues backed his proposed $74 billion cut. Tammy Duckworth was not among them because she sided with the Republican majority instead. While Pentagon budget cutting was being debated, Duckworth, like VoteVets, preferred to fulminate about Trump being a "failed commander in chief" because he did "nothing about reports of Russia putting bounties on the heads of American troops in Afghanistan."[24] Months later, General Frank McKenzie, commander of all remaining troops in Afghanistan, acknowledged that "a detailed review of all available intelligence has not been able to corroborate the existence of such a program."[25]

A WARTIME PRESIDENT

As the economy cratered due to COVID-19, Donald Trump could no longer count on winning a second term based on the stock market being up and unemployment being down. One of the first alarms about this infectious disease threat was sounded by the VA. Dr. Carter Mecher, a senior VA medical officer, had helped develop pandemic emergency plans for the Bush administration. On January 28, 2020, Mecher warned other federal officials that "any way you cut it, this [outbreak] is going to be bad."[26] Mecher recommended strong mitigation efforts, like closing colleges and universities, but these steps were dismissed as overly alarmist and unnecessary. More than a month later, the president was still not even "discouraging large gatherings in any of the cities where the virus had already spread."[27] Yet as COVID-19 cases grew by the thousands in March 2020, Trump shifted gears. He declared himself to be a "wartime president" personally involved in directing military personnel to assist COVID-19 relief efforts because "they're going into war, they're going into a battle."[28] How big was this battle? "This is worse than Pearl Harbor," Trump told the press. "This is worse than the World Trade Center. There has never been an attack like this."[29]

Two months later, the president was flexing his muscles as commander in chief during a far more contentious home front military deployment. Active-duty military personnel, particularly from National Guard units, and veterans of all kinds were drawn into this new crisis situation as it escalated quickly in early June and triggered an unprecedented election-year debate about the military's role in policing civil disturbances. The events of Monday, June 1, proved to be a major detonator. On a conference call that morning, Trump informed state governors that he was placing Army general Mark Milley, chairman of the Joint Chiefs of Staff, in charge of the federal response to nationwide protests over the death of George Floyd in Minneapolis and other police brutality cases involving African Americans. Defense Secretary Mark Esper alarmed his listeners on the call by agreeing with Trump that, in cities facing serious unrest, "we need to dominate the battle space"—with active-duty troops if necessary. Soon Trump, with Esper and Milley behind him—the latter dressed in combat fatigues—marched across Lafayette Park in Washington, DC, after it had been brutally cleared of protesters by the National Guard, US Park Police, and other law enforcement agencies.[30] Trump returned to the White House and discussed plans to invoke the rarely used Insurrection Act, a move viewed by congressional Democrats as a formal declaration of war on civilians.

Tammy Duckworth was among the first to respond. The senator from Illinois called Trump "a draft dodging wannabe-tinpot dictator" who threatened to tarnish "the honor of the military." The former Black Hawk helicopter pilot was particularly livid about Army Secretary Ryan D. McCarthy's decision to deploy two Army National Guard helicopters in Washington, DC. On the night of Monday, June 1, they flew low over a peaceful downtown crowd of several hundred, "with the downward blast from their rotor blades sending protesters scurrying for cover and ripping signs from the sides of buildings." As the *New York Times* observed, "These types of maneuvers are well known to Mr. McCarthy, who served in the Army's elite Ranger Regiment during the opening operations of the war in Afghanistan." According to Duckworth, "What we saw on Monday night was our military using its equipment to threaten and put Americans at risk on American soil."[31]

Other veterans in Congress joined the fray on one side or another. Vote-Vets helped round up signers of an open letter warning that "the President and his Pentagon officials are on the verge of ripping the very fabric of our democracy apart." As Duckworth, Seth Moulton, Max Rose, Jason Crow, and others pointed out in this missive, "Our troops did not join the U.S. military to intimidate their fellow citizens on the streets of Washington or Minneapolis." In a one-sentence query to Milley, former Marine and current House member Ruben Gallego demanded, "Do you intend to obey illegal orders from the president?" Common Defense urged all veterans "to speak out with a loud, overwhelming, united voice" against a presidential threat that was "nothing less than fascism."[32]

Meanwhile, on the right, former Army captain Tom Cotton, Duckworth's Senate colleague from Arkansas, strongly urged Trump to supplement National Guard deployments around the country with active-duty military personnel "to restore order in our streets." On Twitter, Cotton called for "no quarter for insurrectionists, anarchists, rioters, and looters." But as David French, fellow conservative and veteran of the war in Iraq, pointed out, even on a real battlefield, "no quarter" orders—which mean showing the enemy no mercy, even if they try to surrender—are considered a war crime.[33]

A string of former generals, admirals, and White House military advisers in the Obama and Bush administrations quickly made it clear which side they were on.[34] Their public statements reflected two concerns—that Trump's invocation of the Insurrection Act of 1807 and use of the military would severely damage the latter's relationship to the public and create serious morale problems within the enlisted ranks. These prominent veterans were acutely aware that "more than 40 percent of active-duty and reserve personnel are now people of color, and orders to confront protesters demonstrating against a criminal justice system that targets black men troubled many."[35]

If anyone needed a reminder of that demographic reality, it was provided by Kaleth O. Wright, chief master sergeant in the Air Force. This top enlisted airman took to Twitter to express his anger and dismay over the Floyd case and other fatal encounters with the police. "Just like most of the Black Airmen and so many others in our ranks . . . I am outraged at watching another Black man die on television before our very eyes," he wrote. "I am George Floyd . . . I am Philando Castile, I am Michael Brown, I am Alton Sterling, I am Tamir Rice."[36]

In Washington, DC, where the National Guard unit deployed under the command of the federal government is 60 percent nonwhite, there was already palpable unease among citizen soldiers forced to confront friends, neighbors, relatives, and former classmates protesting in the streets. Echoing Wright, former Marine infantry officer Kyle Bibby described his own lifelong awareness "that any interaction with police could all too easily lead to detention, injury, or death. The police don't care that I've gone to war to protect this country—I could be the next George Floyd solely due to the color of my skin." In a letter to Common Defense supporters, Bibby warned that "deploying the military would only further escalate the situation and lead to more chaos and violence."[37]

As Bibby predicted, the Trump administration's later use of paramilitary units from the Department of Homeland Security and other federal agencies in Portland, Oregon, helped inflame the situation there. Among the many targets of militarized policing in Portland was Navy veteran Christopher David, who like Bibby was a graduate of Annapolis. After peacefully approaching several unidentified but heavily armed federal agents, David was pepper-sprayed and beaten in an unprovoked assault viewed 7 million times on YouTube. In solidarity with him and other Portland protesters, local progressive veterans formed a "wall of vets" outside the federal courthouse, which became the site of nightly protests for more than three months.[38] Common Defense began to work with Portland veterans and others in a national campaign called "No War on Our Streets." Its goal was to curb local and state law enforcement agency use of $7.4 billion worth of military gear obtained from the Pentagon since 1990.

"It was our equipment first," noted Bibby, who served in Afghanistan. "We understand it better than the police do. . . . It's important that we have veterans ready to stand up and say: 'These weapons need to go.'"[39] Unfortunately, other veterans who showed up at Black Lives Matter protests—and brought their personal weapons with them—did not sympathize with that cause. They belonged to various right-wing militia groups around the country, which have an estimated fifteen thousand to twenty thousand members. Former military personnel helped create some of these paramilitary groups, and veterans "may now make up at least 25 percent of their rosters."[40] Oath Keepers, a group that recruits both veterans and police officers, was founded by Stewart Rhodes, a lawyer and former Army paratrooper who once worked for ex-congressman Ron Paul. In the wake of postelection protests at the US Capitol, Rhodes and his comrades found themselves under belated law enforcement scrutiny and, in some cases, federal indictment for riotous activity of their own.[41]

A CAMPAIGN TURNING POINT?

As domestic clashes continued, one of the best-known Marine veterans in the country—whose active-duty nickname was "Mad Dog"—joined the debate. Former secretary of defense James Mattis was particularly exercised by President Trump's creation of "a bizarre photo op" in Lafayette Park "with military leadership standing alongside." In a stinging rebuke of his former boss—and of Mark Esper, his successor at the Pentagon—Mattis insisted that "we must reject any thinking of our cities as a 'battlespace' that our uniformed military is called upon to 'dominate.' . . . Militarizing our response, as we witnessed in Washington, D.C., sets up a conflict—a false conflict—between the military and civilian society. . . . Keeping public order rests with civilian state and local leaders who best understand their communities and are answerable to them."[42]

Three days after Trump vowed to unleash the Armed Forces if governors and mayors failed to quell protesters, Esper was backpedaling fast. Citing his own past experience in the Army and National Guard, the defense secretary now emphasized that active-duty forces should be used in a law enforcement role only "as a matter of last resort, and only in the most urgent and dire of situations." At a press briefing on June 3, Esper assured the nation that "we are not in one of those situations now."[43] Esper then ordered thousands of active-duty troops previously dispatched to bases near the capital back to Fort Bragg in North Carolina and Fort Drum in New York. On June 4 the president reportedly spent much of the day privately complaining about Esper, who, along with Milley, was now perceived as an obstacle to his wishes.[44] White House aides ultimately convinced Trump that "he would risk more criticism from military officials if he were to dismiss the defense secretary, fueling a rising revolt among retired officers in the thick of a re-election campaign."[45]

By June 7, Army Secretary McCarthy announced that National Guard troops from out of state would be withdrawn from the District of Columbia over the next few days because the protests had become peaceful.[46] National Guard members would remain on duty, but only as backup for civilian law enforcement. A chastened General Milley issued a mea culpa for his camo-clad march through Lafayette Park earlier in the week. "I should not have been there," he admitted in a commencement address at the National Defense University. "My presence in that moment and in that environment created a perception of the military involved in domestic politics."[47]

SYMBOLS OF WHITE SUPREMACY

One further sign of military opinion—and political momentum—shifting against Trump was the public response to Major General Paul Eaton's (ret.) call to remove the names of "racist traitors" from military bases like Fort Benning, which he once commanded. National Guard member Max Rose, the new congressman from New York, sent a letter to DOD Secretary Esper similarly demanding that all "U.S. military bases and property be named after men and women who've served our nation with honor and distinction, not sought to tear it apart to uphold white supremacy."[48] Making further amends for his controversial Lafayette Park photo op with Trump, General Milley informed Congress that the Joint Chiefs of Staff now frowned on the idea of honoring "officers who turned their back on their oath."[49]

Republicans in Congress started surrendering on the issue too. For example, when the White House tried to lobby Republican congressman Don Bacon, the former Air Force brigadier general from Nebraska responded:

"We're the party of Lincoln, the party of emancipation; we're not the party of Jim Crow. We should be on the right side of this issue."[50] From his command post in the White House, President Trump continued to lay claim to white southern voter terrain and issued, via Twitter, his standard defiant response. As long as he remained in office, he said, "our history as the Greatest Nation in the World will not be tampered with by renaming these Magnificent and Famous Military Installations."[51]

In June 2020, Trump visited one such installation that overlooks the Hudson River. The US Military Academy at West Point still boasted a Robert E. Lee Barracks, a Lee Gate, and a Lee Road, intersected by a Beauregard Place—named after a former commander who left his post to join the Confederacy, led the attack on Union troops at Fort Sumter in South Carolina, and then became one of Lee's top generals. In what he clearly viewed as an opportunity to use the military as a reelection campaign prop, Trump insisted that the class of 2020 be recalled from their homes around the country, where they had been dispersed earlier in the spring after a COVID-related shutdown of the campus. He refused to deliver his commencement address remotely, insisting that the 1,100 graduating cadets—17 of whom had tested positive for the virus—be arrayed in front of him. In his speech he recycled campaign rhetoric from four years earlier about "ending an era of endless wars" in which the US tried to be "policeman of the world" by sending its "troops to solve ancient conflicts in faraway lands."[52] It was a graduation day send-off full of cognitive dissonance for new military officers destined to serve in "faraway lands" because neither Trump nor Joe Biden favored any real change in America's global policing role.

It didn't take a tepid reception by West Point cadets to convince VoteVets that Trump's support among veterans, active-duty personnel, and military families was "soft and receding." To ensure victory over the incumbent, Jon Soltz announced that his group was "putting together the most comprehensive data-driven veteran and military family get-out-the-vote operation the Democratic Party has ever seen."[53] VoteVets believed that effort would have greater impact if there were a veteran on the ticket.

As Joe Biden began to narrow down his possible running-mate choices in mid-July 2020, Tammy Duckworth's name edged up that list. Unfortunately for Duckworth, one of her unique biographical features turned out to be a potential legal liability in the minds of Biden advisers. The fact that Duckworth was born overseas to a Thai mother and a US serviceman father was deemed to be the likely basis for a distracting right-wing legal challenge to her eligibility: "Campaign lawyers feared that it would take just one partisan judge in one swing state to throw the whole Democratic ticket off the ballot."[54]

THE VOTER SUPPRESSION THREAT

Regardless of who was on the ballot with Biden, the Trump administration was determined to make mail balloting more difficult in 2020. This form of voter suppression required accelerated efforts to undermine the US Postal Service (USPS), with the longer-range goal of privatizing it. However, when Republicans took election-year steps in this direction, they reminded a pandemic-stricken nation that veterans—not to mention millions of other Americans—rely heavily on public provision of essential services.[55]

Since 2018, the White House had been eager to sell off the post office to private corporations, thereby enriching investor-owned businesses at the expense of the public and forcing customers to rely on FedEx or UPS instead. Just like at the VA, Trump's assault on a heavily unionized workforce was part of this privatization strategy. As Detroit Postal Workers leader and former Marine Keith Combs told us: "They want to eliminate our collective bargaining rights, which would jeopardize all those benefits we've won for veterans and other employees. They also want to cut delivery days, close local post offices, and raise prices, which would hurt customers."

After passage of the $2.2 trillion stimulus package known as the Coronavirus Aid, Relief, and Economic Security (CARES) Act, the Trump administration had no problem creating a $500 billion fund to aid private corporations, with little congressional oversight. But it would only extend a $10 billion line of credit to the USPS, which soon had hundreds of frontline employees testing positive for COVID-19, thousands in self-quarantine, and scores dying—among them military veterans serving their country once again in a civilian capacity. The USPS's projected pandemic-related revenue loss of $13 billion meant it could run out of money by September 2020, putting 630,000 jobs at risk. This would leave millions of postal service customers, particularly in rural areas, with fewer delivery options for items like the 4 million mail-order prescriptions the USPS delivers every day. It would, for the Trump administration, conveniently disrupt census-taking and presidential election balloting by mail. According to Combs, any USPS cash crunch would "also endanger a benefit for military service members—deeply discounted shipping rates on packages they get overseas," which can be sent by their family members with free packaging materials at the same rate as a domestic shipment.

Faced with these multiple threats, postal workers like Combs and their organizational allies began mobilizing against Trump's midpandemic bid to force the USPS into bankruptcy in order to more quickly privatize mail service. As part of the resulting "US Mail Not for Sale" campaign, VoteVets reminded its own supporters that the "USPS employs nearly 100,000 veterans, making it one of their top federal employers. . . . It has preferential hiring practices for veterans—especially disabled vets—and in many places across the U.S. is the top employer for veterans of color . . . [as customers], disabled veterans, senior veterans, and others depend on the mail to get the benefits they EARNED through their service."[56]

By late July, Republicans in the Senate were still trying to block emergency funding for the USPS, and Trump's newly installed postmaster general, Louis DeJoy, was ordering operational changes that impeded normal delivery.[57] Before DeJoy, a North Carolina businessman worth $110 million, left his logistics company to become postmaster general, he donated more than $2 million to Trump's own reelection effort, the Republican National Committee, and 2020 Senate candidates like Mitch McConnell, Martha McSally, and Thom Tillis.

One of the longest-serving veterans in the House, Representative Peter DeFazio, responded by calling for DeJoy's resignation before his "nefarious collective efforts" suppressed "millions of mail-in ballots and threatened the voting rights of Americans, setting the stage for breach of our Constitution."[58] Aroused by daily news reports on their controversial new boss and his election-related tampering with the USPS, tens of thousands of postal workers rallied around the country in late August. By this point in the summer, the number of their coworkers testing positive for COVID-19 had tripled to nearly ten thousand nationwide. More than eighty had died of the virus, and about fifty thousand had been forced to take "time off at some point during the pandemic because they were sick, or had to quarantine or care for family members."[59]

In Manchester, New Hampshire, Vietnam veteran and longtime American Postal Workers Union member Roger Bleau joined a rally demanding safe working conditions and an end to Republican sabotage of the agency's mission. In a speech to the crowd of several hundred, Bleau told a personal story about why mail delivery was so important to him, even before his thirty-seven-year career at the USPS. "When I was in Vietnam for a year, I was depressed and sometimes suicidal," Bleau confessed. "But mail from home saved my life. . . . Now I get my meds through the post office from the VA." A self-described liberal Democrat, Bleau believed that Trump was dishonoring veterans in multiple ways and was particularly disgusted by his pardoning of Navy SEAL Eddie Gallagher. But Bleau knew from interactions with Republican-leaning neighbors, Facebook friends, and even some USPS retirees that not all veterans agreed with him.

VETERANS FOR TRUMP

Among them were Veterans for Trump, like ex-Marine Al Baldasaro, a former New Hampshire state legislator, and CVA alumnus Darin Selnick, both of whom acted as official campaign surrogates for the president, plastering YouTube, Fox, and other media channels with supportive messages and responses to political attacks. In 2016 Baldasaro was a GOP convention delegate for Trump and campaign adviser on veterans affairs. He attracted Secret Service scrutiny after a radio interview in which he declared, "Hillary Clinton should be put in the firing line and shot for treason."[60] An allied group not officially connected to Trump's 2020 campaign sponsored its own Vets for Trump Facebook page and MAGA Meetups. It was led by Thomas Speciale, an Afghan War veteran who was badly defeated in a Virginia primary race for the US Senate.[61] Speciale was confident that Trump remained just as popular among veterans as he was during his first presidential campaign. As he explained to us, "Trump's rebuilt the military, he fired eight thousand underperforming VA employees, he's fixed the department overall."

When the Republican National Convention met a week later, several veterans whose political star was more ascendant than Speciale's made the case for Trump in 2020. One speaker was Arkansas senator Tom Cotton, who claimed that "Joe Biden has aided and abetted China's rise for 50 years with terrible trade deals"—and that China, the trade war winner, had then "unleashed a plague on the world." The other was Sean Parnell, a *Fox News* favorite seeking to regain the western Pennsylvania congressional seat held by Conor Lamb since 2018. A former Army Ranger, Parnell described how he returned from combat duty in Afghanistan only to find that the "party of my grandfather, a lifelong union Democrat, had turned against the very people it professed to represent." According to Parnell, the party's ranks were now full of "hedge fund managers, Hollywood celebrities, tech moguls and academia—bloated with contempt for middle America."[62]

Biden's riposte to Parnell and other Republican convention speakers who claimed that he was soft on urban rioters took the form of a video address to the National Guard Association of the United States. Noting that his late son, Beau, had served in the Delaware Guard, Biden promised his audience:

"As president, I'll never put you in the middle of politics or personal vendettas. I'll never use the military as a prop or as a private militia to violate rights of fellow citizens. That's not law and order. You don't deserve that."[63]

LOSERS AND SUCKERS

A *Military Times* poll in midsummer 2020 showed positive movement in Biden's direction among military voters. Forty-one percent of the active-duty personnel surveyed said they were voting for him, while 37 percent still favored Trump. In 2017, 46 percent of the troops polled by *Military Times* had a favorable opinion of the president, versus only 37 percent who didn't like him. Three years later, half of the respondents (49.9 percent) now held an unfavorable view of him, compared to about 38 percent who still liked him. Among officers the disapproval rate was even higher—59 percent; more than half of those expressed strong disapproval.

Nearly three-quarters of those surveyed—officers and enlisted personnel—disagreed with Trump's proposed use of the military to help police American cities where there was civil unrest.[64] Even in Florida, where one-third of the state's electorate was part of veteran or military households—which voted disproportionately for Trump in 2016—the president was leading Biden by just four points—50 percent to 46 percent, according to a Monmouth Institute poll.[65] Both of these polls were conducted before Trump's standing among veterans and active-duty troops took another hit when the *Atlantic* disclosed that he had repeatedly referred to them in private as "suckers" and "losers."[66]

The "losers and suckers" controversy gave additional momentum to "dump Trump" appeals directed at veterans by the Republican-backed Lincoln Project. Advised by Fred Wellman, an Army veteran, this group conducted a virtual town hall in September 2020 that attracted ten thousand participants. Speakers criticized the president for his repeated displays of disrespect for the military and diversion of funds from the Pentagon budget to pay for the Mexican border wall instead of improving housing conditions on military bases. "The majority of veteran and active duty members are Republicans," Wellman acknowledged. "But we just ask them why our military is living in moldy housing and Gold Star families treated like this?" To defeat Trump, Wellman believed, a 10 percent swing among vet voters was not required. "One to four percent is all we need," he insisted.[67]

To reach this goal or an even higher level of veteran defection from the Trump camp, VoteVets raised $2 million for a GOTV drive targeting former military personnel in sixteen battleground states, focusing mainly on those able to vote for Amy McGrath, M. J. Hegar, Cal Cunningham, and Mark Kelly. "In 47 days," VoteVets predicted, "we have a chance to take back the Senate by replacing just four Traitor Trump-enabling Republicans with any of these incredible Democrats running against them—which means *we could do it with our VoteVets endorsed veteran candidates alone.*"[68] Common Defense focused its own turnout activities on veterans in Maine, Pennsylvania, North Carolina, and Arizona.

In Arizona participants in its Veterans Organizing Institute who became "deep canvassers" for a group called Vets Forward knocked on the doors of former military personnel to persuade them to choose Mark Kelly over Martha McSally. More than one hundred Vets Forward volunteers from every part of Arizona also signed an open letter declaring McSally unworthy of replacing John McCain in the Senate because of her subservience to Trump.[69] After much internal discussion among seven hundred activists around the country, Common Defense decided to make a formal endorsement of Biden. However, when its leaders met with Biden campaign officials to discuss the timing of this announcement, they learned that their offer of support had been declined. Apparently the aggressiveness of past Common Defense campaigns to impeach Trump and end forever wars had made some Biden advisers wary about being too closely associated with the group.

WINNERS AND LOSERS

As Election Day neared, Biden and Trump held two face-to-face debates, in which the subject of veterans came up. In the first Biden angrily pointed out that his late son, Beau, who received the Bronze Star for his Army National Guard service in Iraq, "was not a loser. He was a patriot and the people left behind there were heroes." Trump immediately steered the conversation back toward Biden's other son, Hunter, whose short career as a directly commissioned officer had not ended gloriously. "I don't know Beau," the president retorted. "I know Hunter. Hunter got thrown out of the military. He was dishonorably discharged . . . for cocaine use."[70] Trump took credit for "fixing of the VA, which was a mess" and made the claim—astounding, even for him—that "308,000 people died" there because "they didn't have proper health care" before his presidency. Now, he boasted, the VA was getting "a 91% approval rating" because "we take care of our vets."[71]

When all the ballots were counted, in an election with the highest turnout rate in more than a century, exit polls showed that Biden had benefited from a swing in his favor among veterans in the range that Fred Wellman had predicted was "all we need." Trump once again led among veterans 54 percent to 44 percent, but that was a 6-percentage-point drop in his level of support from four years earlier and, for the Democratic candidate, an 11-point improvement over Hillary Clinton's performance among vet voters.[72] A later analysis of voting data found big swings toward Biden in a number of communities with military bases and high veteran populations, including Colorado Springs, Colorado—home of the US Air Force Academy—and Bremerton, Washington—which hosts Naval Base Kitsap.[73] This trend also played out in mail balloting from military bases abroad. As a batch of these votes were being counted in Michigan—and running heavily in favor of Biden—one Trump poll watcher already poised to claim election fraud was further confounded. "I had always been told that military personnel tended to be more conservative," he said, "so this stuck out to me as the day went on."[74]

Biden's coattails did not extend to three of the four service candidates running for US Senate seats, despite much backing from the Democratic Party establishment and its big-donor class. As a result, there was no new "squad" in the Senate with military credentials and moderate politics taking their oath in the Capitol in January 2021. Instead, the original squad of four progressive House Democrats first seated two years earlier were all returned to office and claimed two additions to their left-leaning team from successful first-time House races in New York and Missouri. In Arizona Navy veteran and former astronaut Mark Kelly beat incumbent Republican Martha McSally. Among corporate donors, McSally was favored over Kelly by the agribusiness, defense, and energy industries, but Kelly did better among donors from finance and the tech industry. According to the Center for Responsive Politics, his Silicon Valley firm donations were nearly eight times greater—$3.96 million versus $502,870 by mid-October 2020.[75]

In Kentucky, Amy McGrath lost badly to Mitch McConnell. Despite $90 million being poured into her campaign, she earned just over 38 percent of the vote, only 3 percentage points better than Senate candidate Marquita Bradshaw's showing in Tennessee, where the African American activist struggled to raise money in both her Democratic primary and general election contests.[76] The closing volleys in Texas between Republican John Cornyn and M. J. Hegar included an exchange over whether the latter swore too much in public. In a fundraising appeal to supporters, the self-described "badass Texas woman" in the race pled guilty as charged. "I'm pissed off," Hegar wrote, "because John Cornyn doesn't do SHIT for the people of Texas, and it's time to replace him." Unfortunately, not enough Texans agreed, and Cornyn breezed to victory with nearly 54 percent of the vote.

A more serious breach of southern decorum helped torpedo Lieutenant Colonel Cal Cunningham's challenge to Republican Thom Tillis in North Carolina, which became one of the most expensive Senate races ever. More than $282 million was raised and spent either by the candidates directly or outside groups; Cunningham raised twice as much as his opponent in direct donations. Like most veterans turned politicians, Cunningham "leaned heavily on his character and biography, playing up his military service and presenting himself as an inoffensive moderate."[77] If concepts like "honor" and "duty" are central to your service candidacy, sexting with the spouse of a fellow veteran is not advised. Press coverage of this mistake by Cunningham proved to be a major distraction for the married father of two during the final days of his campaign. After Tillis won, Senate Minority Leader Chuck Schumer told Democratic Party donors that he regretted recruiting Cunningham, because his failure to "keep his zipper up" harmed the party's chances of regaining the Senate (which it did anyway, in January 2021, when two nonveterans won runoff elections in Georgia).[78]

Biden's top-of-the-ticket victory in Michigan did help the Democrats hold on to one of their two Senate seats there. Republican John James, who branded himself as the Black candidate with a red, white, and blue message, lost narrowly. In Iowa fellow conservative Joni Ernst, the combat veteran who publicly recounted her experience with military sexual assault, was elected to serve another term. Jason Crow, the Army Ranger and Bronze Star recipient from Colorado who partnered with Republican Liz Cheney to slow down any troop withdrawal from Afghanistan under Trump, comfortably won reelection against a nonveteran. With help from VoteVets, Pennsylvania Democrat Conor Lamb won a second term after besting his right-wing Republican challenger, Sean Parnell—Trump's favorite "warrior"—by just twenty thousand votes. Peter DeFazio, one of the Democrats' longest-serving veterans, narrowly won his bid for an eighteenth term against Alek Skarlatos, the only Oregon National Guard member ever to star in a Clint Eastwood movie. (By late 2021, both Parnell and Skarlatos were angling for 2022 rematches against their Democratic opponents. In Pennsylvania, both Parnell and Lamb sought their respective party's nomination for an open Senate seat, until Parnell withdrew because of a messy divorce. In Oregon, Skarlatos announced another challenge to DeFazio, amid adverse publicity about financial transfers, back and forth, between his campaign treasury and a nonprofit under his control, which delivered little of its promised advocacy for veterans.[79] DeFazio decided to retire.)

Despite his National Guard service during the pandemic and sympathy for ending the US occupation of Afghanistan, Army veteran Max Rose was defeated in New York City's most conservative congressional district after just one term. His Republican opponent, a female State Assembly member, claimed that Rose's appearance at a Staten Island protest over George Floyd's death made him a supporter of defunding the police—which he was not. Nicole Malliotakis got 56 percent of the vote, in a district that increased its 2016 turnout for Trump by 33 percent four years later. That upset did not deter Brittany Ramos DeBarros, the Afro-Latina combat veteran and About Face leader profiled in chapter 5. She announced her intention to compete with Rose for the Democratic nomination in the 2022 midterm elections by championing an agenda considerably to the left of his.[80]

After all the November results were certified, ninety-one veterans were scheduled to land on Capitol Hill in January 2021—seventy-four serving in the House and seventeen in the Senate. Their overall representation in the 117th Congress—17 percent—would be the lowest percentage since World War II.[81] Reflecting a continuing influx of Iraq and Afghanistan veterans, nearly 30 percent of underrepresented millennials in Congress had military service on their résumé.[82]

More than two-thirds of the veterans in Congress were still Republicans, including Arkansas senator Tom Cotton, the supporter of martial law in 2020 rumored to have presidential ambitions in 2024. In Texas voters reelected Congressman Dan Crenshaw, a GOP convention speaker and another rising star in the party. In 2021 Cotton and Crenshaw were joined on Capitol Hill by a right-wing Navy veteran from Texas—Ronny Jackson, the former White House doctor who lionized his last presidential patient, Donald Trump, and denounced his previous one, Barack Obama, as a "Deep State traitor."

In their postelection strategizing about how to regain control of the House in November 2022, Republicans planned to "take a page out of the Democrats 2018 playbook," according to Representative Don Bacon (R-NE), a retired Air Force general. As Bacon noted, in major party competition for viable service candidates, "we've got a built-in advantage [because] about two-thirds of our veterans tend to be Republican."[83] At a big donor event, held during the summer of 2021, House Minority Leader Kevin McCarthy unveiled some of his top Republican congressional primary picks for the following year. They included "two former Navy SEALS, a female Army Reserve judge advocate general and an African American former Army helicopter pilot, all of them united in their disdain for Democrats and their dismay at the U.S. withdrawal from Afghanistan."[84]

One leading Republican target in Virginia was US representative Elaine Luria, a former naval commander, who got elected and reelected to Congress by defeating the same Navy SEAL twice. Among her potential 2022 Republican challengers was state senator Jen Kiggans, who promised to better represent Luria's constituents because she was both a Navy veteran and a Navy wife (in a swing district where one in five residents are veterans, active-duty military personnel, or their relatives).[85]

In January 2021, veterans returning to Congress as Democrats tended to be With Honor Fund favorites like Luria, Lamb, Crow, Moulton, and Sherrill, all reliable supporters of the Pentagon. Former peace candidate for president Tulsi Gabbard was no longer one of their colleagues because she chose not to run again from Hawaii. Gabbard's departure deprived Congress of one of the only post-9/11 veterans willing to force the serious debate on US military policy that most 2020 presidential contenders managed to avoid. Who might become a future House critic of regime change wars, in the wake of Gabbard's lonely crusade against them, was not immediately clear. One deterrent to embracing that role was the perception, among Gabbard's fellow veterans, that becoming a dissenter would make them losers, rather than winners, too.

CONCLUSION

RETHINKING VETERANS AFFAIRS

To care for him who shall have borne the battle,
and for his widow, and his orphan.
—OFFICIAL MOTTO OF US DEPARTMENT
OF VETERANS AFFAIRS, 1959

In the wake of Joe Biden's 2020 victory over Donald Trump, there was much popular rejoicing about the possibility of positive personnel and policy changes in Washington, DC. With weeks left in Trump's presidency, all the major VSOS suddenly found the courage to demand leadership change at the VA, even before Biden was sworn in.[1]

What triggered this eleventh-hour exercise in performative outrage was a damning Inspector General's report about Secretary Robert Wilkie's handling of a sexual assault complaint made by a VA patient in Washington, DC. The victim was Navy veteran Andrea Goldstein, a senior policy adviser to House Veterans Affairs Committee chair Mark Takano, who was physically accosted by an outside contractor working on VA property. Instead of making "meaningful efforts to determine what corrective measures" were "needed in response to this complaint," the IG found that Wilkie, his staff, and some Republican allies in Congress tried to force "the media to focus on the complainant" for the political purpose of discrediting her.[2] This was partisan behavior, disgraceful in any administration. Yet there was zero chance that Trump was going to ditch one of his most dutiful cabinet members for "losing the trust and confidence of American veterans," when the president himself had just experienced Election Day slippage of the same sort. Furthermore, the VSOs had never sought Wilkie's dismissal for leadership failures, of much larger scale and impact, earlier in Trump's term.[3]

Biden's own relationship with the VSOs got off to a bumpy start, when they were excluded from his VA transition team and prominent veterans involved in his campaign got top jobs unrelated to veterans affairs. Vietnam veteran John Kerry was handed the broader brief of saving the planet from climate change as a special ambassador. Pete Buttigieg, much beloved by VoteVets, became secretary of transportation. Tammy Duckworth, the original fighting Democrat from Illinois, chose to stay in the Senate, where she became a key critic of "the federal government's practice of deporting undocumented immigrants who served in the military."[4]

Several other candidates with military backgrounds or relevant VA experience didn't become VA secretary either. Biden's surprise choice to run the VA was fifty-one-year-old Denis McDonough, a former congressional staffer, national security adviser to President Obama, and—during Obama's second term—his White House chief of staff.

"We were expecting a veteran, maybe a post-9/11 veteran," huffed Joe Chenelly, executive director of AMVETS. "Maybe a woman veteran. Or maybe a veteran who knows the VA exceptionally well."[5] IAVA founder Paul Rieckhoff[6] and Pam Campos-Palma, from Vets for the People, expressed similar alarm. A former high-ranking VA official shared the far more relevant concern that McDonough "had no deep understanding or experience running any healthcare or benefits system, much less the largest in the country."

At his confirmation hearing, McDonough pledged to "build strong partnerships" with the VSOs and paid tribute to "the men and women of the VA—dedicated, highly skilled professionals, many of them veterans themselves—who deserve our profound respect and support." As secretary, he promised to focus relentlessly on "providing our veterans with timely world-class health-care" and equally "timely access to their benefits." By Veterans Day 2021, under pressure from VSOs, members of Congress, and public figures like Jon Stewart, a champion of burn pit victims, the VA announced that it was "piloting a comprehensive military exposure model to consider possible relationships of in-service environmental hazards to medical conditions."

"We are seeking more information from veterans, more evidence from more sources, and looking to take every avenue possible to determine where a potential presumptive illness based on military service location may exist in a more expedient and holistic manner," McDonough said. He further encouraged all veterans "who may have been impacted to file a claim even if it was previously denied," a remedial step considered necessary, but insufficient by some burn pit compensation campaigners.[7]

To overcome a growing number of backlogged claims—more than 600,000 to be exact—the Biden administration hired and trained 2,000 new VBA employees.[8] Despite these and other positive moves, the White House had filled only one of the VA's top three leadership positions by late 2021. For McDonough's deputy secretary, Biden chose Donald Remy, a Black veteran who'd previously served as chief operating officer and chief legal officer at the nonprofit National Collegiate Athletic Association. Like McDonough, Remy had no experience dealing with either veterans' benefits or healthcare.

During the prolonged search for a new undersecretary for health (USH), many longtime VA caregivers hoped for a candidate like Dr. Ken Kizer, the bold Clinton-era reformer. "What we need at the VHA is more than just another manager, what we need is a visionary leader," said physician Andrew Pomerantz, who spent three decades pioneering the VA's integration of mental health and primary care. Yet, instead of moving ahead quickly with a strong nominee for this key position, President Biden continued the Trump-era practice of filling it with an acting or interim undersecretary. To one former VA official, this lack of urgency reflected White House disinterest in restoring the VHA's luster as the nation's leading public healthcare system and innovator. Instead, he observed, "their attitude seems to be, 'Just don't produce any embarrassing headlines.'"

At his own confirmation hearing, Secretary McDonough avoided conflict with privatization hawks, like Senator Jerry Moran (R-KS), by assuring them that VHA outsourcing through its Community Care Network would continue. "Let me be clear," he told Moran, "community care will be a key part of how the department cares for our veterans—full stop."[9] During the previous twenty months, the VHA's own recorded "monthly encounters" with patients had shrunk by 25 percent. During that same 2019–20 timeframe, outsourced care increased to 34 percent of all care delivered to veterans at taxpayer expense.[10] Under McDonough's leadership, this trend continued unabated, as promised. In 2021, the VHA allocated $18 billion, or 20 percent of its entire clinical budget, for outsourced care—an amount greater than three years' worth of equivalent spending under the Choice Act.[11]

PRIVATE SECTOR FAILINGS

Despite McDonough's pledge to partner with the "dedicated, highly skilled professionals" providing frontline VA care, there was little initial evidence he was responding to their workplace concerns. In the fall of 2021, two respected organizations representing them—the Association of VA Psychologist Leaders (AVAPL) and the Nurses Organization of Veterans Affairs (NOVA)—shared the alarming results of membership surveys about MISSION Act implementation and its impact on their patients.

The vast majority of NOVA survey participants were unable to assess whether outside providers knew anything about the military service–related conditions they have signed up to treat as part of the Community Care Network.[12] A 2018 RAND survey similarly showed that only 2.3 percent of New York clinicians were prepared to treat veterans.[13] (Under Trump, the VA responded to this troubling dearth of knowledge by partnering with a private company, PsychArmor, to offer online crash courses about service-related conditions.)

RNS surveyed by NOVA also reported that many veterans were waiting between one and four months for mental health, medical, and surgical appointments in the private sector. When those appointments were made, VHA nurses failed to receive required follow-up information in a timely manner or at all. VHA psychologists identified similar problems with "community care" oversight. More than 90 percent of the clinicians polled noted that their private-sector counterparts failed to follow the VHA's explicit treatment recommendations. When these same VHA psychologists tried to evaluate the progress of outsourced care, on a case-by-case basis, 94 percent said they didn't receive treatment plan updates.

All of the respondents complained about not getting progress notes when private-sector providers requested authorization for additional paid sessions with veterans. Based on the information they did receive, 79 percent reported clinical practices by VHA mental health contractors that would have been questioned if used in-house.[14] One anguished clinician told us she was losing sleep over her patients with PTSD who'd been referred to poorly trained private-sector clinicians. In one troubling case, she said, the VA was asked to okay payment for a psychotherapy session conducted via text. Sadly, when some in-house practitioners tried to protect veterans from deficient outside treatment, their angry patients accused them of taking away their "choice."

In September 2021, the authors learned that, in some VA medical centers, veterans were waiting up to four months for private mental health appointments via telehealth (the easiest to get). One solution would have been scheduling those patients for VA telehealth sessions instead. This was impossible, however, due to a double standard embedded in the Trump administration's MISSION Act access standards. Under those Robert Wilkie–written rules, private-sector telehealth counted as "access" but in-house telehealth appointments didn't. A major contributor to private-sector care delays was non-VA patients, who postponed medical appointments at the height of the pandemic, rescheduling them when conditions improved. This influx exposed the real-world constraints on ever-expanding VA outsourcing. As one VA union leader told us, "we have huge delays in care in the private sector because there just aren't enough providers out there to accommodate a huge flood of VA patients."

Even before the COVID-19 pandemic, the rest of the US healthcare system was suffering from nationwide shortages of primary care and mental health providers, insufficient acute care and psychiatric hospital beds, and cutbacks in rural healthcare services.[15] An increasing number of mental health professionals are unwilling to accept insurance, whether private or public, thus limiting their services to patients who can afford to pay out of pocket.[16] The financial viability of many medical practices, including those focusing on primary care, was further undermined by the pandemic, which led several professional organizations representing doctors to seek federal assistance.[17]

Because of the coronavirus crisis, non-VA hospitals and medical practices also lost huge amounts of revenue due to canceled procedures and appointments. Even though more healthcare workers were needed during the pandemic, hospitals all over the country laid off or furloughed staff, cut their pay and hours, or both. By some estimates as many as 40 percent of all private hospitals were expected to emerge from the pandemic in serious financial difficulty. This was particularly true in rural areas, where 179 hospitals had already closed between 2005 and 2014.[18] In 2019, rural hospital closings hit a record high, worsening the shortage of primary care providers in the surrounding areas.[19] The pandemic further threatened the future of one in four of those remaining.[20]

Even big cities have seen closures of major hospitals. At Philadelphia's Hahnemann University Hospital, a wealthy owner decided that the best way to recoup their investment was not to serve poor and working-class patients but to sell the land and buildings to developers. The *New Yorker* chronicled this hospital's 2019 death, noting that more than a fifth of all hospitals are run for profit, a trend "linked to price hikes, an increase in unnecessary procedures, and the destabilization of health-care networks" in the community.[21]

MISSION ACT MOMENTUM

Faced with a private healthcare system in bad shape—and reshaped for the worse, due to COVID-19—the Biden administration had good reason to rethink the diversion of billions of tax dollars from the VA to costly, less-qualified, and not-even-more-accessible outside providers. Yet reversing or even slowing the momentum of partial privatization implemented by a previous administration is no easy task, as the trajectory of Medicare Advantage has demonstrated over the past decade and a half. When Barack Obama first ran for president in 2008, he was sharply critical of Medicare Advantage, a costly and wasteful scheme enacted by his predecessor, George W. Bush. In a campaign debate with Senator John McCain, Obama pledged to repeal the program, which McCain, consistent with his later stance on VA privatization, strongly favored. Once in office, Obama focused instead on the challenge of getting the Affordable Care Act (ACA) passed, albeit without any public option that would have created unwanted competition for private insurers.

"Despite having overhead costs almost seven times that of traditional Medicare (13.7 versus 2%), Medicare Advantage plans have grown rapidly," report David Himmelstein and Steffie Woolhandler, Harvard Medical School faculty and leaders of Physicians for a National Health Program. "They now cover more than one-third of Medicare beneficiaries, up from 13 percent in 2005."[22] Advantage plans are projected to cover nearly half of all Medicare beneficiaries by 2029, if current enrollment trends continue. As other critics noted during the first year of the Biden administration, the Centers for Medicare and Medicaid were still implementing a Trump-era scheme to move millions of Medicare beneficiaries "into mostly commercial, for-profit plans, called Direct Contracting Entities," that would "further waste taxpayer money" and "fully privatize Medicare."[23] Via its political spending and lobbying in Washington, the private insurance industry was thus insuring that no president, including Biden, would ever do what Obama promised he would but didn't: restore the primacy of "original Medicare."[24]

Passage of the Choice Act, which McDonough assisted with as Obama's chief of staff, and then congressional enactment of its successor, the MISSION

Act, has created an equivalent fait accompli. Since 2014, as shown earlier in this book, the VHA has been partially converted into a Medicare-style payer of bills submitted by other healthcare providers. During his campaign for the presidency in 2020, Biden made no public criticism of this trend, unlike Obama, with his 2008 campaign critique of Medicare Advantage (which was followed, unfortunately, by no later reform or reversal of that program). Once powerful private interests acquire a new federal revenue stream, they seek to preserve and expand it, which is why private hospital chains and medical practices will try to convert even more VA patients into new "customers," as postpandemic conditions permit.

Promoters of VA privatization will surely mobilize such interested parties as part of a broader legal and public relations strategy to keep the MISSION Act intact. In August 2021, for example, former Trump appointees, including CVA alumnus and ex–White House adviser Darin Selnick, launched the Veterans 4 America First Institute. They are challenging, from the outside, what they depict as an intransigent VA bureaucracy, trying to thwart wider outsourcing.[25] The group filed a lawsuit against the Biden administration, seeking release of VA records which allegedly show that patients are being placed on wait lists for private care, rather than getting quick private-sector referrals.[26]

In the hopes of manufacturing a Biden-era "scandal" about wait times, Selnick and his allies also planted news stories that blamed callous and selfish VA administrators for actions which "basically defeat the whole purpose of the MISSION Act."[27] One example of such "investigative reporting" was a long November 2021 article in *USA Today*. Its major sources were Selnick, three Republican House members, four dissatisfied VA patients in San Diego, and officials of the Kadima Institute, a private treatment center in La Jolla with a proprietary interest in providing more, rather than less, community care.

Extrapolating from the contested facts of four local cases, the reporter claimed that veterans throughout the country were "caught in the crossfire of the VA's battle to retain patients and funding," which took the form of "overruling [its own] doctors' judgments and preventing them from sending their patients outside." The article was produced in partnership with Inewsource, a "data-driven, nonpartisan newsroom" in San Diego. In a side-bar piece, Inewsource dispensed detailed advice to veterans on how to get non-VA care and vigorously object if their "government is overruling medical decisions."[28]

To maintain and renovate existing hospitals and construct new ones to meet current and future needs, the VA requires an estimated $70 to $80 billion in new capital spending. In the Biden administration's initial infrastructure spending proposal in 2021, $18 billion was earmarked for modernization of these facilities. By the end of that year, Congress was still debating Biden's "Build Back Better Act," which reduced this allocation to $5 billion.

Those determined to privatize the VA want to keep that new capital spending as small as possible. And they have a key tool in the form of a little-known provision of the MISSION Act, which mandated the creation of an Asset and Infrastructure Review (AIR) Commission. Its recommendations may lead to facility closures across the country and prevent the VA from making necessary infrastructure improvements that would help reduce any delays in care and enhance the delivery of healthcare services.

Similar to the Defense Department's Base Realignment and Closure (BRAC) process, the AIR Commission is tasked with developing a list of facilities to close, consolidate, repurpose, or improve. To be implemented, its recommendations would then need White House approval and a single up-or-down vote by Congress that would limit the ability of individual members to defend particular VA facilities in their own districts. Like the Choice Act–created Care Commission, the AIR Commission had a preordained private-sector tilt. One slot on the commission was reserved for a private healthcare industry representative. Another member had to have experience with federal capital asset management and construction, architecture, and "strategic partnerships," which means VA relationships with the private sector. (One leading Republican-backed candidate for this slot was former congressman Phil Roe, a privatization booster during his tenure as chair of the House Veterans Affairs Committee.)

VSOs were allocated three slots, which could be helpful or not depending on who secured those White House appointments. No position on the commission was reserved for anyone with experience in population and/or public health, or rural health, even though more than 20 percent of veterans live in rural areas. No labor representation was mandated, despite the fact that VA hospital or clinic closures would impact thousands of federal employees.

Before Trump left office, his administration helped shape the commission's criteria for determining which VA facilities should remain open and which could potentially be closed and sold to private hospital chains or real estate developers for their underlying property value. The MISSION Act mandated that the VA conduct local "market assessments" of its own capacity to care for veterans and parallel private-sector capacity. VA sources reported that this data collection process was both secretive and flawed. According to one congressional staffer, the "physical capacity" of non-VA facilities was assessed, in part, by just counting the number of cars in their parking lots.

There was insufficient information about the ability of private hospitals or doctors to accept VA patients or how quickly they could, what additional staffing would be necessary, or what the VA would pay for these outside services. In a 2021 report on the Veterans Community Care Program, the Congressional Budget Office (CBO) filled in part of this picture. The report confirmed that private-sector wait times, in both urban and rural areas, were usually longer than at the VA. The quality of its outsourced care was a big question mark, largely because overseeing and coordinating care provided by private doctors and hospitals was so difficult for VHA staff. Nevertheless, CBO analysts favored an expanded division of labor between VA and non-VA caregivers. "If VHA was able to rely on the private sector to treat veterans in areas of the country where delays occurred, it could ensure timely care for veterans in existing VHA hospitals and clinics."[29] If veterans' access to community care was further increased, according to the CBO, "the VHA would save money by not making costly investments in new or larger facilities, equipment, and personnel in an era when the nation's population of veterans is shrinking."

Nowhere did the report suggest possible alternatives to facility closings and program consolidations. Instead, it seemed to be laying the groundwork for future AIR Commission recommendations of the same sort. As discussed below, these other options include making it possible for currently excluded veterans, as well as their family members, to utilize VA care. Similarly, as part of the VHA's fourth mission, Americans who are under- or uninsured could also be cared for in VA facilities.

INSOURCING RATHER THAN OUTSOURCING

The best way to protect the VA's existing patients, and all veterans, is to end wholesale outsourcing of their VA care and begin insourcing it. This means curtailing the use of expensive private-sector care, except when the VA can't provide necessary services in-house. Any objective weighing of the costs and benefits of treatment at the VA versus elsewhere reveals that the former is far better and safer, as numerous studies have confirmed. One of the latest, published in 2021 by three Stanford-affiliated economists, documented the "survival benefit" of the VHA's model of coordinated care. The researchers tracked over 400,000 ambulance calls made by veterans who had both Medicare and the VA. When veterans were taken to a non-VA emergency room, their risk of death over the following twenty-eight days doubled, while the cost to the taxpayer increased by 21 percent.[30] The results of this study—and other comparative research on chronic disease treatment and suicide prevention—were crystal clear: "Outsourcing more services to the private sector is not only irresponsible public policy but may actually cost veterans their lives."[31]

To insource more care, the new VA leadership must continue filling thousands of vacancies left open by Trump as part of his administration's conscious strategy of creating conditions that would discredit the VHA and justify further outsourcing and eventual facility closures. In the postpandemic healthcare labor market, a salaried job, with good benefits, providing care to veterans will be increasingly attractive to the many doctors, nurses, and other healthcare professionals who are new graduates or recently displaced by upheavals in their industry.

To support this effort and better plan for the VA's future, Congress must change how the VA budget is developed. Current budget calculations are based, in large part, on prior utilization. If staffing shortages lead to delays in care and other services, however, this triggers referrals to the private sector, which in turn leads to lower VA utilization, a dynamic baked into both the MISSION and Scott Hannon Acts. Lower utilization is then conveniently used to justify reduced budget allocations. The spiral circles ever downward, and money that could be used to expand VA staffing and services is instead directed to private-sector companies and providers. The only way to reverse this trend is to base budget calculations on a comprehensive model that effectively projects care needs—and veteran preference—into the future.

Even if some VA facilities aren't operating at full capacity today, they will be needed in the future as veterans of the first Gulf War and post-9/11 conflicts get older. While the total number of veterans may be declining, their healthcare needs are not. These needs were further clarified when we exited Afghanistan, when a report from Brown University's Costs of War Project found that healthcare spending on post-9/11 vets will reach $2.5 trillion by 2050, making it the most expensive budget item in the War on Terror. It also revealed that this war's unique nature—long, ethically questionable, and fought by men and women sent on repeated deployments—has created the most disabled generation of veterans in American history.[32]

Many veterans will also seek access to VA care because of lingering economic impacts of COVID-19, like losing their private medical coverage or paying more for it. Plus, all Americans have a big stake in maintaining and expanding the VA's "fourth mission" capacity in anticipation of future pandemics, in which the weaknesses and flaws of the larger US healthcare system will once again be exposed if the crisis of 2020–21 does not lead to its fundamental reform.

EXPANDING VA SERVICES

Before Kayla Williams rejoined the VA as its new assistant secretary of the Office of Public and Intergovernmental Affairs in 2021, she offered some rare creative thinking about how the VA, under progressive leadership, could expand rather than contract for the benefit of underserved nonveterans. "Could there be enhanced partnerships with DOD, Federally Qualified Health Centers, or the Indian Health Service?" Williams asked. "Are there ways to allow VA providers to see Medicaid patients in facilities seeing dramatic reductions in the number of veteran patients? What kinds of innovative solutions exist to increase efficiency while maintaining these vitally important facilities—and capacity—nationwide?" Rather than closing VA facilities, she urged lawmakers to "explore innovative opportunities to enhance their usefulness to local communities."[33]

In 2016, Phillip Longman, author of *Best Care Anywhere: Why VA Health Care Would Work Better for Everyone*, proposed that the VHA offer "a *public option* for health care to a wider range of veterans as well as nonveterans in communities where health care choices are currently limited."[34] As Longman told us, "The VA model of care continues to outperform the rest of the U.S. healthcare system based on key metrics, including patient safety, wait times, cost-effectiveness, avoidance of racial disparities, and adherence to evidence-based protocols of care. Rather than shuttering under-utilized VA facilities, we should be opening them up to as many Americans as possible."

A logical first step in expanding VA care would be to include veterans with bad paper discharges. This could happen if more VSOs backed legal challenges by Swords to Plowshares and other groups to the long-standing military practice of issuing other-than-honorable discharges to soldiers with service-related mental or physical health problems, including those arising from sexual assault. On Capitol Hill, Senators Bernie Sanders and Richard

Blumenthal (D-CT) joined this fight in October 2021, when they wrote to Secretary McDonough urging him to revise the VA's "outdated character of discharge regulations" and finally "uphold Congress's intent to exclude former service members only on the basis of severe misconduct."[35]

A second step would be allowing the VA to serve veterans' families. Psychiatrist Harold Kudler, who served as the VA's chief consultant for mental health, believes there is a strong clinical argument for including family members as patients. "When someone serves in the military, their family serves along with them," he told us. "Clinical experience shows that you can't effectively treat a veteran in a vacuum. Their families are affected by the challenges which the veteran faces and are in a unique position to help the veteran overcome those challenges." As Kudler notes, this holistic approach is already the basis for the VA's home-caregiver program, which received expanded funding through the MISSION Act. With "careful thought," he believes, it will be possible to provide broader coverage in a way that doesn't "sacrifice veteran's healthcare as we also meet the needs of their families."

Another just and logical expansion would be to cover the two-thirds of all VA employees who are not veterans themselves—just as the patients of large private health systems like Kaiser Permanente include their own staff. Whether employed as housekeeping, clerical, or clinical staff, many VHA caregivers have devoted their lives to helping veterans. They do so because they are motivated by the public service mission of the agency, even if that means, for some, working for less pay than in the private sector. VHA healthcare professionals have pioneered models of coordinated care that are unavailable outside their own workplace, and some have done research and teaching that benefits the entire nation. They're already part of a unique culture of healthcare system solidarity between providers and patients; what better way to make those bonds even stronger than by further erasing any distinction between the two?

Finally, the VA could continue to fulfill its fourth mission, post-pandemic, by welcoming nonveteran patients disadvantaged by the widespread shortage of primary care and mental health providers. In many urban areas, the national shortage of primary care providers (PCPS)—exacerbated by COVID-19 conditions—has made it nearly impossible to find a PCP who is accepting new patients. The same is true for patients seeking a psychotherapist or other mental health provider (unless they can pay out of pocket).

There's already precedent for such fourth-mission assistance. In late 2021, the VA hospital in White River Junction opened its doors to civilians in response to a critical scarcity of inpatient mental health treatment options in

Vermont.[36] "The VA has an enormous amount of skill and experience in the area of mental healthcare," said Emily Hawes, Vermont's commissioner of mental health. "We are fortunate that they are willing to help us out."

VSO ROADBLOCKS

Such daring ideas have a fraught history, which suggests that their latest advocates will need to be skilled navigators of political minefields in Washington, DC. In 1996, for example, the Legion actually encouraged Congress to pass legislation allowing all veterans and their families to have access to VA care.[37] Steve Robertson, the Legion's then–legislative director, was a proponent of this "GI Bill of Health." According to Robertson, if it had been enacted, "every veteran and their family members could have bought into the VHA like an HMO." Sadly, other VSOs helped scuttle the Legion's proposal because it expanded eligibility far beyond patients who met existing rules. The VFW was even more obstructive when a VA secretary tried to open up two underutilized VA facilities in rural Virginia and Alabama to nonveterans in the area who lacked access to healthcare. The proponent of that pilot project was Republican appointee Edward J. Derwinski, who had secured over $1 billion in annual increases for 171 VA hospitals. Nevertheless, Derwinski was forced to resign when the VFW threatened to withhold its endorsement of President George H. W. Bush's 1992 reelection effort if Derwinski remained in his cabinet.[38]

In both instances the organizational fear that a nonveteran—even a veteran's spouse—might be treated ahead of someone who served in uniform proved fatal. This knee-jerk reaction was similar to the VFW and DAV's initial response to the Legion's advocacy of the original GI Bill, during World War II. Back then, the Legion's organizational rivals worried that spending millions of dollars to educate able-bodied veterans would leave less money to care for those with actual war wounds, old or new. This crippling shortsightedness persists today. It also explains the refusal by most VSOs to help former soldiers with other-than-honorable discharges because, as one Legion official told us, veterans with bad paper "made bad choices and they have to suffer the consequences."

DEMANDING MORE FOR WHOM?

If VSOs can break with their own worst traditions and embrace their better past stances on extending VA health coverage to more veterans and their families, the next hills to climb will be harder even with their help. Movements for universal, publicly funded healthcare—Medicare for All—and free public higher education have gained traction in recent years because millions of poor and working-class Americans who didn't serve in the military or who are families and friends of active-duty and former service members desperately need the same health security and access to affordable college education that some, but not all, veterans currently have. Just as more labor unions have embraced these demands—even though their dues-payers are better off than most workers—more VSOs need to do the same.

Why would veterans' groups, long devoted to benefit expansion on a members-only basis, suddenly embrace universalization of two essential social programs? The first reason is demographic and thus pragmatic: the veteran population in the US is projected to shrink by one-third over the next twenty-five years. As Kayla Williams asked an audience of fellow GI Bill beneficiaries at the SVA national convention in 2020: "Does it make sense for us—as a dwindling percentage of the population—to just ask for more?" Her question was posed on the eve of a pandemic and resulting economic crisis that exposed huge holes in the social safety net for many friends, neighbors, family members, and fellow taxpayers of the nation's 19 million veterans. "To maintain public good will toward them," Williams warned, "veterans will have to give back to their communities, not just demand more benefits that are not available to others."

In blunter fashion, former Marine pilot Carl Forsling reminded *Task and Purpose* readers that the average nonveteran "doesn't have a retirement plan and has no idea how he's going to send his kids to college," while former career soldiers have good pension coverage, an early retirement option, and now a transferable post-9/11 GI Bill. "Whether you think your pay and benefits are sufficient or not," Forsling wrote, "they're provided by the continuing support of the American taxpayer. If they think veterans are a bunch of insufferable whiners, their gratitude and good will is going to run out."[39]

These concerned voices within the veteran community gained greater resonance after millions of civilians were faced with life-threatening workplace hazards due to COVID-19. As *New York Times Magazine* reporter and former Marine C. J. Chivers noted, soldiers in uniform were "forced to yield part of the warm spotlight they've long enjoyed" to frontline healthcare workers "who protect the American public without banners, medals, hymns, or tuition support."[40] In Independence, Oregon, Dan Greig, an American Legion post officer, gave a Memorial Day speech that linked the service of "fallen veterans" to the present-day heroism of "health-care professionals who are saving others." Like Greig, former defense secretary Jim Mattis publicly acknowledged that "it is not only our troops who are willing to offer the ultimate sacrifice for the safety of the community. Americans in hospitals, grocery stores, post offices, and elsewhere have put their lives on the line in order to serve their fellow citizens and their country." Some of those workers in the private sector even received (short-lived) "hero pay" for doing what was now suddenly deemed "essential work."

Acting on this belated recognition of valorous civilians, Gretchen Whitmer, the Democratic governor of Michigan, announced "a plan to make essential pandemic workers in her state eligible for free college." According to employment researcher Michelle Miller-Adams, Whitmer's goal was to reward "staff members of hospitals and nursing homes, grocery store clerks, sanitation workers, police officers, delivery people, and others working on the front lines." Other advocates of this approach favored a much broader "national federally funded program that will enable any adult without a degree to return to college or earn a comparable credential without paying tuition," because "many other workers [in Michigan and other states] who have lost their jobs[,] or will lose them in the coming recession, will need new skills to navigate the post-pandemic labor market." The model for such legislation would, of course, be the original GI Bill, which "powered the American economy after World War II by providing returning men and women of the armed services with affordable higher education." In the wake of widespread pandemic-created joblessness, "a federal guarantee of training for adult workers could accelerate an economic recovery now—and at relatively low cost."[41]

UNIVERSALIZING BENEFITS

Will Fischer, the former director of the AFL-CIO's Union Veterans Council, is one GI Bill beneficiary who favors universalizing such benefits. Fischer served in Iraq as a Marine before becoming the second person in his family "to graduate from college and do so without the yoke of student debt," thanks to the GI Bill. Now he'd like to see all student debt canceled and public higher education, including vocational schools, made tuition-free because all working-class people "would benefit, without question, from such legislation." Fischer makes the additional argument that limiting free higher education to veterans confronts young people with an unacceptable choice between being forced "to put on a uniform and participate in never-ending U.S. wars or take on crushing debt."[42]

Labor-oriented veterans like Fischer are following in the footsteps of the late Tony Mazzocchi, a visionary survivor of the Battle of the Bulge. After returning home from World War II, Mazzocchi battled powerful employers as a local and then national leader of the Oil, Chemical, and Atomic Workers Union. In 1970 he was a key architect of labor's campaign for the Occupational Safety and Health Act, which now provides workplace protections for 130 million Americans. Not content with that historic achievement, Mazzocchi later tried to put free higher education onto the national political agenda. He was inspired by his own liberating experience as a working-class veteran able to attend college due to "one of the most revolutionary pieces of legislation in the 20th century."[43] Mazzocchi believed that an all-inclusive twenty-first-century version of that original GI Bill could similarly plant the "seeds of the good life" for millions of Americans by allowing them to get post–high school degrees without accumulating ruinous personal debt.

In his two presidential campaigns, Bernie Sanders, a friend and ally of Tony Mazzocchi, finally succeeded in popularizing the idea that public higher education should be free for all. As the presidential race tightened in 2020, the pressure of Sanders's candidacy pushed his only remaining opponent, Joe Biden, to announce that he favored making public colleges and universities free for students from families earning less than $125,000 per year.[44] Amid the looming economic crisis created by COVID-19—and after Sanders suspended his campaign—Biden unveiled an additional "student debt forgiveness plan which would eliminate student debt for low-income and middle-class people who attended public colleges and universities, and other institutions that serve students of color."[45] After Biden was elected, he also proposed spending $109 billion over ten years to make community colleges free for all.[46]

But not everyone expressed confidence that the White House would actually pursue such reforms. As former Army Ranger and Veterans for Peace activist Rory Fanning pointed out, reducing college costs would be "a huge threat to the U.S. war machine" because thousands of soldiers would lose their incentive to stay in the military or enlist in the first place.[47] Sure enough, nine months into Biden's presidency, his "heavily promoted plan to offer tuition-free community college" was dropped from his proposed spending on social programs, after objections from Senators Joe Manchin (D-WV) and Kyrsten Sinema (D-AZ).

In early 2021, the Biden administration did cancel about $2.3 billion in loans for students who were disabled or defrauded by for-profit colleges. But the new president balked at canceling up to $10,000 in student local debt per borrower for millions of others.[48] However, as noted in chapter 3, when the new Democrat-controlled Congress eliminated the 90/10 rule loophole that incentivized GI Bill fraud, that much-needed change was postponed until 2023, a delay that Student Veterans of America called "a bitter pill to swallow."[49]

MEDICARE FOR ALL

During his 2020 campaign for the presidency, Biden was also opposed to Medicare for All, another Sanders plan he deemed "unaffordable." Nevertheless, union members and all workers, including those employed at the VA, still have a big stake in pushing the Biden administration to go beyond its more limited goal of expanding healthcare coverage under the ACA. Medicare for All will only become more politically feasible when it has much broader and stronger support among Americans with job-based insurance coverage, which millions of them lost, along with their jobs, during the pandemic. VA union members, since they're already helping to make a single-payer system work—and work well—are uniquely positioned to be convincing Medicare for All advocates.

National Nurses United (NNU) has long been labor's leading promoter of Medicare for All, while also resisting privatization as a threat to its twenty thousand VA members. NNU backs Sanders for president and spends heavily on legislative work and public education related to healthcare reform. It hosts an impressive website that highlights news and information about what nursing work is like in other nations with national healthcare systems.[50] Yet there could be far more utilization of the VA as a homegrown model for socialized medicine in the union's exemplary single-payer campaign work. Likewise, Physicians for a National Health Program (PNHP), a longtime ally of NNU, tends to keep single-payer advocacy compartmentalized from the anti-privatization work of its own members employed at the VA. The Labor Campaign for Single Payer, a coalition of unions that hopes to get "healthcare off the bargaining table" and replace our current "profit-driven system with Medicare-for-All," could also help situate the struggles of VA patients and providers within the broader healthcare reform movement. If the much smaller-scale campaign to "Save Our VA" fails, the ambitious goal of creating Medicare for All will be much harder to achieve for all who need it.

Veterans' organizations have, of course, generally been MIA from this movement. Instead, they've mounted their own spotty defense of the VHA, preferring, in most cases, not to even think of veterans' healthcare as "socialized medicine." To their credit, some VSO leaders, locally and nationally, have embraced other causes—like disability rights, mental health parity, gun safety, and suicide prevention—in less vet-centric fashion. As Shaun Castle, deputy executive director of Paralyzed Veterans of America (PVA), points out, his organization played an active role in lobbying for the Americans with Disabilities Act (ADA) of 1990, which aided far more nonveterans than veterans. Later, as a student veteran at the University of Alabama, Castle personally led a successful on-campus campaign for university compliance with ADA requirements for wheelchair access.

Ryan Gallucci, the VFW's deputy national service director, believes that VSOs can help all Americans with psychiatric conditions or substance abuse problems win broader insurance coverage by "making it OK for our society to talk about mental health the same way we talk about physical health problems." Despite VSO wariness of anything smacking of gun control, which helped strip lethal-means training from the Hannon Act, several Florida veterans responded to a 2019 high school massacre in their state by expressing solidarity with the student-led gun law reform campaign it spawned. In a powerful op-ed piece for the *Washington Post*, three former Marines, including Joe Plenzler, then a communications director for the Legion, praised the Parkland students for resisting "pure horror" and "making their voices heard." The coauthors of the piece pledged to "stand alongside them to help amplify their message."[51] Initiatives like this offer a glimmer of hope: in the future, veterans' groups may someday tackle "suicide by gun" in their own ranks in a fashion that supports firearms safety and suicide prevention generally.[52]

HELPING VETERANS AS WORKERS

After four years of legal and political battering by a hostile Republican administration, unions representing VA workers welcomed new leadership in Washington. Like the VSOs, the largest of those labor organizations, AFGE, was given no formal role in Biden's VA transition task force. But after dealing with a VA secretary who regularly flouted federal labor relations norms, union members at the VA welcomed the chance to provide input to his successor in any form. Secretary McDonough accepted AFGE's April 2021 invitation to address a union safety conference, where he described worker representation as "critical to strengthening the VA, critical to making the VA more effective, and critical to improving access and outcomes for our veterans."[53]

AFGE and other unions welcomed President Biden's quick revocation of antiunion executive orders that reduced their official presence in VA workplaces and hindered worker representation. The White House also sacked ten Trump appointees to the Federal Service Impasses Panel (FSIP), who nearly always sided with federal agency management in labor relations disputes. Union officials anticipated that VA contract negotiations would be less difficult than under Trump, a low bar for sure.[54] Even without securing congressional repeal of the 2017 legislation that created a punitive and highly politicized Office of Accountability and Whistleblower Protection (OAWP), VA workers hoped that under a new, more labor-friendly VA secretary the OAWP might actually start weeding out a few bad managers rather than just targeting vulnerable frontline workers (although there was little evidence of that new direction by late 2021). In light of his professed commitment to equity and diversity, Secretary McDonough also faced expectations that he would address AFGE's complaint that "white employees who applied for management positions were selected at double the rate of Black applicants" under the previous administration.[55]

According to Germaine Clarno, an AFGE local leader in Chicago, having a Republican president who never "stopped attacking federal employees by attempting to destroy our union" had one upside: "We got smarter, stronger, resilient." According to Clarno, union members across the country must "keep filing grievances, keep filing unfair labor practice charges, keep mobilizing, and keep organizing." One sign that AFGE members at the VA were absorbing this hard-learned lesson was widespread participation in "Worker Memorial Day" activity in April 2021, which highlighted their workplace risks and sacrifices during the pandemic. In the future, such membership mobilizations will definitely be needed to defend VA facilities at risk due to AIR Commission recommendations.

During Donald Trump's final days in office, the job security of the 13 percent of all veterans who are employed in state and local government was also at risk. As the AFL-CIO's Veterans Council reported, COVID-19 created an economic crisis that eliminated 1.6 million public-sector jobs, "nearly three times more than during the entire Great Recession." Even with an infusion of $250 billion in federal aid in 2020, state and local governments were projected to have a collective revenue shortfall of $500 billion over the next three fiscal years, according to the Brookings Institution. Ignoring pleas even from the US Chamber of Commerce, congressional Republicans objected, before and after the presidential election, to providing additional aid sufficient to prevent massive layoffs and cutbacks in vital public programs.[56] Fortunately, with Democrats controlling both the Senate and House, Biden was able to pass the American Rescue Plan Act in March 2021. It allocated another $350 billion for state, local, and tribal governments to help them maintain services, but didn't necessarily relieve local pressure for union contract concessions.[57]

Veterans' charities would, of course, remain a source of assistance for those most in need due to pandemic-related joblessness, loss of healthcare coverage, or housing insecurity. But if COVID-19 proved anything, it was that private philanthropy is no substitute for a broader social safety net. If charitable donors want to help far more veterans—by keeping them employed, with good benefits—they can start by joining efforts to defend the public sector, in the form of not just the VA but also the postal service. As Vietnam-era veteran, former Texas letter carrier, and now labor lawyer Jay Youngdahl argues, "Any attack on the Postal Service is an attack on the larger community of veterans." If members of the public—not to mention veterans' own support organizations—fail to respond accordingly, the USPS will remain on the same slippery slope to privatization and dismantling that is all too familiar to patients at the VHA, including the thousands of postal workers among them.

The defeat of Donald Trump helped thwart parallel Republican efforts to discredit and defund both agencies. But after the 2020 election, Republican megadonor Louis DeJoy resumed "his push for a major operational overhaul at the Postal Service, brushing aside evidence that his original effort caused massive mail delays across the nation before it was temporarily suspended."[58] The Biden administration couldn't directly fire DeJoy—as Senator Tammy Duckworth and others demanded—because the USPS is an agency formally independent of the executive branch. The postmaster general served at the pleasure of a nine-member board of governors, which, by the end of Trump's single term, still had a majority of four to two favoring DeJoy, along with three vacancies.

While the process of filling those open board slots and deciding DeJoy's future played out in Washington, postal workers around the country tried to make the most of the new allies and broader popular support they gained by effectively handling the biggest pile of mail ballots in US history. "Instead of slashing and burning the USPS, we need to be expanding and strengthening it," said Keith Combs, the African American former Marine who now leads postal workers in Detroit. If Congress let local post offices offer banking services to all customers, particularly those in low-income and rural communities, Combs's fellow veterans would be the first to benefit. As Combs notes, they are four times more likely to use predatory payday lenders than nonveterans. Affordable and reliable check cashing, ATM, bill payment, and money transfer services would boost the bottom line of the second-largest employer of veterans while being very pro-veteran on the consumer end.[59]

In May 2021, members of Congress introduced the Postal Service Reform Act of 2021, bipartisan legislation that "would help put the Postal Service on a sustainable financial footing," according to Michigan senator Gary Peters.[60] Unfortunately, the bill, in its initial form, did not explicitly authorize provision of all the financial services advocated by Combs, despite their potential to generate an estimated $1 billion a year in new revenue.[61] Under its own authority, the usps began a limited trial program, in collaboration with the Postal Workers Union, that allowed customers to cash business and payroll checks in four cities and put the proceeds into a single-use gift card. As the *American Prospect* reported, the initial roll-out was poor in one test site, raising union concerns that DeJoy was "using the promise of postal banking to neutralize criticism of his tenure, without moving the nation any closer to a public option for financial services."[62]

In a worsening job market in 2020 and 2021, few veterans' advocates were much inclined to discourage former comrades from entering the field of law enforcement, the next most popular form of public-sector employment for veterans after the post office. Even Common Defense, which opposes military equipment transfers from the Pentagon to local police departments, fell silent on the problematic veteran-to-police pipeline we described in chapter 2. Always willing to question conventional wisdom, retired colonel Andrew Bacevich noted that in the past it might have made "all the sense in the world for us to vector vets toward the police force." But that was before the post-9/11 generation of veterans returned home with such high rates of PTSD, substance abuse, and suicide. "To the extent that we've got a bunch of damaged young people," Bacevich says, "then maybe the last thing we want to do is put them in a job where they carry a gun in an environment that's going to make things worse."

As noted in chapter 2, more research is needed on how military training and experience may affect police officers' interaction with the public. Police departments also need to employ more standardized and careful screening of applicants who have had combat exposure or service-related injuries that might adversely affect their job performance. Veterans should be rewarded for their service, but not at the risk of jeopardizing the mental health of those with preexisting conditions that might be exacerbated by police work. Nor should veterans' hiring preferences stand in the way of police departments achieving the greater diversity they need, along with other major reforms. At the very least, employment counselors should encourage former soldiers to explore options other than law enforcement where possible. For example, the labor-backed Helmets to Hardhats program has connected many transitioning service members to training and apprenticeship opportunities in the building trades, which put them on a path to good union jobs—with hazards of their own, but none like those in policing. If VSO lobbying on behalf of the DOD-terminated Troops to Teachers program succeeds in Congress, that worthwhile effort should be revived, with more funding and under the auspices of the US Department of Education, its former co-administrator.

CONTINUITY OR CHANGE?

On the eve of the 2020 presidential election, when millions of Americans were being bombarded with appeals to back Joe Biden or Donald Trump, Afghan War veteran Brittany DeBarros sent out a fundraising pitch for her group, About Face, which noted that neither major party had fielded an "anti-war candidate." In DeBarros's view, there was no forgiving Biden for the enormous harm resulting from his initial support for open-ended warfare in the Middle East. "Many of us," she wrote, "deployed under the Obama-Biden administration—where despite all their promises to end occupations—we witnessed their devastating expansion of militarism instead." On the other hand, Trump's four-year record included "doubling down on those wars, by dropping record-breaking numbers of bombs on Afghanistan and beyond," negotiating the largest arms deal in US history, and expanding "terrifying state violence" at home, directed at police brutality protesters. Even if Biden won, DeBarros predicted, "the realities of war and militarism" would remain pretty much the same.[63]

While similarly unenthused about their presidential election choices, other longtime critics of US military spending—and some new ones—expressed hope that the huge financial burden of dealing with COVID-19 would result in a reordering of national priorities.[64] However, as noted in the previous chapter, a modest 10 percent cut in DOD spending, proposed by Bernie Sanders, was overwhelmingly defeated in 2020. When that same $740 billion defense authorization bill was finalized six months later, most Democrats and Republicans again found ample reason to support it and then overrode President Trump's veto of the measure. In the House just thirty-seven Democrats—and a single veteran, Tulsi Gabbard—agreed with Representative Ilhan Omar that it was still "unconscionable to pass a Pentagon budget that continues to fund endless wars during a time of widespread suffering across our country."[65] In the Senate only Sanders and five others voted no.

The Pentagon spending package did provide much-needed military pay raises and additional compensation for Vietnam veterans exposed to Agent

Orange (although no assistance for its Southeast Asian victims).[66] As a concession to civil libertarian concerns, federal officers assigned to domestic policing would, in the future, be required to identify themselves and their agency as opposed to concealing that information, as many did during crowd control duty in Portland and other cities after the killing of George Floyd. The Pentagon was also directed to start stripping the names of Confederate generals from its military bases, a provision that helped trigger Trump's unsuccessful veto.[67]

To run the Pentagon and add further racial diversity to his cabinet, president-elect Biden picked Lloyd Austin III, a recently retired African American four-star general. As a veteran, Austin took the same upwardly mobile path, through the revolving door from the Pentagon to the private sector, as Donald Trump's DOD secretaries. In Austin's case, this landed him on the corporate boards of Nucor, Tenet Healthcare, and Raytheon Technologies, where he collected lucrative director fees on top of an estimated $230,000-a-year pension from the military. Austin also became a partner in Pine Island Capital Partners, whose acquisitions included firms making weapon parts and computer-simulated training systems for the DOD and local police departments. As Danny Sjursen noted, the new Pentagon chief "literally puts both the military and the industrial in the military-industrial complex."[68]

Nevertheless, at his confirmation hearing, General Austin referenced some of the "toxic workplace" conditions we described in chapter 1 and acknowledged the urgent need "to rid our ranks of racists and extremists" who might later on, as veterans, become militia members. "We owe our people a working environment free of discrimination, hate and harassment," he declared.[69] In response to some military personnel and veterans being involved in the January 6, 2021, assault on Capitol Hill, Austin ordered a sixty-day stand-down, during which active-duty troops participated in discussions designed to discourage extremism and "reinforce military values." He spoke at a Pride Month celebration at the Pentagon and revoked a Trump-imposed ban on diversity training for the military, much to the chagrin of Republican veterans in Congress like Senator Tom Cotton and Representative Dan Crenshaw.[70]

In May 2021, the DOD also created an "extremism task force" charged with making recommendations about possible changes in the military justice system. But, as one critic predicted, "if the military's handling of sexual assault is any indication of how this 'task force' will confront right-wing extremism, then we can assume there will be plenty of talk without much action to root out the problem."[71] Early in the Biden administration, the Fort Hood scandal (described in chapter 1) seemed to have persuaded enough members of Congress that sexual assault in the military required independent investigation and prosecution. By May 2021, sixty Democrats and Republicans in the Senate favored a bill cosponsored by Kirsten Gillibrand (D-NY) and retired National Guard lieutenant general Joni Ernst (R-IA), a sexual assault survivor. If approved by the House as well, decision-making power about such cases and other felonies, including some hate crimes, would be removed from commanding officers and assigned "to a specially trained team of uniformed prosecutors."[72] In the Senate, two veterans on the Armed Services Committee, Rhode Island Democrat Jack Reed and Oklahoma Republican James Inhofe, fought to narrow the scope of the legislation, limiting it to sexual assault cases only.[73]

Their deference to the Pentagon was emboldened by General Austin's own resistance to broader changes in the military justice system sought by Gillibrand.[74] In November 2021, as the Pentagon proposed its own reforms, to be phased in over nine years, a bipartisan group of eight senators, including Gillibrand and Ernst, vigorously objected in a letter. "The men and women who serve in our military cannot continue to operate another day, let alone another decade, under a chain of command that is unwilling or incapable of taking decisive action to address this epidemic," they wrote. (A month later, Congress passed a watered-down version of military justice reform that did not strip commanders of their control over court-martials but did empower new "special victim prosecutors" to handle cases involving sexual assault, rape, murder, and domestic violence. Gillebrand called the compromise a "disservice to our service members.")[75]

AN AFGHAN WITHDRAWAL

President Biden's withdrawal of US ground forces from Afghanistan drew mixed reactions from veterans. The sudden collapse of the Afghan government in August 2021 was followed by an emergency airlift of 120,000 US allies and the death of thirteen soldiers while protecting Kabul Airport. Helping to provide political cover for the White House were veterans' organizations on the left and right. They included Common Defense, VoteVets, Concerned Veterans for America, and even the American Legion, which also expressed support for bringing combat troops home. In Congress, Jason Crow, the former Army Ranger who joined Republican Liz Cheney's effort to block President Trump's Afghan withdrawal plan, was more receptive to Biden's "decision to finally bring our longest war to an end," although he criticized the administration's refugee evacuation planning.[76]

Republican veteran Dan Crenshaw, a House member from Texas, told Fox News viewers that the chaotic exit was the result of "relying on hollow slogans like 'Bring the troops home' and 'No more endless wars.'" At a September 25, 2021, "Save America" rally in Perry, Georgia, former president Trump denounced his successor for "the most appalling display of incompetence by an American president in history." Trump left thirteen seats at the rally empty to commemorate the "great young warriors murdered" while defending Kabul Airport. In a dramatic preview of his likely use of veterans and military personnel as political props in any third campaign for the presidency in 2024, Trump also welcomed an active-duty Marine to the stage "who bravely served in Kabul during the withdrawal."[77]

In reality, during President Biden's first year in office, most of his other foreign and military policy decisions reflected little change in the status quo. The White House initially put a temporary freeze on the arms sales to Saudi Arabia and the United Arab Emirates, which were fast-tracked by Trump administration secretary of state Mike Pompeo on behalf of Raytheon, as reported in chapter 2. The company's new CEO, Greg Hayes, took the long view of this order flow interruption. During an "earnings call" with Wall Street analysts, he predicted that peace "was not going to break out in the Middle East anytime soon" and the region would remain a source of "solid growth" for Raytheon products. Hayes didn't have long to wait before Biden approved the transfer of weaponry with a "defensive purpose."[78]

Under Biden, the flow of surplus military equipment through the "Pentagon-to-police" pipeline also continued, with few strings attached regarding its domestic use. During the first quarter of 2021, the Defense Logistics Agency reported that nearly $34 million worth of military gear went to local police agencies, almost triple the dollar amount during the last quarter of 2020, under Trump.[79] In September 2021, twenty-two House Democrats, including veterans Conor Lamb and Jared Golden, joined nearly all their Republican colleagues in killing an amendment to the National Defense Authorization Act (NDAA) for 2022 that would have curtailed the flow of weaponry to local police.

By a 316 to 113 vote, the House then approved the NDAA itself, which lavished $778 billion on the Pentagon. Per usual, veterans on the Armed Services Committee who favored such spending—like Golden, Mikie Sherrill, Seth Moulton, and Elaine Luria—had been recent recipients of generous campaign funding from military contractors.[80] In the fall of 2021, over the objections of Bernie Sanders and few others, the Senate was about to join this bipartisan push for Pentagon funding that was $37 billion more than Donald Trump's last budget. (Sanders was particularly outraged by the fact that the NDAA included a $10 billion "handout" to Blue Origin, a space exploration company started by Amazon founder and With Honor Fund donor Jeff Bezos.)[81]

As multiple critics noted, President Biden's Afghan troop withdrawal had produced no "peace dividend." Instead, billions more were allocated to nuclear weapons modernization, "a new Cold War" with China, and ongoing military operations involving 170,000 troops in nearly 160 foreign countries.[82]

SEEKING PEACE AND NEW PRIORITIES

The persistent but always outgunned foes of such military spending needed far more fresh troops to nudge the White House in a better direction. On the education and publicity front, several new institutions shaped, in part, by veterans or military family members helped amplify the voices of foreign-policy critics with military credentials. Among the groups supporting anti-war lobbying and legislation by doing research, writing, and media outreach were the Quincy Institute for Responsible Statecraft, the Eisenhower Media Network (EMN), and the Costs of War Project.

Named after John Quincy Adams and cofounded by Andrew Bacevich, the Quincy Institute is promoting "ideas that move U.S. foreign policy away from endless war and toward vigorous diplomacy in the pursuit of international peace."[83] This think tank attempt to lay the "foundation for a new foreign policy centered on diplomatic engagement and military restraint" has drawn financial backing from both George Soros and Charles Koch. Befitting such odd-couple billionaire funders, the Quincy Institute seeks to create common intellectual ground for anti-interventionists on both ends of the political spectrum. As Bacevich told us when the institute was launched in 2019, "I'm optimistic that we're going to make a dent at least in the foreign policy consensus. That won't necessarily send the military-industrial complex fleeing or surrendering, but it will have some impact." Assessing the Biden administration two years later, Bacevich found it "difficult to profess even modest optimism" because the new president appeared so intent on "clinging to a calcified and militarized conception of national security" that could "put his entire presidency at risk."[84]

Like the Quincy Institute, the nonprofit Eisenhower Media Network (EMN), started by Danny Sjursen, is dedicated "to educating Americans about the social, political, and financial destructiveness of the military industrial complex." EMN has assembled an impressive roster of former military officers and civilian experts on national security issues who can offer media outlets an alternative perspective often missing from much of their day-to-day reporting and commentary. By making such credible sources available to writers, editors, and producers of podcasts, TV and radio shows, national magazines, and newspapers, EMN hopes to reach "broad cross-partisan audiences" beyond the already engaged readers or listeners with progressive movement leanings.[85]

Another invaluable resource for antiwar campaigners are publications and reports from the Costs of War Project. Based at Brown University, this research center was cofounded by Andrea Mazzarino, a social worker and military spouse who has done clinical work with PTSD sufferers.[86] The project has recruited fifty scholars, legal experts, human rights advocates, and healthcare professionals to help calculate and publicize the ongoing financial and human toll of military conflict in Iraq, Afghanistan, and other nations. The project estimates that post-9/11 wars have cost $6.4 trillion, killed more than 800,000 combatants and civilians on all sides, and temporarily or permanently displaced 37 million people from their homes.[87]

In addition to remaining a stalwart defender of the VA, Veterans for Peace greeted the transition from Trump to Biden with no cessation of its rallies, vigils, commemorative events, and civil disobedience actions involving veterans and their supporters. While Joe Biden was nominating yet another Raytheon man to be his secretary of defense, VFP members and their local allies, like the Sunrise Movement, were in Asheville, North Carolina, holding a Raytheon-related die-in. Its target was the Raytheon subsidiary Pratt & Whitney, which planned to open a new manufacturing plant with the help of $27 million in county tax incentives. "Reject Raytheon" campaigners called for public investment in clean energy and infrastructure, healthcare, and education rather than any local expansion of military contracting, which, VFP argues, would have less employment impact.

About Face has continued its own agitation against military contractors, their political influence, and costly weapons deals while also building new connections with the Black Lives Matter movement via a solidarity network called Vets for Black Lives. Like VFP, About Face also frequently joins forces with Native Americans against environmental threats. During the lame-duck session of Congress in late 2020, Common Defense joined a coalition of fifty other groups trying to help Texas congressman Joaquin Castro, a signer of its "End the Forever War Pledge," become the new chair of the

House Foreign Affairs Committee.[88] That effort was defeated, but Common Defense, along with the Quincy Institute, continued to lobby for better appointments to national security positions in the Biden administration.

When Kyrsten Sinema, a Senate Veterans Affairs Committee member with 500,000 veterans among her constituents in Arizona, helped block White House plans to strengthen Medicare, Common Defense orchestrated exemplary protests against her. Five former members of the military serving on Sinema's veterans advisory council resigned. One of these former supporters was Air Force veteran Sylvia Gonzalez Andersh, who accused Sinema of "answering to big donors" in Big Pharma "rather than your own people."[89] In early polling of Arizona Democrats disgruntled with Sinema, Congressman Ruben Gallego, a Latino combat veteran and Common Defense favorite, scored highest among her potential 2024 primary opponents.[90]

Elsewhere in the country, Common Defense continued its bridge-building with organized labor, attracting more union participants to its Veterans Organizing Institutes. This singular solidarity with the labor movement was a continuing reminder of what other VSOs, old and new, could do if they were more focused on working-class veterans employed by the VA, the postal service, or in the private sector. As noted earlier, in chapter 3, even self-proclaimed "veteran-friendly" employers have engaged in unlawful interference with union organizing efforts involving veterans and other workers on their payroll. When such corporate misconduct occurs, more advocates for veterans need to join the fray, on the labor rather than management side.

CIVIL WAR LESSONS, THEN AND NOW

On January 20, 2021, President Joe Biden mounted the back steps of the US Capitol to take the oath of office and give a speech that focused, of necessity, on binding up the nation's political wounds. Just two weeks before, those steps had been stormed by what Biden called "a riotous mob," which tried to "use violence to silence the will of the people." Due to that unprecedented disruption of presidential election certification, Biden's inaugural ceremony was protected by twenty-six thousand National Guard members from all fifty states and three territories. This was more security than Abraham Lincoln had as the Civil War neared its end in 1865, when he too gave an inaugural address, in the very same spot, about "caring for *those* who have borne the battle and their widows and orphans."

Launching or coming under an attack was not a first-time experience for some of the veterans on both sides of the January 6 barricades. Inside the besieged Capitol Building, Democrats Jason Crow, Conor Lamb, and Tammy Duckworth were among those who either helped evacuate terrified colleagues or, later on, raised questions about the military's failure to weed out some of those responsible for the assault. After rioters were finally cleared from the Capitol, thirty-five Republican veterans did what they demanded: voted against certification of Biden as president.[91] One rare Republican dissenter, who voted to impeach Trump over the events of January 6, was Illinois House member Adam Kinzinger, a former Air Force pilot and now Air National Guard lieutenant colonel.

Kinzinger further enraged Trump backers and endangered his own political future because he felt "duty bound to conduct a full investigation into the worst attack on the Capitol since 1814 and to make sure it can never happen again." While serving on that investigative committee in October 2021, the conservative six-term congressman announced he would not run for reelection the following year. Peter Meijer, an Iraq War veteran just elected to the House from Illinois, was also among the ten Republicans voting to impeach Trump; he faced multiple 2022 primary challengers vying for the former president's endorsement.

As their later testimony revealed, veterans serving on the Capitol Police were among those traumatized by the Trump-inspired attack. More than 140 officers suffered injuries due to being beaten, tased, tear-gassed or crushed on January 6. Sergeant Aquilino Gonell, a former Army infantryman, confessed to feeling greater fear that day "than in my entire deployment in Iraq."[92] To assist "siege survivors," the VA sent several of its mobile vet centers to Capitol Hill to provide "free, easily accessible mental health resources and counseling." It was a familiar assignment for VA caregivers skilled at "addressing stress, fatigue, grief, trauma and other thoughts or feelings individuals may be experiencing."[93] Hopefully, being treated by the VA was an educational experience for any nonveterans on Capitol Hill previously involved in bipartisan efforts to undermine it. By the end of January 2021, two uniformed defenders of the Capitol had committed suicide, despite the availability of such help.

If Abraham Lincoln were alive today and advising current policy makers, he would remind them that his second inaugural address also called for achieving "a just and lasting peace among ourselves and with all nations." Doing that requires real change in the interrelated fields of veterans' and military affairs, not just virtuous symbolic gestures like making the VA motto gender-neutral or renaming military bases after heroes rather than traitors. A series of costly and disastrous post-9/11 conflicts have created a new generation of scarred survivors of both enemy and friendly fire. They may be smaller in number, as a percentage of the population, because we now have an all-volunteer force, policing the world with fewer boots on the ground. But many who served share one thing in common with the majority of Americans who did not. Their hopes for a better life have been narrowed or foreclosed by the continuing expense of these conflicts. Our society has paid too high a price for foreign occupations and interventions, which have, of course, inflicted their greatest damage on the much poorer nations directly impacted. Veterans and nonveterans alike need national leaders willing to pursue alternatives to war or at least recognize that the full cost of war has rarely been considered, or properly calculated, by architects of the forever warfare that continues today.

NOTES

PREFACE AND AUTHORS' NOTE AND ACKNOWLEDGMENTS

1. Bernie Sanders, *Our Revolution* (New York: St. Martin's, 2016), 66. In recognition of his services to veterans, as chair of the Senate Veterans Affairs Committee, Sanders was a 2014 recipient of the American Legion's "Patriot Award," presented annually by the nation's largest veterans' organization.

2. Formal interview requests were made but declined or ignored by former VA secretary Robert Wilkie; Steven Cohen, founder of the Cohen Veterans Network; former American Legion legislative director Lou Celli; and Pete Conaty of Pete Conaty & Associates.

INTRODUCTION

1. In this book, we sometimes employ the generic term *soldier* to refer to any past or present military personnel. We are aware that only the Army has "soldiers" and that members of other military branches—the Navy, Marines, Air Force, and our new Space Force—prefer to be labeled more precisely, which we do when we describe the military background or rank of particular veterans from those branches quoted and profiled in the book.

2. Richard Severo and Lewis Milford, *The Wages of War: When America's Soldiers Came Home—from Valley Forge to Vietnam* (New York: Simon & Schuster, 1989), 64–79.

3. Severo and Milford, *Wages of War*, 130.

4. Severo and Milford, *Wages of War*, 183.

5. Severo and Milford, *Wages of War*, 264–79.

6. Michael J. Bennett, *When Dreams Came True: The G.I. Bill and the Making of Modern America* (Washington, DC: Brassey's, 1996), 17.

7. For more on this GI antiwar movement, see the personal testimonies of participants collected by Ron Carver, David Cortright, and Barbara Doherty in *Waging Peace in Vietnam: US Soldiers and Veterans Who Opposed the War* (New York: New Village Press, 2019).

8. Carver, Cortright, and Doherty, *Waging Peace*, 4.

9. Carver, Cortright, and Doherty, *Waging Peace*, 4.

10. Katherine Schaeffer, "The Changing Face of America's Veteran Population," Pew Research Center, April 5, 2021, https://www.pewresearch.org/fact-tank/2021/04/05/the -changing-face-of-americas-veteran-population/.

11. Carver, Cortright, and Doherty, *Waging Peace*, 11.

12. Jennifer Mittelstadt, *The Rise of the Military Welfare State* (Cambridge, MA: Harvard University Press, 2015), 33.

13. Mittelstadt, *Rise*, 9, 4.

14. Abraham Lincoln, "Transcript of President Abraham Lincoln's Second Inaugural Address (1865)," www.ourdocuments.gov, https://www.ourdocuments.gov/doc.php ?flash=false&doc=38&page=transcript, accessed November 24, 2020.

15. Allen C. Guelzo, *Abraham Lincoln: Redeemer President* (Grand Rapids, MI: Wm. B. Eerdmans, 1999).

16. Andrew J. Bacevich, *Breach of Trust: How Americans Failed Their Soldiers and Their Country* (New York: Metropolitan Books, 2013), 62.

17. US Department of Defense, "2018 Demographics: Profile of the Military Community," iii.

18. Helene Cooper, "African-Americans Are Highly Visible in the Military, but Almost Invisible at the Top," *New York Times*, May 25, 2020, https://www.nytimes.com /2020/05/25/us/politics/military-minorities-leadership.html.

19. Lori Robinson and Michael E. O'Hanlon, "Women Warriors: The Ongoing Story of Integrating and Diversifying the American Armed Forces," Brookings Institution, May 2020, https://www.brookings.edu/essay/women-warriors-the-ongoing-story-of -integrating-and-diversifying-the-armed-forces/.

20. CFR.org editors, "Demographics of the U.S. Military," Council on Foreign Relations, July 13, 2020, https://www.cfr.org/backgrounder/demographics-us-military.

21. Matt Kennard, *Irregular Army: How the US Military Recruited Neo-Nazis, Gang Members, and Criminals to Fight the War on Terror* (New York: Verso, 2015), 11.

22. Luke Goldstein, "Posse Profiles: Veteran Dennis White '19 Talks Progressive Politics and Journey from West Virginia to Wesleyan," *Wesleyan Argus*, October 13, 2017, http://wesleyanargus.com/2017/10/13/posse-profiles-veteran-dennis-white-19 -talks-progressive-politics-and-journey-from-west-virginia-to-wesleyan/.

23. Kathy Roth-Douquet and Frank Schaeffer, AWOL: *The Unexcused Absence of America's Upper Classes from Military Service—and How It Hurts Our Country* (New York: HarperCollins, 2006).

24. Jim Golby, Lindsay P. Cohn, and Peter D. Feaver, "Thanks for Your Service: Civilian and Veteran Attitudes after Fifteen Years of War," in *Warriors and Citizens: American Views of Our Military*, ed. Kori Schake and Jim Mattis (Stanford, CA: Hoover Institution, 2016), 105–7.

25. CFR.org editors, "Demographics."

26. CFR.org editors, "Demographics," 96–99.

27. Lawrence J. Korb, "Caring for U.S. Veterans: A Plan for 2020," Center for American Progress, December 4, 2019, https://www.americanprogress.org/issues/security /reports/2019/12/04/478034/caring-u-s-veterans-plan-2020/.

28. Heidi Peltier, "The Growth of the 'Camo Economy' and the Commercialization of the Post-9/11 Wars," research paper, Brown University Costs of War Project, June 30, 2020, https://watson.brown.edu/costsofwar/papers/2020/growth-camo-economy-and-commercialization-post-911-wars-0.

29. Stacy Bannerman, *Homefront 911: How Families of Veterans Are Wounded by Our Wars* (New York: Arcade, 2015), xvi.

30. Christine A. Elnitsky, Michael P. Fisher, and Cara L. Blevins, "Military Service Member and Veteran Reintegration: A Conceptual Analysis, Unified Definition, and Key Domains," *Frontiers in Psychology* 8 (2017): 369, https://doi.org/10.3389/fpsyg.2017.00369.

31. Elliot Ackerman, *Places and Names: On War, Revolution, and Returning* (New York: Penguin Press, 2019), 76–77.

32. Daniel Sjursen, *Patriotic Dissent: America in the Age of Endless War* (Berkeley: Heyday, 2020), 26.

33. James Hatch and Christian D'Andrea, *Touching the Dragon: And Other Techniques for Surviving Life's Wars* (New York: Knopf, 2018), 40.

34. Hatch and D'Andrea, *Touching the Dragon*, 223.

35. Kayla Williams, *Plenty of Time When We Get Home: Love and Recovery in the Aftermath of War* (New York: W. W. Norton, 2014), 60.

36. Jason Kander, *Outside the Wire: Ten Lessons I've Learned in Everyday Courage* (New York: Hachette, 2018), 170.

37. Erik Edstrom, "On Memorial Day, Veterans Count Who We've Lost, Knowing There Will Be More to Count Next Year," NBC News, May 25, 2020, https://www.nbcnews.com/think/opinion/memorial-day-veterans-count-who-we-ve-lost-knowing-there-ncna1213251.

38. For more on the role of veterans and military voters in the 2016 presidential election, see Jasper Craven, "Democrats Are Ignoring One Key Voting Group: Veterans," *New York Times*, October 10, 2018, https://www.nytimes.com/2018/10/10/magazine/veterans-democrats-midterm-elections.html.

39. Interview with Robert Wilkie, *Fox News @ Night*, April 24, 2019, https://www.foxnews.com/entertainment/today-on-fox-news-april-24-2019.

40. Ruth Igielnik, Kim Parker, and Anthony Cilluffo, "Trump Draws Stronger Support from Veterans Than from the Public on Leadership of U.S. Military," Pew Research Center, July 10, 2019, https://www.pewsocialtrends.org/2019/07/10/trump-draws-stronger-support-from-veterans-than-from-the-public-on-leadership-of-u-s-military/.

41. See interviews conducted by Jennifer Steinhauer, "Trump's Actions Rattle the Military World: 'I Can't Support the Man,'" *New York Times*, June 12, 2020, https://www.nytimes.com/2020/06/12/us/politics/trump-polls-military-approval.html.

42. Veterans for Responsible Leadership, home page, https://vfrl.org, accessed February 6, 2021.

43. Paige Williams, "The Veterans Organizing to Stop Trumpism," *New Yorker*, December 18, 2020, https://www.newyorker.com/news/news-desk/the-veterans-organizing-to-stop-trumpism?.

44. Tom Dreisbach and Meg Anderson, "Nearly 1 In 5 Defendants in Capitol Riot Cases Served in the Military," NPR, *All Things Considered*, January 21, 2021, https://

www.npr.org/2021/01/21/958915267/nearly-one-in-five-defendants-in-capitol-riot
-cases-served-in-the-military.

45. Dave Philipps, "Navy SEAL in Capitol Mob Sank into Extremist Ideas," *New York Times*, January 27, 2021, https://www.nytimes.com/2021/01/26/us/navy-seal-adam-newbold-capitol.html.

46. For profile of Lee, see David Kirkpatrick, Mike McIntire, and Christiaan Triebert, "Before Capitol Riot, Thousands Made Small Donations Online," *New York Times*, January 17, 2021, https://www.nytimes.com/2021/01/16/us/capitol-riot-funding.html.

47. See two revealing *New Yorker* profiles by Ronan Farrow, "Air Force Combat Veteran Breached the Senate," January 9, 2021, https://www.newyorker.com/news/news-desk/an-air-force-combat-veteran-breached-the-senate, and "A Former Marine Stormed the Capitol as Part of a Far-Right Militia," January 14, 2021, https://www.newyorker.com/news/news-desk/a-former-marine-stormed-the-capitol-as-part-of-a-far-right-militia?utm_.

48. Catie Edmondson, "Newly Elected Republicans Embody Their Party's Split in the Aftermath of a Riot," *New York Times*, January 13, 2021, https://www.nytimes.com/2021/01/12/us/politics/house-freshman-republicans-impeachment.html.

49. Since 2008, veterans who served in combat after November 11, 1998, including in the Iraq and Afghanistan Wars, have been eligible for five years of VHA care, without regard to their income or service-related condition. See VA Press Release entitled "Five Years of VA Health Care for Combat Veterans," February 26, 2008, https://www.va.gov/opa/pressrel/pressrelease.cfm?id=1454.

50. Terri Tanielian et al., "Ready to Serve: Community-Based Provider Capacity to Deliver Culturally Competent, Quality Mental Health Care to Veterans and Their Families," RAND Corporation, 2014, https://www.rand.org/pubs/research_reports/RR806.html.

51. Veterans also serve other veterans as employees of the VA's lesser-known and less visible National Cemetery Administration. See Jasper Craven, "Veterans Who Bury Their Own," *New York Times*, May 31, 2021, https://www.nytimes.com/2021/05/30/opinion/memorial-day-calverton-cemetery.html.

52. Daniel Zwerdling, "At VA Hospitals, Training and Technology Reduce Nurses' Injuries," NPR, February 25, 2015, https://www.npr.org/2015/02/25/387298633/at-va-hospitals-training-and-technology-reduce-nurses-injuries.

53. Suzanne Gordon, *Wounds of War: How the VA Delivers Health, Healing, and Hope to the Nation's Veterans* (Ithaca, NY: Cornell University Press, 2018), 139–41.

54. Linda J. Bilmes, "The Long-Term Costs of United States Care for Veterans of the Afghanistan and Iraq Wars," Watson Institute, Brown University, August 18, 2021, https://watson.brown.edu/costsofwar/files/cow/imce/papers/2021/Costs%20of%20War_Bilmes_Long-Term%20Costs%20of%20Care%20for%20Vets_Aug%202021.pdf.

55. Veterans of Foreign Wars, "VFW: VA Health Care Trending in Right Direction," September 27, 2019, https://www.vfw.org/media-and-events/latest-releases/archives/2019/9/vfw-va-health-care-trending-in-right-direction.

56. Ron Kovic, *Born on the Fourth of July* (New York: McGraw-Hill, 1976).

57. Gordon, *Wounds of War*, 29–34.

58. Barbara Starfield, Thomas A. Parrino, Elwood Headley, Carol Ashton, and Kenneth Kizer, "Primary Care in VA Primer," Management Decision and Research Center, Health Services Research and Development Service, in collaboration with Foundation for Health Services Research, http://www.hsrd.research.va.gov/publications/internal/pcprim.htm, accessed October 4, 2021.

59. David Stires, "Technology Has Transformed the VA," *Fortune*, May 11, 2006, http://archive.fortune.com/magazines/fortune/fortune_archive/2006/05/15/8376846/index.htm.

60. "The Best Medical Care in the US," *Bloomberg Businessweek*, July 16, 2006, https://www.bloomberg.com/news/articles/2006-07-16/the-best-medical-care-in-the-u-dot-s-dot.

61. Amy C. Edmondson, Brian R. Golden, and Gary J. Young, "Turnaround at the Veterans Health Administration (A)," Harvard Business School Case 608-061, *Harvard Business Review*, July 2007 (revised January 2008), http://www.hbs.edu/faculty/Pages/item.aspx?num=34818.

62. US Department of Veterans Affairs, "Veterans Health Administration," https://www.va.gov/health/, accessed December 1, 2020.

63. M. Penn et al., "Comparison of Wait Times for New Patients between the Private Sector and United States Department of Veterans Affairs Medical Centers," *JAMA Network Open* 2, no. 1 (2019): e187096, doi:10.1001/jamanetworkopen.2018.7096, https://jamanetwork.com/journals/jamanetworkopen/fullarticle/2720917; Carrie M. Farmer and Terri Tanielian, "Ensuring Access to Timely, High-Quality Health Care for Veterans: Insights from RAND Research" (Santa Monica, CA: RAND Corporation, 2019), https://www.rand.org/pubs/testimonies/CT508.html.

64. United States Government Accountability Office, "Prescription Drugs: Department of Veterans Affairs Paid About Half as Much as Medicare Part D for Selected Drugs in 2017," December 2020, https://www.gao.gov/assets/gao-21-111.pdf.

65. Gordon, *Wounds of War*, 13–16.

66. Gordon, *Wounds of War*, 368–71.

67. US Department of Veterans Affairs, "Eligibility for VA Disability Benefits," https://www.va.gov/disability/eligibility/.

68. In October 2021, Senator Bernie Sanders tried to reduce the maddening complexity of this system by introducing a bill that would radically reduce the number of locally based eligibility thresholds and, thus, "expand eligibility, particularly for veterans in rural areas." See Press Release from Office of Bernie Sanders, "Sanders Introduces Legislation to Expand Veterans Dental and Health Care," October 20, 2021, https://www.sanders.senate.gov/press-releases/news-sanders-introduces-legislation-to-expand-veterans-dental-and-health-care/.

69. US Department of Veterans Affairs, "VA Priority Groups," https://www.va.gov/health-care/eligibility/priority-groups/, accessed November 28, 2020.

70. See Adam W. Gaffney, David Himmelstein, and Steffie Woolhandler, "Lack of Care for Those Who Serve: Healthcare Coverage and Access among US Veterans," a 2019 study conducted by Public Citizen and Harvard Public Health School, https://www.citizen.org/wp-content/uploads/Lack-of-Care-for-those-Who-Serve-Final-DS.pdf?.

71. US Department of Veterans Affairs, "Verification Assistance Brief: Determining Veteran Status," https://www.va.gov/OSDBU/docs/Determining-Veteran-Status.pdf, accessed November 28, 2020.

72. Swords to Plowshares, "Underserved: How the VA Wrongfully Excludes Veterans with Bad Paper," National Veterans Legal Services Program, 6, https://uploads-ssl.webflow.com/5ddda3d7ad8b1151b5d16cff/5e67da6782e5f4e6b19760b0_Underserved.pdf, accessed October 4, 2021.

73. Veterans Benefits Administration, *Annual Benefits Report*, FY 2020, https://www.benefits.va.gov/REPORTS/abr/docs/2020_ABR.pdf. For a conservative critique of the "disability industrial complex" (aka the VBA), see Daniel Gade and Daniel Huang, *Wounding Warriors: How Bad Policy Is Making Veterans Sicker and Poorer* (Washington: Ballast Books, 2021). The authors argue that disability benefits foster a costly and unhealthy culture of entitlement and dependence among veterans—and should be sharply restricted, not expanded.

74. Paul Starr, "The Meaning of Privatization," *Yale Law and Policy Review* 6 (1988): 6–41, https://www.princeton.edu/~starr/articles/articles80-89/Starr-MeaningPrivatization-88.htm.

75. For further documentation of the downside of privatizing public health, municipal water systems, and other basic services, see Donald Cohen and Allen Mikaelian, *Privatization of Everything: How the Plunder of Public Goods Transformed America and How We Can Fight Back* (New York: New Press, 2021).

76. Starr, "Meaning."

77. Suzanne Gordon, "Fact Checking Fact-Checkers on Privatizing Vets' Health Care," *American Prospect*, December 12, 2016, https://prospect.org/world/fact-checking-fact-checkers-privatizing-vets-health-care/.

78. Concerned Veterans for America, "2021 Policy Agenda," https://cv4a.org/2021-policy-agenda/, accessed January 26, 2021.

CHAPTER 1: A TOXIC WORKPLACE

1. Matthew Cox, "Army Launches New 'Warriors Wanted' Campaign Aimed at Generation Z," *Military.com*, October 19, 2018, https://www.military.com/dodbuzz/2018/10/19/army-launches-new-warriors-wanted-campaign-aimed-generation-z.html.

2. GoArmy, "What's Your Warrior?," YouTube video, https://www.youtube.com/watch?v=7TprgnuYfyQ, accessed July 16, 2020.

3. GoArmy, "Army Career Match," quiz, https://www.goarmy.com/?iom=AFTU-20-980_N_PSEA_71700000059783001_700000001989777_43700049512734346_5870005434485243_%2Bgoarmy&gclid=EAIaIQobChMIoauXw7LS6gIVDdbACh1K3w3EEAAYAiAAEgIfnPD_BwE&gclsrc=aw.ds, accessed July 16, 2020.

4. *The Matrix*, film, directed by Lana Wachowski and Lilly Wachowski, Warner Brothers, 1999.

5. As quoted by Chris Vognar, "Those Who Served Have Their Say," *New York Times*, October 24, 2021, https://www.nytimes.com/2021/10/22/arts/television/american-veteran-pbs.html. See also Greg Cope White's memoir, *The Pink Marine: One Boy's Journey Through Bootcamp to Manhood* (Los Angeles: About Face Books, 2016), which he is developing into a TV series with Norman Lear, of *All in the Family* fame.

6. Midwest Disability, "What Percentage of Soldiers See Combat?," December 13, 2019, https://www.midwestdisability.com/blog/2019/12/what-percentage-of-soldiers -see-combat.shtml.

7. Erving Goffman, *Asylums: Essays on the Social Situation of Mental Patients and Other Inmates* (New York: Doubleday, 1961).

8. Tyler E. Boudreau, *Packing Inferno: The Unmaking of a Marine* (Port Townsend, WA: Feral House, 2008), 78.

9. Dave Grossman, *On Killing: The Psychological Cost of Learning to Kill in War and Society* (New York: Little, Brown, 2009), xxxi.

10. Dennis McGurk, Dave I. Cotting, Thomas W. Britt, and Amy B. Adler, "Joining the Ranks: The Role of Indoctrination in Transforming Civilians to Service Members," in *Military Life: The Psychology of Serving in Peace and Combat*, vol. 2: *Operational Stress*, ed. Amy B. Adler, Carl Andrew Castro, and Thomas W. Britt (Westport, CT: Praeger Security International, 2006), 14–16.

11. McGurk et al., "Joining the Ranks," 39.

12. Erik Edstrom, *Un-American: A Soldier's Reckoning of Our Longest War* (New York: Bloomsbury, 2020), 39.

13. Edstrom, *Un-American*, 35.

14. As journalist Spencer Ackerman reports, gaining legal status for themselves was a big post-9/11 recruitment incentive for "an estimated 130,000 people who became citizens through their U.S. military service." But, under President Trump, "dozens of undocumented recruits in the expedited-citizenship program ended up purged," the military began denying enlistment applications from immigrants without papers, and deportations of veterans who lacked citizenship status greatly increased. See Ackerman, *Reign of Terror: How the 9/11 Era Destabilized America and Produced Trump* (New York: Viking, 2021), 276–77.

15. Edstrom, *Un-American*, 41.

16. Leedjia Svec et al., "Executive Summary on Hazing in the Military," Defense Equal Opportunity Management Institute, Directorate of Research, Technical Report #09-12, January 2012, 16, https://www.researchgate.net/publication/325995996 _Executive_Summary_on_Hazing_in_the_Military.

17. Svec et al., "Executive Summary," 17–18.

18. Svec et al., "Executive Summary on Hazing in the Military," 17–18.

19. Svec et al., "Executive Summary on Hazing in the Military," 16.

20. "Parris Island Hazing Scandal: Three Marines Face Court-Martial," *Marine Corps Times*, December 13, 2016, this URL leads to a search on the Marine Corps Times website that turns up zero results. An article with this title and date (written by Jeff Schogol) appears on DefenseNews: https://www.defensenews.com/news/your-marine -corps/2016/12/13/parris-island-hazing-scandal-three-marines-face-court-martial/.

21. US Department of Veterans Affairs, Military Sexual Trauma, https://www .mentalhealth.va.gov/docs/mst_general_factsheet.pdf, accessed July 29, 2020.

22. Tiia-Triin Truusa and Carl Andrew Castro, "Definition of a Veteran: The Military Viewed as a Culture," in *Military Veteran Reintegration: Approach, Management, and Assessment of Military Veterans Transitioning to Civilian Life*, ed. Carl Andrew Castro and Sanela Dursun (London: Academic Press, 2019), 15–17.

23. Jennifer Mittelstadt, *Rise of the Military Welfare State* (Cambridge, MA: Harvard University Press, 2015), 9–10.

24. Jasper Craven, "Inside Haley Britzky's Exposé of Shoddy Military Housing," Battle Borne, February 25, 2021, https://battleborne.substack.com/p/inside-haley -britzkys-expose-of-shoddy.

25. John Ismay, "Military Families Say Base Housing Is Plagued by Mold and Ne- glect," *New York Times*, December 13, 2019, https://www.nytimes.com/2019/12/13/us /military-base-housing-mold.html.

26. Daarel Burnette II, "School Quality a Critical Family Issue for Military," *Educa- tion Week*, September 24, 2019, https://www.edweek.org/policy-politics/school-quality -a-critical-family-issue-for-military/2019/09.

27. Phillip Carter, Amy Schafer, Katherine Kidder, and Moira Fagan, "Lost in Trans- lation: The Civil-Military Divide and Veteran Employment" (Washington, DC: Center for a New American Security, 2017), 8.

28. *Military.com*, "More Military Families Struggle with Debt," https://www.military .com/money/personal-finance/credit-debt-management/more-military-families -struggle-with-debt.html, accessed October 4, 2021.

29. Daniel Gade and Daniel Huang, *Wounding Warriors: How Bad Policy Is Making Veterans Sicker and Poorer* (Washington: Ballast Books, 2021), 374.

30. Jane C. Timm, "Fact Check: Trump Brags to Troops about 10 Percent Pay Raise He Didn't Actually Give Them," NBC News, December 27, 2018, https://www.nbcnews .com/politics/donald-trump/fact-check-trump-brags-troops-about-10-percent-pay -raise-n952336.

31. Wikipedia, "United States Military Pay," last edited September 19, 2021, https://en.wikipedia.org/wiki/United_States_military_pay.

32. Jennifer Steinhauer, "Pandemic Leaves More Military Families Seeking Food Assistance," *New York Times*, December 16, 2020, https://www.nytimes.com/2020/12 /16/us/politics/coronavirus-military-hunger.html.

33. Navy Cyberspace, "2019 US Military Basic Pay Charts," https://www.navycs.com /charts/2019-military-pay-chart.html, accessed December 22, 2020.

34. *Military.com*, "2020 Active Duty Pay," https://www.military.com/sites/default /files/2020-07/2020_ad_pay.pdf, accessed October 4, 2021.

35. Carter et al., "Lost in Translation," 15.

36. *Military.com*, "More Military."

37. Samantha Reeves, "5 Reasons Members of the Military Go into Debt," https:// www.veteransunited.com/money/5-reasons-members-of-the-military-go-into-debt/, accessed March 2, 2016.

38. Samuel R. Cook, "Financial Instability: Suicide's Weapon of Choice" (United States Army War College, 2013), 12, https://apps.dtic.mil/dtic/tr/fulltext/u2/a589131 .pdf, accessed July 12, 2019.

39. Kenneth T. MacLeish, *Making War at Fort Hood: Life and Uncertainty in a Mili- tary Community* (Princeton, NJ: Princeton University Press, 2013), 218.

40. Amy Bushatz, "Military and Food Stamps," February 18, 2018, https://www .military.com/paycheck-chronicles/2014/02/18/military-and-food-stamps.

41. Steinhauer, "Pandemic."

42. *Military.com*, "10 Reasons to Hire Vets," https://www.military.com/hiring
-veterans/resources/10-reasons-to-hire-vets.html, accessed October 4, 2021.

43. David Vine, *Base Nation: How U.S. Military Bases Abroad Harm America and
the World* (New York: Skyhorse, 2017), 135–44.

44. US Department of Veterans Affairs, Office of Academic Affiliations, "Military
Health History Pocket Card for Clinicians," Veterans Health Administration, https://
www.va.gov/oaa/pocketcard/overview.asp.

45. Research Advisory Committee on Gulf War Veterans Illness, "Gulf War Ill-
ness and the Health of Gulf War Veterans," November 2008, https://www.va.gov
/RAC-GWVI/docs/Committee_Documents/GWIandHealthofGWVeterans_RAC
-GWVIReport_2008.pdf.

46. Veterans Healthcare Policy Institute, "A Fresh Look at Veterans, Toxic Exposures, and Access to VA Care and Benefits," November 2, 2021, https://www
.veteranspolicy.org/post/a-fresh-look-at-veterans-toxic-exposures-and-access-to-va
-care-and-benefits.

47. James H. Binns, House Committee on Veterans Affairs, Testimony, https://
archives-veterans.house.gov/witness-testimony/mr-james-h-binns, accessed November 19, 2021.

48. MacLeish, *Making War*, 57.

49. Robin L. Toblin, Phillip J. Quartana, Lyndon A. Riviere, Kristina Clarke Walper,
and Charles W. Hoge, "Chronic Pain and Opioid Use in US Soldiers after Combat
Deployment," *JAMA Internal Medicine* 174, no. 8 (2014): 1400–1401, doi:10.1001/ja-
mainternmed.2014.2726, http://jamanetwork.com/journals/jamainternalmedicine
/fullarticle/1885986.

50. Rita Rubin, "VA Efforts to Reduce Opioid Overdose Deaths in At-Risk Veterans," *JAMA* 322, no. 24 (2019): 2374, doi:10.1001/jama.2019.20562, https://jamanetwork
.com/journals/jama/article-abstract/2757798.

51. Tara Copp, "DOD: At Least 126 Bases Report Water Contaminants Linked to
Cancer, Birth Defects," *Military Times*, April 26, 2018, https://www.militarytimes.com
/news/your-military/2018/04/26/dod-126-bases-report-water-contaminants-harmful
-to-infant-development-tied-to-cancers/.

52. Kayla Williams, "Health Issues Facing Women Veterans," in *Invisible Veterans*, ed.
Kate Hendricks Thomas and Kyleanne Hunter (Santa Barbara, CA: Praeger, 2019), 30.

53. Sonner Kehrt, "Exposed: Burn Pits May Force the Military to Acknowledge
Generations of Poisoned Veterans," *War Horse*, August 12, 2021, https://thewarhorse
.org/military-poisoned-toxic-exposure-burn-pits-secret-testing/.

For a detailed account of the Uzbekistan base hazards, see Ken Olsen, "The Casualties of K2," *American Legion Magazine*, March 2021, https://www.legion.org/magazine
/251860/march-american-legion-magazine-shines-light-k2-toxic-exposure.

54. Joseph Hickman, *The Burn Pits: The Poisoning of America's Soldiers* (New York:
Hot Books, 2016), xiv, 27.

55. Hickman, *Burn Pits*, 30–31, 92–93.

56. Hickman, *Burn Pits*, 27–29.

57. Steve Beynon, "VA Secretary Wants More Vets Sickened by Burn Pits to File Claims, but Many Are Still Being Turned Away," *Military.com*, April 28, 2021, https://www.military.com/daily-news/2021/04/28/va-secretary-wants-more-vets-sickened-burn-pits-file-claims-many-are-still-being-turned-away.html.

58. Louis Jacobson, "Chris Matthews Says Cheney Got $34 Million Payday from Halliburton," Politifact, May 24, 2010, https://www.politifact.com/factchecks/2010/may/24/chris-matthews/chris-matthews-says-cheney-got-34-million-payday-h/.

59. Robert H. Bauman and Dina Rasor, *Shattered Minds: How the Pentagon Fails Our Troops with Faulty Helmets* (Lincoln, NE: Potomac Books, 2019), xx.

60. Bauman and Rasor, *Shattered Minds*, 68, 271. Qualifying for VA treatment for brain damage becomes more difficult when the DOD fails to record and report "concussive events," as was the case after a January 2020 missile attack in Iraq that left 100 soldiers with head injuries. See Meghann Myers, "CENTCOM Didn't Properly Document Brain Injuries after 2020 Iraq Barrage," *Military Times*, November 2, 2021, https://www.militarytimes.com/news/pentagon-congress/2021/11/03/centcom-didnt-properly-document-brain-injuries-after-2020-iraq-barrage/.

61. Jean A. Langlois, Wesley Rutland-Brown, and Marlena M. Wald, "The Epidemiology and Impact of Traumatic Brain Injury: A Brief Overview," *Journal of Head Trauma Rehabilitation* 21, no. 5 (2006): 375–78, http://citeseerx.ist.psu.edu/viewdoc/download?doi=10.1.1.471.3907&rep=rep1&type=pdf.

62. Centers for Disease Control and Prevention, "Severe Hearing Impairment among Military Veterans," July 22, 2011, https://www.cdc.gov/mmwr/preview/mmwrhtml/mm6028a4.htm.

63. Roxana Tiron, "Vets Tormented by Hearing Loss Face 3M Earplug Mass Lawsuit," Class Action News, *Bloomberg Government*, February 6, 2020, https://about.bgov.com/news/vets-tormented-by-hearing-loss-face-3m-in-earplug-mass-lawsuit/.

64. Nate Raymond, "3M Hit with $8.2 Million Verdict in Fourth Military Earplug Trial," Reuters, October 1, 2021, https://www.reuters.com/legal/litigation/3m-hit-with-82-million-verdict-fourth-military-earplug-trial-2021-10-01/.

65. J. L. Thomas, J. E. Wilk, L. A. Riviere, D. McGurk, C. A. Castro, and C. W. Hoge, "Prevalence of Mental Health Problems and Functional Impairment among Active Component and National Guard Soldiers 3 and 12 Months following Combat in Iraq," *Archives of General Psychiatry* 67, no. 6 (2010): 614–23, https://www.ncbi.nlm.nih.gov/pubmed/20530011.

66. Jeffrey A. Lieberman, "Solving the Mystery of Military Mental Health: A Call to Action," *Psychiatric Times*, December 18, 2018, https://www.psychiatrictimes.com/view/solving-mystery-military-mental-health-call-action.

67. Veterans Disability Info, "How to Reclaim VA Benefits with a Personality Disorder Diagnosis," August 1, 2016, https://www.veteransdisabilityinfo.com/blog.php?article=va-benefits-denial-based-on-personality-disorder-diagnosis-appeal-the-claim_328. See also Todd C. Leroux, "US Military Discharges and Pre-

existing Personality Disorders: A Health Policy Review," *Administration and Policy in Mental Health* 42, no. 6 (2014): 748–55, https://blogs.uw.edu/brtc/files/2014/12 /Leroux-2014-US-military-discharges-for-PDs.pdf.

68. Abigail H. Gewirtz, Stephen J. Cozza, and Kenneth W. Kizer, "The Need for Clinicians to Recognize Military-Connected Children," *JAMA Pediatrics*, August 10, 2020, https://jamanetwork.com/journals/jamapediatrics/article-abstract/2769286.

69. Erin P. Finley, *Fields of Combat: Understanding PTSD among Veterans of Iraq and Afghanistan* (Ithaca, NY: Cornell University Press, 2011), 83.

70. Military Authority, "The Infantryman's Creed," http://www.militaryauthority. com/wiki/military-creeds/us-army-the-infantrymans-creed.html.

71. Mary Jennings Hegar, *Shoot like a Girl: One Woman's Dramatic Fight in Afghanistan and on the Home Front* (New York: Berkley, 2017), 262.

72. Disabled American Veterans, "Women Veterans: The Journey Ahead," foreword, January 2019, https://www.dav.org/wp-content/uploads/2018_Women-Veterans -Report-Sequel.pdf.

73. Disabled American Veterans, "Women Veterans," 10.

74. US Department of Veterans Affairs, "Women Veterans Health Care: Facts and Statistics about Women Veterans," https://www.womenshealth.va.gov/womenshealth /latestinformation/facts.asp, accessed October 4, 2021.

75. US Department of Veterans Affairs, "National Center for Veterans Analysis and Statistics Report on Minority Veterans," March 2017, vi, https://www.va.gov/vetdata /docs/SpecialReports/Minority_Veterans_Report.pdf.

76. US Department of Veterans Affairs, "National Center," 10.

77. Disabled American Veterans, "Women Veterans," 11, 10.

78. Geoff Ziezulewicz, "Tinder, Sailor, Hooker, Pimp: The U.S. Navy's Sex Trafficking Scandal in Bahrain," *Military Times*, June 16, 2020, https://www.militarytimes .com/news/your-military/2020/06/16/tinder-sailor-hooker-pimp-the-us-navys-sex -trafficking-scandal-in-bahrain/.

79. Michael Winerip, "Revisiting the Military's Tailhook Scandal," *New York Times*, May 13, 2013, https://www.nytimes.com/2013/05/13/booming/revisiting-the-militarys -tailhook-scandal-video.html.

80. Disabled American Veterans, "Women Veterans," 6.

81. Disabled American Veterans, "Women Veterans," 34.

82. Sexual Assault Prevention and Response Office (SAPRO), *Annual Report on Sexual Harassment and Violence at the Military Service Academies: Academic Program Year 2018–2019* (Washington, DC: Department of Defense, 2020), 13.

83. Caitlin M. Kenney, "Pentagon: Reports of Sexual Assault, Harassment in the Military Have Increased," *Stars and Stripes*, April 30, 2020, https://www.stripes.com /news/us/pentagon-reports-of-sexual-assault-harassment-in-the-military-have -increased-1.627966.

84. Jennifer Steinhauer, "A #MeToo Moment Emerges for Military Women after Soldier's Killing," *New York Times*, July 11, 2020, https://www.nytimes.com/2020/07/11 /us/politics/military-women-metoo-fort-hood.html.

85. Elizabeth Landers and Zachary Cohen, "GOP Senator Reveals She Was Sexually Assaulted When She Served in the Military," CNN, March 7, 2019, https://www.cnn.com/2019/03/06/politics/martha-mcsally-rape-sexual-assault-survivor/index.html.

86. Kayla Epstein, "Republican Sen. Joni Ernst Says She Is a Survivor of Sexual Assault," *Washington Post*, January 24, 2019, https://www.washingtonpost.com/politics/2019/01/24/republican-sen-joni-ernst-says-she-is-survivor-sexual-assault/.

87. Kristen J. Leslie, "Betrayal by Friendly Fire," in *War and Moral Injury: A Reader*, ed. Robert Emmet Meagher and Douglas A. Pryer (Eugene, OR: Cascade Books, 2018), 249.

88. Protect Our Defenders, "Military Sexual Assault Fact Sheet," https://www.protectourdefenders.com/factsheet/, accessed October 4, 2021.

89. Manny Fernandez, "A Year of Heartbreak and Bloodshed at Fort Hood," *New York Times*, September 9, 2020, https://www.nytimes.com/2020/09/09/us/fort-hood-deaths-army.html.

90. Acacia Coronado, "Army Secretary: Fort Hood Has High Rates of Murder, Assault," Associated Press, August 6, 2020, https://apnews.com/article/army-texas-sexual-assault-racial-injustice-d85cd06dd8eefaba1b633ad44f4264ce.

91. Christina Morales, "'An Empty Presence in My Chest': Vanessa Guillen's Family Calls for Change in the Military," *New York Times*, July 6, 2020, https://www.nytimes.com/2020/07/06/us/fort-hood-soldier-vanessa-guillen-remains-found.html.

92. Sarah Mervosh and John Ismay, "Army Finds 'Major Flaws' at Fort Hood: 14 Officials Disciplined," *New York Times*, December 8, 2020, https://www.nytimes.com/2020/12/08/us/fort-hood-officers-fired-vanessa-guillen.html.

93. As quoted by Melinda Wenner Moyer, "A Poison in the System: The Epidemic of Military Sexual Assault," *New York Times Magazine*, August 8, 2021, https://www.nytimes.com/2021/08/03/magazine/military-sexual-assault.html.

94. Kayla Williams, *Plenty of Time When We Get Home* (New York: W. W. Norton, 2014), 66–68.

95. *Military.com*, "2012 Military Suicides Hit Record High of 349," January 14, 2013, https://www.military.com/daily-news/2013/01/14/2012-military-suicides-hit-record-high-of-349.html.

96. Kenneth T. MacLeish, "Imagining Military Suicide" (Vanderbilt University, February 26, 2013), https://watson.brown.edu/costsofwar/files/cow/imce/papers/2013/Imagining%20Military%20Suicide.pdf.

97. C. Todd Lopez, "DOD Releases Report on Suicide among Troops, Military Family Members" (US Department of Defense, September 26, 2019), https://www.defense.gov/Explore/News/Article/Article/1972793/dod-releases-report-on-suicide-among-troops-military-family-members/.

98. Lolita Baldor and Robert Burns, "Military Suicides Rise 15% as Senior Leaders Call for Action," Associated Press, September 20, 2021, https://apnews.com/article/coronavirus-pandemic-health-army-lloyd-austin-aa9971be75f6a78d9b6530d6ff3d6d72.

99. US Department of Veterans Affairs, "National Veteran Suicide Prevention Annual Report" (Office of Mental Health and Suicide Prevention), 3, 16, https://www.mentalhealth.va.gov/docs/data-sheets/2019/2019_National_Veteran_Suicide_Prevention_Annual_Report_508.pdf, accessed December 8, 2020.

100. Matthew Hoh, "Was It Just? America and Her Suicidal Combat Veterans," *CounterPunch*, July 9, 2021, https://www.counterpunch.org/2021/07/09/was-it-just-america-and-her-suicidal-combat-veterans/.

101. "New Report Details Unusually High Rate of Suicides among Post-9/11 War Service Members," press release, Brown University Costs of War Project, June 21, 2021, https://www.commondreams.org/newswire/2021/06/21/new-report-details-unusually-high-rate-suicides-among-post-911-war-service.

102. US Department of Veterans Affairs, "National Veteran."

103. Lara Seligman and Dan Diamond, "Esper Eyes $2.2 Billion Cut to Military Health Care," *Politico*, August 16, 2020, https://www.politico.com/news/2020/08/16/esper-eyes-22-billion-cut-military-health-care-395578.

104. Jared Serbu, "DOD Plans to Cut 18,000 Uniformed Health Positions, but No Clear Plan to Replace Them," Federal News Network, April 5, 2019, https://federalnewsnetwork.com/defense-main/2019/04/dod-plans-to-cut-18000-uniformed-health-positions-but-no-clear-plan-to-replace-them/.

105. US Department of Defense, "Audit of the Department of Defense's Sustainment, Restoration, and Modernization of Military Medical Treatment Facilities," DODIG-2020-103 (Office of the Inspector General, July 8, 2020), https://www.dodig.mil/reports.html/Article/2269756/audit-of-the-department-of-defenses-sustainment-restoration-and-modernization-o/.

106. Travis Tritten, "The Pentagon Is Failing to Screen Most Transitioning Troops for Suicide Risk, Watchdog Says," *Military.com*, November 12, 2021, https://www.military.com/daily-news/2021/11/12/pentagon-failing-screen-most-transitioning-troops-suicide-risk-watchdog-says.html.

107. Tritten, "The Pentagon Is Failing." As this report noted, Navy veteran Gil Cisneros, the Biden administration's new undersecretary of defense for personnel and readiness, pledged to improve the DOD's performance by working with the VA to introduce a single baseline military exit exam and ensure better sharing of its results between the two agencies.

108. Swords to Plowshares, "Underserved: How the VA Wrongfully Excludes Veterans with Bad Paper," National Veterans Legal Services Program, 6, https://uploads-ssl.webflow.com/5ddda3d7ad8b1151b5d16cff/5e67da6782e5f4e6b19760b0_Underserved.pdf, accessed October 4, 2021.

109. Dana Montalto, "Op-Ed: How the VA Has Illegally Denied Healthcare to Thousands of Veterans," *Los Angeles Times*, May 31, 2021, https://www.latimes.com/opinion/story/2021-05-31/veterans-healthcare-denied-access. OutVets, which represents LGBTQ military veterans, was one of several advocacy groups behind a 2020 study documenting the extent of the bad paper problem. See *Turned Away: How VA Unlawfully Denies Health Care to Veterans with Bad Paper Discharges*, https://www.legalservicescenter.org/wp-content/uploads/Turn-Away-Report.pdf.

110. Swords to Plowshares, "Underserved," 13–14.

111. Dave Philipps, "Suit Calls Navy Board Biased against Veterans with PTSD," *New York Times*, March 3, 2018, https://www.nytimes.com/2018/03/02/us/navy-ptsd-lawsuit.html.

1. Elizabeth McLaughlin, "America's Veterans Said to Be Disproportionately Affected by Government Shutdown," ABC News, January 9, 2019, https://abcnews.go .com/beta-story-container/Politics/americas-veterans-disproportionately-affected -government-shutdown/story?id=60260832.

2. US Department of Veterans Affairs, "Sec. Wilkie to Govt. Union: Stop Exploiting Veteran Suicide" (news release), Office of Public and Media Relations, January 14, 2019, https://www.va.gov/opa/pressrel/includes/viewPDF.cfm?id=5178.

3. Tim Marcin, "Donald Trump Calls Thousand Oaks Shooter a 'Sick Puppy' after California Shooting Left 12 Dead," *Newsweek*, November 9, 2018, https://www .newsweek.com/donald-trump-thousand-oaks-shooting-sick-puppy-1209379.

4. Jerry Lembcke, *The Spitting Image: Myth, Memory, and the Legacy of Vietnam* (New York: NYU Press, 2000), 4.

5. Chris Vognar, "Those Who Served Have Their Say," *New York Times*, October 24, 2021, https://www.nytimes.com/2021/10/22/arts/television/american-veteran-pbs.html.

6. Kristen L. Rouse, "Hiring and Retaining Veterans and Reservists as Employees," NYC Veterans Alliance, January 19, 2017, https://www.nycveteransalliance.org/cter_keynote.

7. Daniel Gade and Daniel Huang, *Wounding Warriors: How Bad Policy Is Making Veterans Sicker and Poorer* (Washington: Ballast Books, 2021), 27.

8. David Vine, *Base Nation: How U.S. Military Bases Abroad Harm America and the World* (New York: Skyhorse, 2017), 152; Mark L. Gillem, *America Town: Building the Outposts of Empire* (Minneapolis: University of Minnesota Press, 2007), 160.

9. US Bureau of Labor Statistics, "Military Careers," *Occupational Outlook Handbook*, https://www.bls.gov/ooh/military/military-careers.htm?view_full, accessed October 4, 2021.

10. Daniel Sjursen, *Ghost Riders of Baghdad: Soldiers, Civilians, and the Myth of the Surge* (Lebanon, NH: University Press of New England, 2015), 217.

11. Andrew Van Dam, "What Are the Odds of a Former Fighter Pilot Being at the Controls of Your Plane?," *Washington Post*, April 20, 2018, https://www.washingtonpost .com/news/wonk/wp/2018/04/20/the-odds-youll-be-flown-by-a-former-fighter -pilot-like-southwests-shults-have-plummeted/. As Van Dam reports, fifty years ago, 80 percent of the pilots working in private-sector aviation had military backgrounds. In recent years, that number has dropped to 30 percent because of greater pilot retention by the Navy and Air Force, leaving commercial airlines with a smaller pool of military-trained pilots to draw upon.

12. Boris Groysberg, Andrew Hill, and Toby Johnson, "Which of These People Is Your Future CEO? The Different Ways Military Experience Prepares Managers for Leadership," *Harvard Business Review*, November 2010.

13. Anthony DiFlorio, "Why Is Comcast Hiring More Than 20 Battalions of Military Veterans?," *The Hill*, https://thehill.com/changing-america/respect/diversity-inclusion /485645-comcast-will-hire-2100-veterans-battling, accessed October 4, 2021.

14. House of Representatives, "150th Anniversary of West Point Association of Graduates," *Congressional Record* 165, no. 43 (March 11, 2019), https://www.congress .gov/congressional-record/2019/03/11/house-section/article/H2631-1.

15. Danny Sjursen, "Trump's Own Military Mafia," *TomDispatch*, April 9, 2020, https://www.tomdispatch.com/blog/176686/tomgram%3A_danny_sjursen%2C _trump%27s_own_military_mafia_.

16. Mark Green (@RepMarkGreen), "ICYMI: Socialized Medicine Will Not Only Entail a Massive Government Expansion into the Private Life of Every American: It Will Also Place a Tremendous Burden on the Backs of American Taxpayers," Twitter, October 27, 2020, 3:09 p.m., https://twitter.com/RepMarkGreen?ref_src=twsrc%5Egoo gle%7Ctwcamp%5Eserp%7Ctwgr%5Eauthor.

17. Thomas Gibbons-Neff, "No Questions about US Wars in Defense Chief's Confir-mation Hearing," *New York Times*, July 16, 2019, https://www.nytimes.com/2019/07/16 /us/politics/esper-confirmation-defense.html.

18. Mandy Smithberger, "Brass Parachutes: The Problem of the Pentagon Revolving Door," POGO, November 5, 2018, https://www.pogo.org/report/2018/11/brass-parachutes/.

19. *Military.com*, "Top 20 Employers of Veterans," https://www.military.com/veteran-jobs /career-advice/job-hunting/top-20-employers-of-veterans.html, accessed October 4, 2021.

20. Ryan Bort, "Trump's Pick for Defense Secretary Is as Swampy as You'd Expect," *Rolling Stone*, July 17, 2019, https://www.rollingstone.com/politics/politics-news/trump -defense-secretary-mark-esper-859988/.

21. Michael LaForgia and Edward Wong, "War Crime Risk Grows for US over Saudi Strikes in Yemen," *New York Times*, September 14, 2020, https://www.nytimes.com /2020/09/14/us/politics/us-war-crimes-yemen-saudi-arabia.html.

22. Drew DeSilver, "How Veterans and Non-veterans Fare in the US Job Market," Pew Research Center, September 17, 2019, https://www.pewresearch.org/fact-tank /2019/09/17/how-veterans-and-non-veterans-fare-in-the-u-s-job-market/; Jasper Craven and Suzanne Gordon, "As the Veteran Suicide Crisis Persists, Washington Turns to Snake Oil and Swamp Creatures," Popular Resistance, September 30, 2020, https://popularresistance.org/as-the-veteran-suicide-crisis-persists-washington-turns -to-snake-oil-and-swamp-creatures/.

23. *Military.com*, "Top 20 Employers of Veterans."

24. Joyce Hahn, Henry Hyatt, Hubert Janicki, Erika McEntarfer, Seth Murray, and Lee Tucker, "Veteran Employment Outcomes," US Census, April 24, 2020, https://lehd .ces.census.gov/doc/VEO_Tech_Doc.pdf.

25. David Cooper and Dan Essrow, "1 in 5 Veterans Would Benefit from Raising the Federal Minimum Wage to $15," Economic Policy Institute, November 7, 2017, https:// www.epi.org/publication/1-in-5-veterans-would-benefit-from-raising-the-federal -minimum-wage-to-15-workers-at-the-federal-minimum-wage-are-paid-less-today -than-during-the-vietnam-war/.

26. Charles Szypszak, *Military Leadership Lessons for Public Service* (Jefferson, NC: McFarland & Company, 2016), 30.

27. Feds Hire Vets, "Veterans' Preference," https://www.fedshirevets.gov/job-seekers /veterans-preference/, accessed August 19, 2020.

28. US Postal Service, "Transitioning Military," https://about.usps.com/careers /career-opportunities/transitioning-military.htm, accessed October 4, 2021.

29. US Postal Service, "Transitioning Military"; Cooper and Essrow, "1 in 5 Veterans."

30. Paul Prescod, "Defend the Post Office, Defend Black Workers," *Jacobin*, July 3, 2019, https://www.jacobinmag.com/2019/07/post-office-black-workers-bernie-sanders -usps.

31. Postal Reporter, "One Way to Honor Vets? Protect the Postal Service," November 6, 2019, http://www.postal-reporter.com/blog/one-way-to-honor-vets-protect-the -postal-service/.

32. Leo Shane III, "DOD Killed Off Troops to Teachers Program That Helped Thousands: Advocates Want to Revive It," *Military Times*, October 14, 2021, https://www .militarytimes.com/education-transition/2021/10/14/dod-killed-off-troops-to-teacher -program-that-helped-thousands-advocates-want-to-revive-it/.

33. Sean Mclain Brown, "Why Veterans Should Consider Careers in Law Enforcement," American Legion, November 29, 2018, https://www.legion.org/careers/244034 /why-veterans-should-consider-careers-law-enforcement.

34. Simone Weichselbaum and Beth Schwartzapfel, "When Warriors Put On the Badge," Marshall Project, March 30, 2017, 4, https://www.themarshallproject.org/2017 /03/30/When-Warriors-Put-On-The-Badge.

35. Weichselbaum and Schwartzapfel, "When Warriors," 15.

36. Weichselbaum and Schwartzapfel, "When Warriors," 14.

37. Weichselbaum and Schwartzapfel, "When Warriors," 9, 8.

38. Jennifer M. Reingle Gonzalez, Stephen A. Bishopp, Katelyn K. Jetelina, Ellen Paddock, Kelley Pettee Gabriel, and M. Brad Cannell, "Does Military Veteran Status and Deployment History Impact Officer Involved Shootings? A Case-Control Study," *Journal of Public Health* 41, no. 3 (2019): 245–52, https://doi.org/10.1093/pubmed /fdy151.

39. International Association of Chiefs of Police (IACP), "Employing Returning Combat Veterans as Law Enforcement Officers," September 2009, 14, 16.

40. IACP, "Employing Returning Combat Veterans," 29, 11.

41. Kathleen Belew, *Bring the War Home: The White Power Movement and Paramilitary America* (Cambridge, MA: Harvard University Press, 2018), 189–93.

42. Luke Barr, "Record Number of US Police Officers Died by Suicide in 2019, Advocacy Group Says," *ABC News*, January 2, 2020, https://abcnews.go.com/Politics /record-number-us-police-officers-died-suicide-2019/story?id=68031484.

43. Suzanne Gordon, *Wounds of War: How the VA Delivers Health, Healing, and Hope to the Nation's Veterans* (Ithaca, NY: Cornell University Press, 2018), 39–41.

44. Weichselbaum and Schwartzapfel, "When Warriors."

45. Peter Singer, *Corporate Warriors: The Rise of the Privatized Military Industry* (Ithaca, NY: Cornell University Press, 2008), 16.

46. William Hartung, "Profits of War: Corporate Beneficiaries of the Post-9/11 Pentagon Spending Surge," September 13, 2021, 12–13, https://watson.brown.edu /costsofwar/papers/2021/ProfitsOfWar.

47. Ori Swed and Thomas Crosbie, "The Demographics of America's Private Military Contractors," Pacific Standard, March 14, 2019, https://psmag.com/social-justice /the-demographics-of-private-military-contractors.

48. Singer, *Corporate Warriors*, 247.

49. Singer, *Corporate Warriors*, 257.

50. Combat Veterans to Careers, "5 Reasons Veterans Struggle to Transition to the Civilian Workforce," January 24, 2019, https://combatveteranstocareers.org/5-reasons -veterans-struggle-transitioning-to-the-civilian-workplace/.

51. Daniel Gade, "Veterans Need Help Becoming Civilians Again," *Wall Street Journal*, November 11, 2021, https://www.wsj.com/articles/our-veterans-need-help -becoming-civilians-again.

52. Natalie Gross, "Study: Companies Still Don't Understand Veterans," *Military Times*, July 26, 2018, https://rebootcamp.militarytimes.com/news/employment/2018 /07/26/study-companies-still-dont-understand-veterans/.

53. Phillip Carter, Amy Schafer, Katherine Kidder, and Moira Fagan, "Lost in Translation: The Civil-Military Divide and Veteran Employment" (Washington, DC: Center for a New American Security, 2017), 10.

54. C. Jeffrey Waddoups, "Did Employers in the United States Back Away from Skills Training during the Early 2000s?," *ILR Review*, December 9, 2015, https:// journals.sagepub.com/doi/abs/10.1177/0019793915619904?journalCode=ilra.

55. Dwyer Gunn, "US Employers Say They Can't Find Skilled Workers," *Marker*, September 9, 2019, https://marker.medium.com/u-s-employers-say-they-cant-find -skilled-workers-d9d812c174e1.

56. Combat Veterans to Careers, "5 Reasons."

57. Carter et al., "Lost in Translation," 14.

58. US Department of Housing and Urban Development, "2019 Annual Homelessness Assessment Report (AHAR) to Congress," 54, https://www.huduser.gov/portal /sites/default/files/pdf/2019-AHAR-Part-1.pdf.

59. National Coalition for Homeless Veterans, "Background and Statistics," http:// nchv.org/index.php/news/media/background_and_statistics/.

60. US Department of Housing and Urban Development, "2019 Annual Homelessness Assessment Report," 55–56.

61. Andrea K. Finlay et al., "Use of Veterans Health Administration Mental Health and Substance Use Disorder Treatment after Exiting Prison: The Health Care for Reentry Veterans Program," *Administration and Policy in Mental Health* 44, no. 2 (2017): 177–87, https://www.ncbi.nlm.nih.gov/pmc/articles/PMC4916025/.

62. Jennifer Bronson et al., "Veterans in Prison and Jail, 2011–12," US Department of Justice, Justice Outreach Programs, Bureau of Justice Statistics, December 2015, https://www.bjs.gov/content/pub/pdf/vpj1112.pdf.

63. Jonathan Shay, *Odysseus in America: Combat Trauma and the Trials of Homecoming* (New York: Scribner's, 2002).

64. Jonathan Shay, *Achilles in Vietnam: Combat Trauma and the Undoing of Character* (New York: Scribner, 1994), 5.

65. Shay, *Achilles*, 4–10.

66. Harold G. Koenig et al., "Assessment of Moral Injury in Veterans and Active Duty Military Personnel with PTSD: A Review," *Psychiatry*, June 28, 2019.

67. Marie Carlson, Maurice Endlsey, Darnell Motley, Lamise N. Shawahin, and Monnica T. Williams, "Addressing the Impact of Racism on Veterans of Color: A Race-Based Stress and Trauma Intervention," *Psychology of Violence* 8, no. 6 (2018): 748–62, http:// www.monnicawilliams.com/articles/Carlson_RaceTraumaVeterans_2018.pdf.

68. Brett T. Litz, Nathan Stein, Eileen Delaney, Leslie Lebowitz, William P. Nash, Caroline Silva, and Shira Maguen, "Moral Injury and Moral Repair in War Veterans: A Preliminary Model and Intervention Strategy," *Clinical Psychology Review* 29, no. 8 (2009): 695–706, https://icds.uoregon.edu/wp-content/uploads/2015/03/Litz-et-al -2009-Moral-Injury-and-Moral-Repair-in-War-Veterans.pdf.

69. Kristen J. Leslie, "Betrayal by Friendly Fire," in *War and Moral Injury: A Reader*, ed. Robert Emmet Meagher and Douglas A. Pryer (Eugene, OR: Cascade Books, 2018), 248.

70. Shay, *Odysseus*, 21–22.

71. Megan Stack, "The Veterans Struggling to Save Afghan Allies," *New Yorker*, August 30, 2021, https://www.newyorker.com/news/news-desk/the-veterans-struggling -to-save-afghan-allies.

72. Carter et al., "Lost in Translation," 6.

73. For more on "the veteran as immigrant," see Tiia-Triin Truusa and Carl Andrew Castro, "Definition of a Veteran: The Military Viewed as a Culture," in *Military Veteran Reintegration: Approach, Management, and Assessment of Military Veterans Transitioning to Civilian Life*, ed. Carl Andrew Castro and Sanela Dursun (London: Academic Press, 2019), 14–15.

74. Commonwealth Club of San Francisco, "The Art and Soul of Combat Veterans," audio recording of event held on November 1, 2013, https://www.commonwealthclub .org/events/archive/podcast/art-and-soul-combat-veterans.

75. Truusa and Castro, "Definition of a Veteran," 16.

76. Military Friendly, "School of Visual Arts," https://www.militaryfriendly.com /school-of-visual-arts/; US Department of Veterans Affairs, "Yellow Ribbon Program," https://www.va.gov/education/about-gi-bill-benefits/post-9-11/yellow-ribbon -program/ (both accessed October 6, 2021).

77. Dave Grossman, *On Killing: The Psychological Cost of Learning to Kill in War and Society* (New York: Little, Brown, 2009), 179.

78. Shay, *Achilles*, 53.

79. J. J. Jackson, F. Thoemmes, K. Jonkmann, and U. Trautwein, "Military Training and Personality Trait Development: Does the Military Make the Man, or Does the Man Make the Military?," *Psychological Science* 20, no. 10 (2012): 1–8, https://journals .sagepub.com/doi/abs/10.1177/0956797611423545.

80. Jeffrey L. Thomas, Joshua E. Wilk, Lyndon A. Riviere, Dennis McGurk, Carl A. Castro, and Charles W. Hoge, "Prevalence of Mental Health Problems and Functional Impairment among Active Component and National Guard Soldiers 3 and 12 Months following Combat in Iraq," *Archives of General Psychiatry* 67, no. 6 (2010): 614–23, https://pubmed.ncbi.nlm.nih.gov/20530011/.

81. M. Jakupcak, D. Conybeare, L. Phelps, S. Hunt, H. A. Holmes, B. Felker, M. Klevens, and M. E. McFall, "Anger, Hostility, and Aggression among Iraq and Afghanistan War Veterans Reporting PTSD and Subthreshold PTSD," *Journal of Traumatic Stress* 20, no. 6 (2007): 945–54.

82. Jennifer M. Gierisch, "Intimate Partner Violence: Prevalence among US Military Veterans and Active Duty Servicemembers and a Review of Intervention Approaches" (US Department of Veterans Affairs, Health Services Research and De-

velopment Service, March 2013), 26, https://www.hsrd.research.va.gov/publications /esp/partner_violence-REPORT.pdf. Gierisch defines IPV as the "experience of emotional, physical, or sexual abuse," which "encompasses a range of physical, sexual, or psychological harms or stalking behavior by a current or former partner across a continuum of severity."

83. Gierisch, "Intimate Partner Violence," 27–29.

84. Gierisch, "Intimate Partner Violence," 31.

85. Gierisch, "Intimate Partner Violence," 43.

86. Gierisch, "Intimate Partner Violence," 31, 33.

87. Rachel Kimerling et al., "Prevalence of Intimate Partner Violence among Women Veterans Who Utilize Veterans Health Administration Primary Care," *Journal of General Internal Medicine* 31, no. 8 (2016): 888–94, https://www.ncbi.nlm.nih.gov /pmc/articles/PMC4945568/.

88. Blue Star Families, "Here's What Military Spouses Say about Domestic Violence," October 22, 2018, https://bluestarfam.org/2018/10/heres-what-military-spouses -say-about-domestic-violence/.

89. Stacy Bannerman, *Homefront 911: How Families of Veterans Are Wounded by Our Wars* (New York: Arcade, 2015), 90.

90. Bannerman, *Homefront 911*, xiii

91. Bannerman, *Homefront 911*, xvi.

92. Bannerman, *Homefront 911*, 236.

93. Elahe Izadi, Dan Lamothe, and Emily Wax-Thibodeaux "FBI: El Paso Clinic Victim Was VA Doctor Who Had Filed Complaint against Alleged Killer," *Washington Post*, January 7, 2015, https://www.washingtonpost.com/news/post-nation/wp/2015 /01/06/doctor-shot-presumed-shooter-found-dead-at-el-paso-va-clinic/?utm_term= .cff081511b6f.

94. US Attorney's Office, District of Colorado, "Man Who Held Nurse Practitioner Hostage at VA Hospital Charged and Arrested," December 8, 2015, https://www.justice .gov/usao-co/pr/man-who-held-nurse-practioner-hostage-va-hospital-charged-and -arrested.

95. Gordon, *Wounds of War*, 138–41.

96. David Swanson, "Yet Another Mass Shooter Was a Military Veteran," *Counter-Punch*, March 4, 2020, https://www.counterpunch.org/2020/03/04/yet-another-mass -shooter-was-a-military-veteran/.

97. Meghan Keneally, "Why the Link between Veterans and Mass Shootings Is More Complicated Than You Think," *ABC News*, November 15, 2018, https://abcnews.go.com /US/link-veterans-mass-shootings-complicated/story?id=59057321.

98. Belew, *Bring the War Home*, 209–34.

99. Wikipedia, "Yountville Shooting," last edited September 24, 2021, https://en .wikipedia.org/wiki/Yountville_shooting.

100. Toyin Owoseje, "California Shooting: Gunman Ian Long Wanted to Join U.S. Marines 'So He Could Kill for His Country,'" *Independent*, November 12, 2018, https://www.independent.co.uk/news/world/americas/california-shooting-ian-long -thousand-oaks-gunman-marines-borderline-bar-grill-a8629761.html.

101. Bridget Bartlett et al., "Revitalizing Military Recruitment without Restoring the Draft" (Princeton University, Woodrow Wilson School of Public and International Affairs, 2009), 1, 5, http://dc-20788-1635065795.us-east-1.elb.amazonaws.com/sites /default/files/content/docs/news/WWS402GFinalTaskForceReport.pdf.

102. Tom Vanden Brook, "Army Lifts Ban on Waivers for Recruits with History of Some Mental Health Issues," *USA Today*, November 12, 2017, https://www.usatoday .com/story/news/politics/2017/11/12/army-lifts-ban-recruits-history-self-mutilation -other-mental-health-issues/853131001/.

103. A. Winston, A. Thompson, and J. Hanrahan, "Ranks of Notorious Hate Group Include Active-Duty Military," *ProPublica*, May 3, 2018, https://www.propublica.org /article/atomwaffen-division-hate-group-active-duty-military.

104. S. Springer, "Secret Tapes Show Neo-Nazi Group The Base Recruiting Former Members of the Military," NBC *News*, October 15, 2020, https://www.nbcnews.com/news /us-news/secret-tapes-show-neo-nazi-group-base-recruiting-former-members-n1243395.

105. Gordon, *Wounds of War*, 138–39.

106. Rajeev Ramchand et al., "Veterans and COVID-19: Projecting the Economic, Social, and Mental Health Needs of America's Veterans," Bob Woodruff Foundation, March 2020, 3, https://bobwoodrufffoundation.org/wp-content/uploads/2020/04 /BWF_WhitePaper-COVID19-5.0-Final.pdf.

107. Ramchand et al., "Veterans and COVID-19," 5–6.

108. Niraj Chokshi and Ben Casselman, "Airline Job Cuts Could Pressure Congress and Trump on Stimulus," *New York Times*, August 25, 2020, https://www.nytimes.com /2020/08/25/business/american-airline-furlough-19000.html.

109. Niraj Chokshi, "Airlines, Facing Painfully Slow Recovery, Begin Furloughing Thousands," *New York Times*, October 1, 2020, https://www.nytimes.com/2020/09/30 /business/airline-worker-furloughs-coronavirus.html.

110. Ramchand et al., "Veterans and COVID-19," 11.

CHAPTER 3: STOLEN VALOR

Epigraph: Erik Edstrom, "After 18 Memorial Days of the 'War on Terror,' Will We Ever Learn?," *Truthout*, May 12, 2020, https://truthout.org/articles/after-18-memorial-days -of-the-war-on-terror-will-we-ever-learn/?eType=Em.

1. Ben Fountain, *Billy Lynn's Long Halftime Walk* (Edinburgh: Canongate Books, 2012), 187.

2. At least one NFL player, Pat Tillman, did enlist in the Army after 9/11, only to die in Afghanistan from friendly fire, an incident that the Army tried to cover up but that is recounted by his fellow Army Ranger—turned antiwar activist—Rory Fanning in *Worth Fighting For: An Army Ranger's Journey out of the Military and across America* (Chicago: Haymarket Books, 2014).

3. National Football League, Super Bowl LIV, broadcast football game, February 2, 2020, https://www.foxsports.com/nfl/super-bowl-2020.

4. *American Sniper*, film, dir. Clint Eastwood (Warner Brothers Entertainment, 2014).

5. Matthew Cole and Sheelagh McNeill, "'American Sniper' Chris Kyle Distorted His Military Record, Documents Show," *Intercept*, May 25, 2016, https://theintercept

.com/2016/05/25/american-sniper-chris-kyle-distorted-his-military-record
-documents-show/.

6. Anne Morse, "Fake War Stories Exposed," CBS News, 2005, https://www.cbsnews
.com/news/fake-war-stories-exposed/.

7. Raymond Hernandez, "Richard Blumenthal's Words on Vietnam Service Differ
from History," *New York Times*, May 18, 2010, https://www.nytimes.com/2010/05/18
/nyregion/18blumenthal.html.

8. David Wood, "VA Secretary Robert McDonald Falsely Claimed He Served in
'Special Forces,'" *Huffington Post*, February 24, 2015, https://www.huffpost.com/entry
/robert-mcdonald-special-forces_n_6739184.

9. Rachel Monroe, "How to Spot a Military Impostor," *New Yorker*, October 26,
2020, https://www.newyorker.com/magazine/2020/10/26/how-to-spot-a-military
-impostor.

10. Ben Miller and Colleen Campbell, "Addressing the $1.5 Trillion in Federal Stu-
dent Loan Debt," Center for American Progress, 2019, https://www.americanprogress
.org/issues/education-postsecondary/reports/2019/06/12/470893/addressing-1-5
-trillion-federal-student-loan-debt/.

11. Jasper Craven, "Scrutiny of Colleges That Get Billions in GI Bill Money Remains
Mired in Bureaucracy," *Hechinger Report*, March 30, 2020, https://hechingerreport
.org/scrutiny-of-colleges-that-get-billions-in-gi-bill-money-remains-mired-in
-bureaucracy/.

12. Carrie Wofford and James Schmeling, "Betsy DeVos vs. Student Veterans," *New
York Times*, February 18, 2019, https://www.nytimes.com/2019/02/18/opinion/betsy
-devos-student-veterans.html.

13. Natalie Gross, "Vet Groups Are Blasting Trump's Education Secretary.
Here's Why," Reboot Camp, *Military Times*, February 19, 2019, https://rebootcamp
.militarytimes.com/news/education/2019/02/19/vet-groups-are-blasting-trumps
-education-secretary-heres-why/.

14. New York State Attorney General, "Statement by A.G. Schneiderman on $25
Million Settlement Agreement Reached in Trump University Case," press release,
November 18, 2016, https://ag.ny.gov/press-release/2016/statement-ag-schneiderman
-25-million-settlement-agreement-reached-trump.

15. Nancy Kaffer, "What Betsy DeVos Got Wrong about Detroit Schools," *Detroit
Free Press*, November 2, 2019, https://www.freep.com/story/opinion/columnists/nancy
-kaffer/2019/11/02/betsy-devos-detroit-schools-charters/4113145002/.

16. Stacy Cowley, "The Students Are Victims of Fraud, but the Government Won't
Help," *New York Times*, July 10, 2020, https://www.nytimes.com/2020/07/10/business
/student-loans-betsy-devos-borrower-defense.html?searchResultPosition=2.

17. Sarah Butrymowicz and Meredith Kolodner, "For-Profit Colleges, Long Troubled, See Surge amid Pandemic," *New York Times*, June 17, 2020, https://www.nytimes
.com/2020/06/17/business/coronavirus-for-profit-colleges.html.

18. Jasper Craven, "For-Profit Colleges That Get GI Bill Money Need More Oversight,
Veterans Say," PBS, December 11, 2019, https://www.pbs.org/newshour/education/for
-profit-colleges-that-get-gi-bill-money-need-more-oversight-veterans-say.

19. Derek Kravitz and Al Shaw, "Bridgepoint Education: Trump Town," *ProPublica*, March 7, 2018, https://projects.propublica.org/trump-town/organizations/bridgepoint -education.

20. Joan Gardiner, "Platinum Partners," Enlisted Association of the National Guard of the United States, 2018, https://eangus.org/view/affinity-partners/.

21. Andrew Kreighbaum, "Veterans Groups Join Congressional Dems in Pushing to Close Federal Aid 'Loophole,'" *Inside Higher Ed*, August 27, 2019, https://www .insidehighered.com/news/2019/08/27/veterans-groups-join-congressional-dems -pushing-close-federal-aid-loophole.

22. Open Secrets, "Rep. Virginia Foxx—North Carolina District 05," https://www .opensecrets.org/members-of-congress/virginia-foxx/news?cid=N00026166, accessed October 6, 2021.

23. Consumer Financial Protection Bureau (CFPB), "Consumer Financial Protection Bureau Takes Action against Bridgepoint Education, Inc. for Illegal Student Lending Practices," September 12, 2016, https://www.consumerfinance.gov/about-us /newsroom/consumer-financial-protection-bureau-takes-action-against-bridgepoint -education-inc-illegal-student-lending-practices/.

24. Erica L. Green, "Over Veterans' Protests, Trump Vetoes Measure to Block Student Loan Rules," *New York Times*, May 29, 2020, https://www.nytimes.com/2020/05 /29/us/politics/devos-trump-student-loan-rules.html.

25. In 2017 the Trump administration even found a way to make legal challenges to consumer fraud more difficult. Vice President Mike Pence broke a Senate tie and was the deciding vote to repeal a CFPB rule that facilitated class-action litigation against financial predators. As advocates for veterans and active-duty personnel pointed out, forcing plaintiffs in uniform to instead pursue individual arbitration cases when they have few personal financial resources and are often deployed abroad guarantees that fewer claims will be filed.

26. Government Accountability Office, "VA Needs to Ensure That It Can Continue to Provide Effective School Oversight," Report to Congressional Committees, November 2018, https://www.gao.gov/assets/700/695539.pdf.

27. US Department of Veterans Affairs, Office of Inspector General, "VA's Oversight of State Approving Agency Program Monitoring for Post-9/11 GI Bill Students," Report 16-00862-179, December 2018, https://www.va.gov/oig/pubs/VAOIG-16-00862-179.pdf.

28. Aaron Glantz, "University of Phoenix Archives," *Reveal*, March 10, 2020, https:// www.revealnews.org/tag/university-of-phoenix/.

29. Danielle Douglas-Gabriel, "VA Backs Down from Plan to Suspend University of Phoenix and Other Colleges from Accessing GI Bill Benefits," *Washington Post*, July 2, 2020, https://www.washingtonpost.com/education/2020/07/02/va-backs-down-plan -suspend-university-phoenix-other-colleges-accessing-gi-bill-benefits/.

30. Butrymowicz and Kolodner, "For-Profit Colleges."

31. Jasper Craven and Suzanne Gordon, "VA's Mental Health Care Crisis Draws Private Firms Pitching Dubious PTSD Treatments," *Reveal*, August 29, 2018, https:// revealnews.org/article/vas-mental-health-care-crisis-draws-private-firms-pitching -dubious-ptsd-treatments/.

32. Andy Barr, "Rep. Barr Successfully Includes Equine Therapy in Veteran Suicide Prevention Bill," press release, December 5, 2019, https://barr.house.gov/2019/12/rep -barr-successfully-includes-equine-therapy-in-veteran-suicide-prevention-bill.

33. Scott Gordon and Sue Ambrose, "Hope, Hype or Shaky Science? Experts Fault $2.2 Million Veterans Study Involving Spinning Chair," NBC 5, Dallas–Fort Worth, October 1, 2015, https://www.nbcdfw.com/news/local/experts-fault-22-million -veterans-study-involving-spinning-chair/177764/.

34. Revive Centers, "Multi-axis Rotational Device (GyroStim)," March 20, 2020, https://revivecenters.com/multi-axis-rotational-device/.

35. Isaac Arnsdorf, "GOP Senator Pushed VA to Use Unproven 'Brainwave Fre-quency' Treatment," *ProPublica*, October 17, 2018, https://www.propublica.org/article /dean-heller-pushed-va-to-use-unproven-brainwave-frequency-treatment.

36. Suzanne Gordon, "Heller's Penchant for Privatizing Hurts Veterans' Health Care" (guest op-ed), *Nevada Current*, October 29, 2018, https://www.nevadacurrent.com/2018 /10/24/guest-op-ed-hellers-penchant-for-privatizing-hurts-veterans-health-care/.

37. Jasper Craven and Suzanne Gordon, "Is This Hedge-Fund Titan Greasing the Levers for Privatizing the Veterans Health Administration?," *The Nation*, April 12, 2018, https://www.thenation.com/article/archive/is-this-hedge-fund-titan-greasing -the-levers-for-privatizing-the-veterans-health-administration/.

38. Paul Sullivan, "Disgraced Hedge Fund Manager Focuses on Aiding Veterans," *New York Times*, November 4, 2016, https://www.nytimes.com/2016/11/06/giving /disgraced-hedge-fund-manager-focuses-on-aiding-veterans.html.

39. Sarah Kleiner, "Veterans Charity Raises Millions to Help Those Who've Served, but Telemarketers Are Pocketing Most of It," Center for Public Integrity, last modified January 5, 2018, https://publicintegrity.org/politics/veterans-charities /veterans-charity-raises-millions-to-help-those-whove-served-but-telemarketers-are -pocketing-most-of-it/.

40. "'An Intolerable Fraud,'" editorial, *New York Times*, February 8, 2008, https:// www.nytimes.com/2008/02/08/opinion/08fri1.html.

41. See Emma Moore et al., "Funding Flows in the Sea of Goodwill: An Analysis of Major Funders in the Veteran-Serving Nonprofit Space," Center for a New American Security, May 28, 2019, https://www.cnas.org/publications/reports/funding-flows -in-the-sea-of-goodwill. In 2015 Wounded Warrior took in more revenue than the American Legion and the Veterans of Foreign Wars combined.

42. Chip Reid and Jennifer Janisch, "CBS News Investigates Wounded Warrior Proj-ect," CBS News, March 11, 2016, https://www.cbsnews.com/news/cbs-news-investigates -wounded-warrior-project-spending/.

43. Dave Philipps, "Wounded Warrior Project Spends Lavishly on Itself, Insiders Say," *New York Times*, January 27, 2016, https://www.nytimes.com/2016/01/28/us/wounded -warrior-project-spends-lavishly-on-itself-ex-employees-say.html.

44. Wounded Warrior Project, "Wounded Warrior Project Announces Changes to Maximize Impact," news release, August 31, 2016, https://www.woundedwarriorproject .org/featured-campaign/wounded-warrior-project-announces-changes-to-maximize -impact.

45. Lynnsey Gardner, "Charity Watchdog Drops Wounded Warrior Project from Watch List," WJXT Channel 4, October 3, 2016, https://www.news4jax.com/news/2016/10/03/charity-watchdog-drops-wounded-warrior-project-from-watch-list/.

46. Thom Tillis, "Senator Tillis Discusses Why the Independence Fund Matters," video, YouTube, August 31, 2020, https://www.youtube.com/watch?v=IFNudb6cyNk.

47. Nicholas Confessore, "Veterans, Feeling Abandoned, Stand by Donald Trump," *New York Times*, November 2, 2016, https://www.nytimes.com/2016/11/03/us/politics/donald-trump-veterans.html.

48. Jasper Craven, "Trump's Favorite Veterans Charity Has Been Very Good for Its CEO. What Now?," *Mother Jones*, November 13, 2020, https://www.motherjones.com/politics/2020/11/the-independence-fund-donald-trump-veterans/.

49. Jasper Craven and Suzanne Gordon, "As the Veteran Suicide Crisis Persists, Washington Turns to Snake Oil and Swamp Creatures," *Battle Borne*, September 24, 2020, https://battleborne.substack.com/p/as-the-veteran-suicide-crisis-persists.

50. L. Longley, "Boots on the Ground: How Corporate Foundations Are Supporting Veterans," *Inside Philanthropy*, July 5, 2019, https://www.insidephilanthropy.com/home/2019/7/5/boots-on-the-ground-how-corporate-foundations-are-supporting-veterans.

51. US Department of Veterans Affairs, "PREVENTS: Supplemental Materials for the PREVENTS Roadmap," 31, https://www.va.gov/PREVENTS/docs/PREVENTS-Supplemental-Materials-for-the-Roadmap-508.pdf, accessed June 17, 2020.

52. US Department of Veterans Affairs, "PREVENTS," 33–34.

53. Jake Alimahomed-Wilson and Ellen Reese, eds., *The Cost of Free Shipping: Amazon in the Global Economy* (London: Pluto, 2020), 275–81.

54. N. Bose, "Amazon's Surveillance Can Boost Output and Possibly Limit Unions—Study," Reuters, September 15, 2020, https://www.reuters.com/article/us-amazon-com-workers-surveillance/amazons-surveillance-can-boost-output-and-possibly-limits-unions-study-idUSKBN25R2L1.

55. Bernie Sanders, "Navy Veteran Experiences Amazon's Horrific Working Conditions," video, Facebook Watch, July 19, 2018, https://www.facebook.com/senatorsanders/videos/navy-veteran-experiences-amazons-horrific-working-conditions/10157162842017908/.

56. Ben Fox Rubin, "Amazon or the Military: Warehouse Bosses Pressured 3 Workers to Choose," CNET, August 24, 2019, https://www.cnet.com/news/amazon-or-the-military-warehouse-bosses-pressured-3-workers-to-choose/.

57. As quoted in Jodi Kantor, Karen Weise, and Grace Ashford, "The Amazon That Customers Don't See," *New York Times*, June 15, 2021, https://www.nytimes.com/interactive/2021/06/15/us/amazon-workers.html.

58. N. Sturdivant, "Raleigh Military Veteran Finds New Opportunity as He Works to Fulfill Holiday Orders," CBS17.com, December 21, 2020, https://www.cbs17.com/news/local-news/wake-county-news/raleigh-military-veteran-finds-new-opportunity-as-he-works-to-fulfill-holiday-orders/.

59. Annie Palmer, "'Amazon Is Not Taking Care of Us': Warehouse Workers Say They're Struggling to Get Paid Despite Sick Leave Policy," CNBC, April 8, 2020, https://

www.cnbc.com/2020/04/08/amazon-warehouse-workers-say-they-struggle-to-get
-paid-despite-sick-leave-policy.html.

60. J. Conley, "As Retail Giants Enjoy Soaring Profits, Workers Demand Hazard
Pay amid Soaring Pandemic," Common Dreams, November 24, 2020, https://www
.commondreams.org/news/2020/11/24/retail-giants-enjoy-soaring-profits-workers
-demand-hazard-pay-amid-soaring-pandemic?cd-0.

61. T. Bray and C. Hoffman, "We Have a Question for Jeff Bezos and Other Billionaires," *New York Times*, July 29, 2020, https://www.nytimes.com/2020/07/29/opinion
/amazon-union-congress-antitrust.html.

62. J. Greene, "Amazon Warehouse Workers in Alabama File to Hold Unionization Vote," *Washington Post*, November 24, 2020, https://www.washingtonpost.com
/technology/2020/11/23/amazon-warehouse-workers-union/?ut.

63. D. Dayen, "USAA Grabs Coronavirus Checks from Military Families," *American
Prospect*, April 16, 2020, https://prospect.org/coronavirus/usaa-bank-grabs-stimulus
-checks-from-military-families/.

64. Dayen, "USAA Grabs Coronavirus Checks."

65. Jamie Court, "Drug Companies against Prop 61 Repeat Rent-a-Vet Strategy,"
Consumer Watchdog, September 27, 2016, https://consumerwatchdog.org/blog/drug
-companies-against-prop-61-repeat-rent-vet-strategy.

66. Travis Tritten, "House Passes Asbestos Bill over Veterans' Objections," *Stars and
Stripes*, January 8, 2016, https://www.stripes.com/news/house-passes-asbestos-bill
-over-veterans-objections-1.387802.

67. Travis Tritten, "Lobbying Efforts for Asbestos Bill Fueled Infighting among
Vets," *Stars and Stripes*, January 7, 2016, https://www.stripes.com/news/lobbying
-efforts-for-asbestos-bill-fueled-infighting-among-vets-1.387612.

68. Jamie Court, "Drug Companies."

69. Luke Broadwater, "Democrats, Progressive to Moderate, Press Biden to Embrace Medicare Expansion," *New York Times*, May 27, 2021, https://www.nytimes.com
/2021/05/27/us/politics/medicare-expansion-biden.html.

CHAPTER 4: LAST STAND OF THE LEGION POST?

1. Henry Howard, "Post Evolves from a Time of Discrimination," American Legion,
September 11, 2016, https://www.legion.org/membership/234033/post-evolves-time
-discrimination.

2. American Legion, "Preamble to the Constitution," https://www.legion.org
/preamble, accessed December 10, 2020.

3. Jeff Stoffer, "Our WWII Story: We Are Comrades Now," American Legion, August 26,
2020, https://www.legion.org/magazine/250024/our-wwii-story-we-are-comrades
-now.

4. Philip M. Callaghan, "The Road to a Better GI Bill," American Legion, August 1,
2008, https://www.legion.org/education/911gibill.

5. Patricia Kime, "After Decades of Fighting, the Blue Water Navy Benefits Bill
Is Now a Law," *Military.com*, June 26, 2019, https://www.military.com/daily
-news/2019/06/26/after-decades-fighting-blue-water-navy-benefits-bill-now-law
.html.

6. Mike Enzi, "Enzi Statement on the Blue Water Navy Vietnam Veterans Act of 2017," news release, December 17, 2018, https://www.enzi.senate.gov/public/index.cfm /2018/12/blue-water-navy-vietnam-veterans-act-of-2017.

7. Suzanne Gordon and Phillip Longman, "Longman-Gordon Report—VA Healthcare: A System Worth Saving," American Legion, 2017, https://www.legion.org /publications/238801/longman-gordon-report-va-healthcare-system-worth-saving.

8. During his fifty years in the labor movement, one coauthor of this book, Steve Early, participated in countless union meetings held in veterans halls; when he retired from active duty as a national staff member of the Communications Workers of America in 2007, his retirement party was held at a VFW Hall in West Medford, Massachusetts.

9. The traditional VSOs are federally chartered as "Patriotic and National Organizations." Their role in helping members file and pursue claims for veterans' benefits administered by the VA is officially recognized by the VA secretary. See US Department of Veterans Affairs, "Directory of Veterans Service Organizations," https://www.va.gov/vso/.

10. Steven B. Brooks, "Pompeo: Americanism Means Recognizing America as 'an Exceptional Nation,'" American Legion, August 27, 2019, https://www.legion.org/accountable /246899/pompeo-americanism-means-recognizing-america-exceptional-nation.

11. Joe Allen, "The American Legion Is Not Your Friend," Jacobin, August 5, 2019, https://www.jacobinmag.com/2019/08/american-legion-history-world-war-veterans -socialists-red-scare.

12. Allen, "The American Legion."

13. James Mauer, It Can Be Done: The Autobiography of James Hudson Maurer (New York: Rand School Press, 1938).

14. Jasper Craven, "The Exclusionary White Men of the American Legion," New Republic, August 28, 2020, https://newrepublic.com/article/159112/american-legion -racism-sexism-history.

15. Michael J. Bennett, When Dreams Came True: The GI Bill and the Making of Modern America (Washington, DC: Brassey's, 1996), 64.

16. Lauren Katzenberg, "When Veterans Camped for Pay," New York Times, June 20, 2020, 2.

17. Bennett, When Dreams, 61.

18. Daniel A. Sjursen, Patriotic Dissent: America in the Age of Endless War (Berkeley, CA: Heyday, 2020), 90.

19. Bennett, When Dreams, 17.

20. Athan Theoharis, "The FBI and the American Legion Contact Program, 1940–1966," Political Science Quarterly 100, no. 2 (Summer 1985): 271–86.

21. American Veterans Committee records from the George Washington University Special Collections Research Center, https://searcharchives.library.gwu.edu /repositories/2/resources/305, accessed December 22, 2020.

22. Katharine Q. Seelye, "June Willenz, Champion of Women in the Military, Dies at 95," New York Times, May 24, 2020, https://www.nytimes.com/2020/05/24/us/june -willenz-dead.html.

23. Ron Carver, David Cortright, and Barbara Doherty, eds., *Waging Peace in Vietnam: US Soldiers and Veterans Who Opposed the War* (New York: New Village Press, 2019).

24. Nan Levinson, *War Is Not a Game: The New Antiwar Soldiers and the Movement They Built* (New Brunswick, NJ: Rutgers University Press, 2016), 29.

25. Jerry Lembcke, *The Spitting Image: Myth, Memory, and the Legacy of Vietnam* (New York: NYU Press, 2000), 54.

26. S. Brian Wilson, *Don't Thank Me for My Service: My Viet Nam Awakening to the Long History of US Lies* (Atlanta: Clarity, 2018), 247.

27. Levinson, *War Is Not a Game*.

28. John Kerry, *Every Day Is Extra* (New York: Simon & Schuster, 2018), 33.

29. Jasper Craven, "Veterans of Domestic Wars," *The Baffler*, April 28, 2020, https://thebaffler.com/salvos/veterans-of-domestic-wars-craven.

30. David E. Bonior, Steven Champlin, and Timothy Kolly, *The Vietnam Veteran: A History of Neglect* (New York: Praeger, 1984), 46.

31. "Those Who Served," editorial, *Washington Post*, January 9, 1977.

32. Bonior, Champlin, and Kolly, *Vietnam Veteran*, 79.

33. David E. Bonior, *Whip: Leading the Progressive Battle during the Rise of the Right* (Westport, CT: City Point Press, 2018), 98.

34. Bonior, *Whip*, 89–90.

35. Gerald Nicosia, *Home to War* (1997; rpt., Three Rivers Press, 2001), 596.

36. Bonior, Champlin, and Kolly, *Vietnam Veteran*, 114.

37. Jonathan Alter, *His Very Best: Jimmy Carter, a Life* (New York: Simon & Schuster, 2020), 587.

38. Kristi Garbrandt, "Veteran Service Organizations See Declining Numbers," *Willoughby (Ohio) News Herald*, December 18, 2017.

39. Jon R. Anderson, "Vision for a New VFW: The Story of Denver's Post 1," *Military Times*, July 18, 2015, https://www.militarytimes.com/veterans/2015/07/18/vision-for-a-new-vfw-the-story-of-denver-s-post-1/.

40. Patricia Murphy, "Some Young Veterans Abandon the American Legion in Favor of New Organizations," NPR, August 24, 2018, https://www.npr.org/2018/08/24/641705970/some-young-veterans-abandon-the-american-legion-in-favor-of-new-organizations.

41. Craven, "Exclusionary White Men."

42. D. Barnett, "National Commander: Kaepernick's Decision 'Highly Regrettable,'" American Legion, August 30, 2016, https://www.legion.org/commander/233933/national-commander-kaepernicks-decision-highly-regrettable.

43. Ed Lavandera, "Texas Democrat Fights for Survival in GOP Hotbed," CNN, October 8, 2010, https://www.cnn.com/2010/POLITICS/10/08/chet.edwards/index.html.

44. Pete Hegseth, "Government Health Care Equals Disaster," video, YouTube, December 9, 2013, https://www.youtube.com/watch?v=aV23c-FHkXQ.

45. "Obama's Stuck in a VA Echo Chamber," editorial, AZCentral, March 13, 2015, https://www.azcentral.com/story/opinion/editorial/2015/03/12/obama-phoenix-va/70242360/.

46. Jasper Craven, "The Congressman Who Turned the VA into a Lobbying Free-for-All," *Politico*, April 4, 2019, https://www.politico.com/magazine/story/2019/04/04/donald-trump-veterans-affairs-jeff-miller-226483.

47. Stephen Trynosky, *Beyond the Iron Triangle: Implications for the Veterans Health Administration in an Uncertain Policy Environment*, monograph (Fort Leavenworth, KS: School of Advanced Military Studies, 2014), https://cgsc.contentdm.oclc.org/digital/collection/p4013coll3/id/3283.

48. Commission on Care, "Final Report," June 30, 2016, https://s3.amazonaws.com/sitesusa/wp-content/uploads/sites/912/2016/07/Commission-on-Care_Final-Report_063016_FOR-WEB.pdf.

49. Dennis Wagner, "Deaths at Phoenix VA Hospital May Be Tied to Delayed Care," AZCentral, April 10, 2015, https://www.azcentral.com/story/news/politics/2014/04/10/deaths-phoenix-va-hospital-may-tied-delayed-care/7537521/.

50. Alicia Mundy, "The VA Isn't Broken, Yet," *Washington Monthly*, June 24, 2016, https://washingtonmonthly.com/magazine/maraprmay-2016/the-va-isnt-broken-.

51. US Department of Veterans Affairs, "Review of Alleged Patient Deaths, Patient Wait Times, and Scheduling Practices at the Phoenix VA Health Care System," Office of Inspector General, August 26, 2014, ii, https://www.va.gov/oig/pubs/VAOIG-14-02603-267.pdf.

52. Concerned Veterans for America Foundation, "The Care They've Earned," 2014, https://cvafoundation.org/the-care-theyve-earned/.

53. Craven, "Congressman Who Turned the VA."

54. The dismissal of two Phoenix administrators, Sharon Helman and Lance Robinson, was upheld in federal court, although both filed a further appeal. In a separate proceeding, Helman pled guilty to criminal charges of accepting vacations, airline tickets, and other perks from a lobbyist. See Dennis Wagner, "Snafu Forces VA to Reset Probe of Top Phoenix Managers," AZCentral, February 16, 2015, https://www.azcentral.com/story/news/arizona/investigations/2015/02/16/snafu-forces-va-reset-probe-top-phoenix-managers/23479453/.

55. Pew Research Center, "Beyond Distrust: How Americans View Their Government," November 23, 2015, https://www.pewresearch.org/politics/2015/11/23/beyond-distrust-how-americans-view-their-government/.

56. Dennis Wagner, "Arizona-Based VA Contractor Collected 'Tens of Millions' in Over Payments, Federal Audit Says," AZCentral, November 14, 2017, https://www.azcentral.com/story/news/local/arizona-investigations/2017/11/13/va-inspectors-question-millions-dollars-paid-triwest-veterans-healthcare-contract/737341001/.

57. Office of Inspector General, US Department of Veterans Affairs, Veterans Health Administration, "Audit of the Timeliness and Accuracy of Choice Payments Processed through the Fee Basis Claims System," December 21, 2017, ii, https://www.va.gov/oig/pubs/VAOIG-15-03036-47.pdf.

58. Wagner, "Arizona-Based VA Contractor."

59. Isaac Arnsdorf and Jon Greenberg, "The va's Private Care Program Gave Companies Billions and Vets Longer Waits," *ProPublica*, December 18, 2018, https://www.propublica.org/article/va-private-care-program-gave-companies-billions-and-vets-longer-waits.

60. Patricia Kime, "TriWest Settles Overpayment Dispute with va for $180 Million," *Military.com*, January 5, 2020, https://www.military.com/daily-news/2021/01/05/triwest-settles-overpayment-dispute-va-180-million.html.

61. Craven, "Congressman Who Turned the va."

62. TriWest Healthcare Alliance, "TriWest Community Partners," http://www.triwest.com/en/about-triwest/community-outreach/triwest-community-partners/, accessed December 28, 2020.

63. Joe Carlson, "Cleveland Clinic Cases Highlight Flaws in Safety Oversight," *Modern Healthcare*, June 7, 2014, https://www.modernhealthcare.com/article/20140607/MAGAZINE/306079939/cleveland-clinic-cases-highlight-flaws-in-safety-oversight.

64. Mundy, "va Isn't Broken."

65. RAND Corporation, "Assessment B (Health Care Capabilities)," US Department of Veterans Affairs, September 1, 2015, https://www.va.gov/opa/choiceact/documents/assessments/Assessment_B_Health_Care_Capabilities.pdf, xv–xvi.

66. Michael Blecker, "Letter of Dissent," *Stars and Stripes*, June 29, 2016, https://www.stripes.com/polopoly_fs/1.417806.1467833798!/menu/standard/file/Dissent%20Letter%20from%20Commissioner%20Michael%20Blecker%20-%206%2029%2016%20(1)-final.pdf.

67. Darin Selnick and Stewart Hickey, "Commission Report Dissent," June 30, 2016, https://freebeacon.com/wp-content/uploads/2016/07/COC-Commissioners-Report-Dissent-063016-1.pdf.

68. Concerned Veterans for America, "Fixing Veterans' Health Care: A Bipartisan Policy Taskforce," January 2016, https://cv4a.org/wp-content/uploads/2016/01/Fixing-Veterans-Healthcare.pdf.

69. Jeff Steele, "Examining Veterans Choice Program and the Future of Care in the Community," American Legion, June 6, 2017, https://www.legion.org/legislative/testimony/237716/examining-veterans-chouce-program-and-future-care-community.

70. David J. Shulkin, *It Shouldn't Be This Hard to Serve Your Country: Our Broken Government and the Plight of Veterans* (New York: PublicAffairs, 2019), 306.

71. Jerry Moran, "Senators McCain, Moran Introduce Legislation to Reform va into 21st Century Health Care System," December 4, 2017, https://www.moran.senate.gov/public/index.cfm/2017/12/senators-mccain-moran-introduce-legislation-to-reform-va-into-21st-century-health-care-system.

72. Craven, "Exclusionary White Men."

73. Trynosky, *Beyond the Iron Triangle*.

74. J. Craven, "The Life and Death of the Veteran Advocate," *Battle Borne*, October 6, 2020, https://battleborne.substack.com/p/the-life-and-death-of-the-veteran.

Epigraph: Jennifer Steinhauer, "Veterans' Groups Compete with Each Other and Struggle with the VA," *New York Times*, January 4, 2019, https://www.nytimes.com /2019/01/04/us/politics/veterans-service-organizations.html.

1. Student Veterans of America, "About SVA," September 16, 2020, https:// studentveterans.org/about/.

2. Kayla Williams and Lindsay Church, "The 'Big Six' Veteran Service Organizations (VSOS) Have Mostly Chosen Not to Address the Issue of Racism in America and in the Veteran Community in the Midst of the George Floyd Protests," *Task and Purpose*, June 9, 2020, https://taskandpurpose.com/analysis/veteran-service-organizations -black-lives-matter/.

3. Dave Philipps, "Wounded Warrior Project Spends Lavishly on Itself, Insiders Say," *New York Times*, January 27, 2016, https://www.nytimes.com/2016/01/28/us /wounded-warrior-project-spends-lavishly-on-itself-ex-employees-say.html.

4. Steve Early and Suzanne Gordon, "A Common Defense: Mobilizing Veterans in Labor to Beat Trump and the GOP," *Labor Notes*, November 2, 2020, https:// labornotes.org/blogs/2020/10/common-defense-mobilizing-veterans-labor-beat -trump-and-gop.

5. IAVA insiders report that, after one recent data scrub of its email list, the number of IAVA contacts with up-to-date addresses numbered only about 200,000. As its annual revenue declined and staff size contracted, the group gave up its expensive leased office location in Midtown Manhattan and shifted to a smaller WeWork space near Wall Street.

6. Paul Rieckhoff, *Chasing Ghosts* (New York: NAL Caliber, 2007).

7. Nan Levinson, *War Is Not a Game: The New Antiwar Soldiers and the Movement They Built* (New Brunswick, NJ: Rutgers University Press, 2016), 77–78.

8. Carl Hulse, "Iraq Veteran Will Deliver War Critique for Democrats," *New York Times*, May 1, 2004, https://www.nytimes.com/2004/05/01/us/iraq-veteran-will-deliver -war-critique-for-democrats.html.

9. Hulse, "Iraq Veteran."

10. Leo Shane III, "IAVA Attracts the Spotlight—and Detractors," *Stars and Stripes*, September 5, 2012, https://www.stripes.com/iava-attracts-the-spotlight-and-detractors -1.188171.

11. See Dahr Jamail's *The Will to Resist: Soldiers Who Refuse to Fight in Iraq and Afghanistan* (Chicago: Haymarket Books, 2009). For a first-person account of an Army Ranger's fight for conscientious objector (CO) status, see Rory Fanning's *Worth Fighting For: An Army Ranger's Journey out of the Military and across America* (Chicago: Haymarket Books, 2014). Fanning estimates there may have been as many as sixty thousand post-9/11 enlisted men and women who sought CO status.

12. Levinson, *War Is Not a Game*, 77–78.

13. Iraq and Afghanistan Veterans of America (IAVA), "Veteran Advocate," November 12, 2020, https://iava.org/veteran-advocacy/.

14. IAVA, "2012 Impact Report," https://iava.org/iavas-2012-annual-impact-report/, accessed October 7, 2021.

15. "The New Greatest Generation" (cover), *Time*, August 29, 2011, http://content
.time.com/time/covers/0,16641,20110829,00.html.

16. Bryant Jordan, "IAVA Chief Criticizes Sanders as 'Apologist' for Scandal-Riddled
VA," *Military.com*, September 29, 2015, https://www.military.com/daily-news/2015/09
/29/iava-chief-criticizes-sanders-apologist-scandal-riddled-va.html.

17. Richard A. Oppel Jr., "American Legion, Citing Problems, Calls for Veterans
Secretary to Resign," *New York Times*, May 7, 2014, https://www.nytimes.com/2014/05
/08/us/american-legion-citing-problems-calls-for-veterans-secretary-to-resign.html.

18. IAVA, "Veteran Advocate."

19. IAVA, "IAVA Financials," November 23, 2020, https://iava.org/about/iava
-financials/.

20. IAVA, "IAVA's 2018 Impact Report," 18, https://iava.org/iavas-2018-impact
-report/, accessed January 22, 2021.

21. IAVA, "IAVA's Annual Heroes Gala," https://iava.org/heroes-gala/, accessed
December 19, 2020.

22. Jasper Craven and Suzanne Gordon, "VA's Mental Health Care Crisis Draws
Private Firms Pitching Dubious PTSD Treatments," *Reveal*, August 29, 2018, https://
revealnews.org/article/vas-mental-health-care-crisis-draws-private-firms-pitching
-dubious-ptsd-treatments/.

23. Jasper Craven and Suzanne Gordon, "Unhealthy Skepticism," *Washington
Monthly*, July/August 2018.

24. Paul Rieckhoff, letter to Paul Glastris, editor in chief of *Washington Monthly*,
October 18, 2018, authors' personal collection.

25. Rachel Kimerling et al., "Access to Mental Health Care among Women Veterans:
Is VA Meeting Women's Needs?," *Med Care* 53, no. 4, suppl. 1 (2015): S97–S104, https://
pubmed.ncbi.nlm.nih.gov/25767985/.

26. Suzanne Gordon, *Wounds of War: How the VA Delivers Health, Healing, and
Hope to the Nation's Veterans* (Ithaca, NY: Cornell University Press, 2018), 117–29.

27. Kayla Williams, "As VA's National Baby Shower Winds Down, Services for
Women Veterans Will Continue to Ramp Up," *Vantage Point* (US Department of
Veterans Affairs), May 15, 2018, https://www.blogs.va.gov/VAntage/48440/vas-national
-baby-shower-winds-services-women-veterans-will-continue-ramp/.

28. Allison Jaslow, "Cultural Change Needed at VA to Support Women Veterans," *Philadelphia Inquirer*, June 4, 2017, https://www.inquirer.com/philly/opinion
/commentary/20170605_Cultural_change_needed_at_VA_to_support_women
_veterans.html.

29. Emily Wax-Thibodeaux, "VA Employees Wanted a Gender-Neutral Mission Statement. The Agency Refused," *Washington Post*, April 28, 2019, https://www
.washingtonpost.com/news/checkpoint/wp/2018/02/14/va-employees-wanted-a
-gender-neutral-mission-statement-the-agency-refused/.

30. Suzanne Gordon and Jasper Craven, "Trump's War on Veterans," *American
Prospect*, April 7, 2020, https://prospect.org/health/trump-war-on-veterans/.

31. Glassdoor, "IAVA Reviews," https://www.glassdoor.com/Reviews/IAVA-Reviews
-E505674.htm, accessed December 19, 2020.

32. Ward Carroll, "Paul Rieckhoff Wants Vets to Help America 'Bring the Temperature Down,'" *We Are the Mighty*, October 30, 2020, https://www.wearethemighty.com /mighty-trending/paul-rieckhoff-wants-vets-to-help-america-bring-the-temperature -down/.

33. Carroll, "Paul Rieckhoff."

34. IAVA, "Statement of Jeremy Butler, Chief Executive Officer of Iraq and Afghanistan Veterans of America, before the Senate and House Veterans' Affairs Committees," March 7, 2018, https://www.veterans.senate.gov/imo/media/doc/4%20-%20IAVA%20 Testimony%2003.07.19.pdf.

35. VoteVets, "About," https://www.votevets.org/about, accessed January 21, 2021.

36. VoteVets, "PAC Profile," https://www.opensecrets.org/political-action-committees -pacs/C00418897/summary/2020, accessed December 19, 2020.

37. VetVoice Foundation, "About," https://www.vetvoicefoundation.org/about, accessed January 21, 2021.

38. VoteVets, "About."

39. Jennifer Steinhauer, "Two Veterans Groups, Left and Right, Join Forces against the Forever Wars," *New York Times*, March 16, 2019, https://www.nytimes.com/2019/03 /16/us/politics/vote-vets-concerned-veterans-america.html.

40. Jasper Craven, "Two Marine Vets with Divergent Worldviews Team Up to End the Forever Wars," *Battle Borne*, September 8, 2020, https://battleborne.substack.com /p/two-marine-vets-with-divergent-worldviews-15c.

41. Jennifer Steinhauer, "Trump Pentagon Purge Could Accelerate His Goal to Pull Troops from Afghanistan," *New York Times*, November 13, 2020, https://www.nytimes .com/2020/11/13/us/politics/trump-afghanistan-troops.html.

42. Jennifer Steinhauer, "Fox Host's 'America First' Shift Makes an Exception for Trump's Iran Strike," *New York Times*, January 6, 2020, https://www.nytimes.com/2020 /01/06/us/politics/pete-hegseth-trump-fox-news.html.

43. VoteVets, "About."

44. Jasper Craven, "Pete Buttigieg and the Democrats' Veteran Problem," *New Republic*, February 11, 2020, https://newrepublic.com/article/156531/pete-buttigieg -democrats-veteran-problem.

45. Carrie Levine, "'Dark Money': A Pro-veteran Nonprofit's Political Weapon," Center for Public Integrity, June 1, 2016, https://publicintegrity.org/politics/dark -money-a-pro-veteran-nonprofits-political-weapon/.

46. For more on the personal background and antiwar movement activism of Brittany DeBarros, see the longer biographical profile in Michael Messner's *Unconventional Combat: Intersectional Action in the Veterans' Peace Movement* (New York: Oxford University Press, 2021).

47. Anuradha Bhagwati, *Unbecoming: A Memoir of Disobedience* (New York: Atria Books, 2020).

48. Yvonne Sanchez, "Sen. Martha McSally Reveals She Was Raped by Superior Officer while in the Air Force," AZCentral, March 7, 2019, https://www.azcentral.com /story/news/politics/arizona/2019/03/06/martha-mcsally-reveals-she-raped-superior -officer-air-force/3082201002/.

49. Bhagwati, *Unbecoming*, 20.

50. Bhagwati, *Unbecoming*, 202.

51. Candice Bernd, "As Trump Threatens to Send Military into Cities, Some GIS Refuse to Comply," *Truthout*, June 3, 2020, https://truthout.org/articles/as-trump -threatens-to-send-military-into-cities-some-gis-refuse-to-comply/.

52. Brittany DeBarros, "Time's Up Common Defense," *Medium*, February 5, 2019, https://medium.com/timesupprogressives/times-up-common-defense -3a0e0795cfod.

53. DeBarros, "Time's Up."

54. Bhagwati, *Unbecoming*, 270.

55. Bhagwati, *Unbecoming*, 209, 211.

56. Bhagwati, *Unbecoming*, 211.

57. Bhagwati, *Unbecoming*, 212.

58. Angry Americans with Paul Rieckhoff, website, https://www.angryamericans.us/, accessed December 19, 2020.

59. Anuradha Bhagwati, "Donald Trump Is Getting It Right on Veterans Care," *New York Times*, February 4, 2019, https://www.nytimes.com/2019/02/03/opinion/trump -veterans-health-care.html.

60. Rick Porter, "Freida Pinto to Star in Military Drama from Entertainment One," *Hollywood Reporter*, December 19, 2019, https://www.hollywoodreporter.com/live -feed/freida-pinto-star-military-drama-eone-1263769.

61. Bhagwati, *Unbecoming*, 34.

62. Reid Wilson, "DCCC Exec Resigns amid Furor over Minority Representation," *The Hill*, July 29, 2019, https://thehill.com/homenews/campaign/455179-dccc-exec -resigns-amid-furor-over-minority-representation.

63. Sanford School of Public Policy at Duke University, "Allison Jaslow," https://hart .sanford.duke.edu/faculty/allison-jaslow/, accessed January 22, 2021.

64. Pam Campos-Palma, website, https://www.pamcampos.com/workwithme, accessed January 22, 2021.

CHAPTER 6: A VA HEALTHCARE STRUGGLE

1. Suzanne Gordon and Jasper Craven, "Trump's War on Veterans," *American Prospect*, April 7, 2020, https://prospect.org/health/trump-war-on-veterans/.

2. J. Craven, "Sanders-Led Law Hasn't Cured Veterans Health Care Issues," VTDigger, October 16, 2017, from https://vtdigger.org/2017/10/16/sanders-led-law-hasnt -cured-veterans-health-care-issues/.

3. Carrie M. Farmer, Susan D. Hosek, and David M. Adamson, "Balancing Demand and Supply for Veterans' Health Care," RAND Corporation, 13, https://www.rand.org /pubs/periodicals/health-quarterly/issues/v6/n1/12.html; US Department of Veterans Affairs, FY 2021 Budget Submission, February 2021, https://www.va.gov/budget/docs /summary/fy2021VAbudgetInBrief.pdf.

4. Aaron Glantz, "Understaffed Veterans Affairs Scrambles to Confront COVID-19," *Reveal*, March 16, 2020, https://revealnews.org/article/understaffed-veterans-affairs -scrambles-to-confront-covid-19/.

5. US Department of Veterans Affairs, "Concerns with Access and Delays in Outpatient Mental Health Care at the New Mexico VA Health Care System," Report #17-05572-170, Office of Inspector General, July 23, 2019, https://www.va.gov/oig/pubs /VAOIG-17-05572-170.pdf.

6. Courtney Kube and Rich Gardella, "Former Therapist: VA Is Hurting Mental Health Care for Combat Veterans at Its Vet Centers," NBC News, November 4, 2019, https://www.nbcnews.com/health/health-care/former-therapist-va-hurting-mental -health-care-combat-veterans-its-n1075781; J. Greenberg and I. Arnsdorf, "How We Crunched the Numbers on the VA's Private Care Program," *ProPublica*, December 18, 2018, https://www.propublica.org/article/how-we-crunched-the-numbers-on-the-vas -private-care-program.

7. Gale Holland, "Veterans Protest the Gutting of West L.A. PTSD Therapy Groups," *Los Angeles Times*, December 29, 2018, https://www.latimes.com/local/lanow/la-me -ptsd-group-shutdown-20181229-story.html.

8. Carson Gerber, "Kokomo VA Clinic Closes Less Than a Year after Opening," *Kokomo (IN) Tribune*, March 24, 2019, https://www.kokomotribune.com/news/kokomo -va-clinic-closes-less-than-a-year-after-opening/article_e95df948-4cd5-11e9-b220 -a7763ad04263.html.

9. Mary Frost, "Veterans Fear the Worst as Brooklyn VA Hospital Announces Cutbacks," *Brooklyn Eagle*, May 31, 2018, https://brooklyneagle.com/articles/2018/05 /31/veterans-fear-the-worst-as-brooklyn-va-hospital-announces-cutbacks/; Stephen T. Watson, "Advocates Decry Closing of Veterans Affairs Outpatient Program in Amherst," *Buffalo (NY) News*, August 9, 2018, https://buffalonews.com/news/local /advocates-decry-closing-of-veterans-affairs-outpatient-program-in-amherst/article _61f727bd-8f4a-55a1-9533-a86553226b98.html.

10. Lisa Rein, "Exodus from Trump's VA: When the Mission of Caring for Veterans 'Is No Longer a Reason for People to Stay,'" *Washington Post*, May 3, 2018, https:// www.washingtonpost.com/politics/who-wants-to-work-there-now-trumps-ronny -jackson-fiasco-may-be-the-least-of-vas-worries/2018/05/02/e1c64af0-44cf-11e8-8569 -26fda6b404c7_story.html.

11. Jeremy Diamond, "Trump Pledges to Reform VA, Give Vets Access to Private Care," CNN, October 31, 2015, https://www.cnn.com/2015/10/31/politics/donald-trump -veterans-norfolk/index.html.

12. Jasper Craven, "The Congressman Who Turned the VA into a Lobbying Free-for-All," *Politico*, April 4, 2019, https://www.politico.com/magazine/story/2019/04/04 /donald-trump-veterans-affairs-jeff-miller-226483.

13. Joe Davidson, "VA in 'Critical Condition, Requires Intensive Care,' but Improving, Says Boss," *Washington Post*, May 17, 2017, https://www.washingtonpost.com /news/powerpost/wp/2017/05/31/va-in-critical-condition-requires-intensive-care-but -improving-says-boss/.

14. David Shulkin, Shereef Elnahal, Ellen Maddock, and Megan Shaheen, eds., *Best Care Everywhere* (Washington, DC: US Department of Veterans Affairs, 2017).

15. Suzanne Gordon, "Why Is the VA Hiding a PR Goldmine?," *Washington Monthly*, December 8, 2017, https://washingtonmonthly.com/2017/12/08/why-is-the-va-hiding -a-pr-goldmine/.

16. David J. Shulkin, *It Shouldn't Be This Hard to Serve Your Country: Our Broken Government and the Plight of Veterans* (New York: PublicAffairs, 2019), 327.

17. Tom Sullivan, "Q&A: David Shulkin on the VA's 'Superpower,'" *Health Evolution*, October 23, 2019, https://www.healthevolution.com/insider/qa-david-shulkin-on-the -vas-superpower/.

18. Shulkin, *It Shouldn't Be This Hard to Serve Your Country*, 306–7.

19. US Department of Veterans Affairs, "Administrative Investigation: VA Secretary and Delegation Travel to Europe," Office of Inspector General, February 14, 2018.

20. Maegan Vazquez, "Shulkin Says He Was Fired via Trump Tweet," CNN, April 2, 2018, https://www.cnn.com/2018/04/02/politics/shulkin-tweet-fired-cnntv/index.html.

21. Lisa Rein and Josh Dawsey, "Trump Loyalist at VA Forced Out after Collecting Pay but Doing Little Work," *Washington Post*, December 11, 2018, https://www .washingtonpost.com/politics/there-were-times-i-didnt-have-a-lot-to-do-trump -loyalist-at-va-forced-out-after-collecting-pay-but-doing-little-work/2018/12/11 /26e4704a-fcb7-11e8-ad40-cdfd0eodd65a_story.html.

22. Daniel Van Schooten, "'Terrified' of Retaliation inside Veterans Affairs Whistleblower Office," PoGo, March 5, 2020, https://www.pogo.org/investigation/2020/03 /terrified-of-retaliation-inside-veterans-affairs-whistleblower-office/.

23. Jasper Craven, "Abusing Those Who Served," *The Intercept*, July 8, 2019, https:// theintercept.com/2019/07/08/veterans-affairs-police-va/.

24. Jasper Craven, "Trump's War on VA Workers Is Exposing Them to the Coronavirus," *New Republic*, April 15, 2020, https://newrepublic.com/article/157293/trumps -war-va-workers-exposing-coronavirus.

25. Jasper Craven, "Soldier of Fortune," *The Baffler*, July 9, 2020, https://thebaffler .com/latest/soldier-of-fortune-craven.

26. Lawrence Wilkerson, "A Traitor at the VA," *LA Progressive*, May 29, 2020, https:// www.laprogressive.com/traitor-at-the-va/.

27. Veterans of Foreign Wars, "Veterans Choice Program Second Report," May 11, 2015, https://www.vfw.org//media/VFWSite/Files/Advocacy/SecondVeteransChoicePr ogramReport.pdf?la=en.

28. Terri Tanielian et al., "Ready or Not? Assessing the Capacity of New York State Health Care Providers to Meet the Needs of Veterans," RAND Corporation, 2018, https:// www.rand.org/pubs/research_reports/RR2298.html.

29. Nicholas Fandos, "Senate Approval Is Last Hurdle for an Overhaul of Veterans' Health Care," *New York Times*, May 24, 2018, https://www.nytimes.com/2018/05/23/us /politics/veterans-health-care.html.

30. US Department of Health and Human Services, "Report to Congress on the Nation's Substance Abuse and Mental Health Workforce Issues," SAMHSA, January 24, 2013, https://store.samhsa.gov/shin/content/PEP13-RTC-BHWORK/PEP13-RTC -BHWORK.pdf.

31. David Mechanic, "More People Than Ever Before Are Receiving Behavioral Health Care in the United States, but Gaps and Challenges Remain," *Health Affairs* 33, no. 8 (August 2014): 1416–24; T. F. Bishop, M. J. Press, S. Keyhani, and H. A. Pincus, "Acceptance of Insurance by Psychiatrists and the Implications for Access to Mental Health Care," *JAMA Psychiatry* 71, no. 2 (February 2014): 176–81.

32. Mental Illness Policy Org, "About 50% of Individuals with Severe Psychiatric Disorders (3.5 Million People) Are Receiving No Treatment," http://mentalillnesspolicy.org /consequences/percentage-mentally-ill-untreated.html, accessed October 4, 2021.

33. US Department of Veterans Affairs, "State of the VA Fact Sheet," Office of Public Affairs, May 31, 2017, http://www.blogs.va.gov/VAntage/wp-content/uploads/2017/05 /StateofVA_FactSheet_5-31-2017.pdf.

34. Veterans Health Administration, "Pending Appointment and Electronic Wait List Summary—National, Facility, and Division Level Summaries Wait Time Calculated from Preferred Date for the Period Ending: 5/15/2017," https://www.va .gov/HEALTH/docs/DR70_052017_Pending_and_EWL_Biweekly_Desired_Date _Division.pdf, accessed October 7, 2021.

35. US Senate Committee on Veterans Affairs, "Pending Health Care Legislation Committee Hearing," video, July 11, 2017, https://www.veterans.senate.gov/hearings /pending-health-care-legislation-07112017.

36. Veterans Healthcare Policy Institute, "Veterans Deserve Accountability from Private Healthcare Providers," December 18, 2018, https://www.veteranspolicy.org/the-blog -2/2018/12/20/veterans-deserve-accountability-from-private-healthcare-providers.

37. Suzanne Gordon and Steve Early, "Vets and VA Workers Are MIA from Biden Transition," *American Prospect*, November 18, 2020, https://prospect.org/health/vets -and-va-workers-are-mia-from-biden-transition/.

38. Veterans of Foreign Wars, "Veterans Prefer VA Care" (report), September 25, 2015, https://www.vfw.org/media-and-events/latest-releases/archives/2015/9/vfw -report-veterans-prefer-va-care#:~.

39. Phillip Longman and Suzanne Gordon, "Longman-Gordon Report—VA Healthcare: A System Worth Saving," American Legion, September 2017, https://www.legion .org/publications/238801/longman-gordon-report-va-healthcare-system-worth -saving.

40. Disabled American Veterans, "Setting the Record Straight: Reform and Modernization of the VA Health Care System," https://www.dav.org/settingtherecordstraight/, accessed December 20, 2020.

41. Disabled American Veterans, "VSO Letter Supporting VA MISSION Act of 2018," May 7, 2018, https://www.dav.org/learn-more/news/2018/vso-letter-supporting-va -mission-act-of-2018/.

42. Nancy Pelosi, "Pelosi Statement on Passage of VA MISSION Act," May 23, 2018, https://www.speaker.gov/newsroom/51618-3.

43. Bernie Sanders, "Sanders to Vote No on Mission Act," Common Dreams, May 23, 2018, https://www.commondreams.org/newswire/2018/05/23/sanders-vote -no-va-mission-act.

44. Nicholas Fandos, "Senate Sends Major Overhaul of Veterans Health Care to Trump," *New York Times*, May 23, 2018, https://www.nytimes.com/2018/05/23/us /politics/veterans-health-care.html.

45. Donald J. Trump, "Remarks by President Trump at Signing of the VA Mission Act of 2018," https://www.whitehouse.gov/briefings-statements/remarks-president-trump -signing-va-mission-act-2018/, accessed January 9, 2021. Link no longer available.

46. Joe Davidson, "Trump Rejects Parts of va Law He Was 'Very Happy' to Sign," *Washington Post*, June 11, 2018, https://www.washingtonpost.com/news/powerpost /wp/2018/06/11/trump-challenges-parts-of-va-law-he-was-very-happy-to-sign/.

47. Jasper Craven, "Trump's Favorite Veterans Charity Has Been Very Good for Its ceo. What Now?," *Mother Jones*, November 13, 2020, https://www.motherjones.com /politics/2020/11/the-independence-fund-donald-trump-veterans/.

48. US Senate Veterans Affairs Committee, "Tester Leads 28 Senators in Demanding Answers on va Community Care Implementation," January 29, 2019, https:// www.veterans.senate.gov/newsroom/minority-news/tester-leads-28-senators-in -demanding-answers-on-va-community-care-implementation.

49. US Department of Veterans Affairs, "Report to Congress Health Care Standards for Quality (mission Act, Section 104)," March 2019, Appendix B, 2–3.

50. Jasper Craven and Suzanne Gordon, "The va Is Becoming a Temp Agency for Private Hospitals," *American Prospect*, January 30, 2020, https://prospect.org/health /the-va-is-becoming-a-temp-agency-for-private-hospitals/.

51. Abbie Bennett, "No Maximum Wait Time Set by va for Veterans," Connecting Vets, September 28, 2020, https://connectingvets.radio.com/articles/no-maximum -wait-time-set-by-va-for-veterans-community-care.

52. Isaac Arnsdorf, "va Was 'Taken Advantage Of' by Paying Billions in Fees, Secretary Says," *ProPublica*, December 19, 2018, https://www.propublica.org/article/va -secretary-robert-wilkie-testimony-va-mission-act.

53. Isaac Arnsdorf and Jon Greenberg, "The va's Private Care Program Gave Companies Billions and Vets Longer Waits," *ProPublica*, December 18, 2018, https://www .propublica.org/article/va-private-care-program-gave-companies-billions-and-vets -longer-waits.

54. Brad Racino, "Veterans and Their Therapists Decry San Diego va's Handling of Mental Health Care," Inewsource, November 18, 2020, https://inewsource.org/2020/11 /18/veterans-and-therapists-decry-san-diego-vas-mental-health-care/.

55. American Federation of Government Employees, "va Secretary to Congress: Filling 49,000 Vacancies Not a Priority," March 4, 2019, https://www.afge.org/article /va-secretary-to-congress-filling-49000-vacancies-not-a-priority/.

56. Suzanne Gordon and Jasper Craven, "The Best Health System to React to covid-19," *American Prospect*, March 20, 2020, https://prospect.org/coronavirus/the -best-health-system-to-react-to-covid-19/.

57. Clifford Marks, "America's Looming Primary-Care Crisis," *New Yorker*, July 25, 2020, https://www.newyorker.com/science/medical-dispatch/americas-looming -primary-care-crisis.

58. Jennifer Steinhauer, "v.a. Criticized for Effort to Keep Some Veterans Away from Private Care during Outbreak," *New York Times*, March 25, 2020, https://www .nytimes.com/2020/03/25/us/politics/coronavirus-veterans-mission-act-trump.html.

59. Steinhauer, "v.a. Criticized."

60. Leonie Heyworth et al., "Expanding Access through Virtual Care: The va's Early Experience with Covid-19," Commentary, nemj Catalyst, July 1, 2020, https:// catalyst.nejm.org/doi/full/10.1056/cat.20.0327.

61. Chris Serres, "VA Outreach Puts Minnesota Veterans on Vaccine Fast Track," *Minneapolis Star-Tribune*, March 25, 2021, https://www.startribune.com/va-outreach -puts-minnesota-veterans-on-vaccine-fast-track/600038449/.

62. Three months later, 70 percent of the VA's total workforce had provided proof of vaccination status and Secretary McDonough was being pressed to increase that number. See McDonough interview with Steve Inskeep and Quil Lawrence, "The Head of the VA Says the U.S. Failed Some Veterans for 30 Years," NPR, October 22, 2021, https://www.npr.org/2021/10/22/1048289046/the-head-of-the-va-says-the-u-s-failed -some-veterans-for-30-years.

63. Christopher T. Rentsch et al., "Covid-19 by Race and Ethnicity: A National Cohort Study of 6 Million United States Veterans," *PLOS Medicine*, May 17, 2020, https://www.ncbi.nlm.nih.gov/pmc/articles/PMC7273292/.

64. Pam Belluck, "Patients with Long Covid Face Worrisome Risks," *New York Times*, April 22, 2021, https://www.nytimes.com/2021/04/22/health/covid-patients -health-risks-long-term.html.

65. Johnny Diaz, "Two Charged in Coronavirus Outbreak at Veterans' Home That Left 76 Dead," *New York Times*, September 25, 2020, https://www.nytimes.com/2020 /09/25/us/veterans-home-holyoke-covid.html.

66. Joanne Kenen, Allan James Vestal, and Darius Tahir, "Sadness and Death: Inside the VA's State Nursing Home Disaster," *Politico*, August 24, 2021, https:// www.politico.com/news/2021/08/24/veterans-nursing-home-coronavirus-502558. As the inaccurate and misleading headline to this article illustrates, much COVID-related coverage of state veterans' homes wrongly conflated them with VA-run facilities.

67. US Department of Veterans Affairs, "VA Fourth Mission Summary," https://www .va.gov/health/coronavirus/statesupport.asp, accessed November 1, 2021.

68. Linda Ward-Smith, "What VA Nurses Need to See from the Biden Administration," *Morning Consult*, May 6, 2021, https://morningconsult.com/opinions/nurses -week-what-va-nurses-need-to-see-from-the-biden-administration/?.

69. Matt Shuham, "FEMA Diverted Masks from Veterans Hospitals, VA Official Says," *Talking Points Memo*, April 25, 2020, https://talkingpointsmemo.com/news /fema-diverted-masks-from-veterans-hospitals-va-official-says.

70. Sheila Elliott, "Care for Veterans," *Virginian-Pilot* (Norfolk, VA), March 23, 2020, https://www.pilotonline.com/opinion/letters/vp-ed-lets-0323-20200323 -cp7lulpvgveczf6oka6tacbkxi-story.html.

71. Sarah Jaffe, "A Better Health Care System?," *Progressive*, June 10, 2020, https:// progressive.org/magazine/a-better-health-care-system-jaffe/.

72. Christopher Rowland, "Anti-malarial Drug Trump Touted Is Linked to Higher Rates of Death in VA Coronavirus Patients, Study Says," *Washington Post*, April 21, 2020, https://www.washingtonpost.com/business/2020/04/21/anti-malarial-drug -trump-touted-is-linked-higher-rates-death-va-coronavirus-patients-study-says/.

73. Judd Legum, "The Real Scandal Isn't What Trump Said about Veterans. It's What He Did to Them," *Popular Information*, September 8, 2020, https://popular.info/p/the -real-scandal-isnt-what-trump.

74. Joseph Magagnoli, Siddharth Narendran, Felipe Pereira, Tammy Cummings, James W. Hardin, S. Scott Sutton, and Jayakrishna Ambati, "Outcomes of Hydroxychloroquine Usage in United States Veterans Hospitalized with Covid-19," *MedRxiv*, April 21, 2021, https://www.medrxiv.org/content/10.1101/2020.04.16 .20065920v1.full.pdf.

75. Josh Eidelson, "Head of Top U.S. Federal Union Resigns amid Harassment Claims," *Bloomberg*, February 28, 2020, https://www.bloomberg.com/news/articles /2020-02-28/head-of-top-u-s-federal-union-resigns-amid-harassment-claims.

76. Eli Rosenberg, "President of Federal Employee Union AFGE Takes Leave amid Sexual Harassment Investigation," *Washington Post*, October 28, 2019, https://www .washingtonpost.com/business/2019/10/28/president-federal-employee-union-afge -takes-leave-amid-sexual-harassment-investigation/.

77. Russ Read, "VA Blasts Federal Union for Allowing 'a Culture of Sexual Harassment' to Thrive at Highest Levels," *Washington (DC) Examiner*, November 23, 2019, https://www.washingtonexaminer.com/policy/defense-national-security/va-blasts -federal-union-for-allowing-a-culture-of-sexual-harassment-to-thrive-at-highest -levels.

78. Erich Wagner, "Vast Majority of VA Employees Have Either Witnessed or Experienced Racism at Work, Survey Finds," *Government Executive*, August 10, 2020, https://www.govexec.com/management/2020/08/vast-majority-va-employees-have -either-witnessed-or-experienced-racism-work-survey-finds/167583/.

79. Jasper Craven and Suzanne Gordon, "As the Veteran Suicide Crisis Persists, Washington Turns to Snake Oil and Swamp Creatures," *Battle Borne*, September 24, 2020, https://battleborne.substack.com/p/as-the-veteran-suicide-crisis-persists.

80. Dave Philips, "Gun Divide Poses Another Hurdle in Fight to Reduce Veterans' Suicides," *New York Times*, October 15, 2020, https://www.nytimes.com/2020/10/15/us /veterans-suicides-guns-firearms.html.

81. Code of Federal Regulations, "Petition for Rulemaking to Amend 38 C.F.R. §§ 3.12(A), 3.12(D), 17.34, 17.36(D) Regulations Interpreting 38 U.S.C. § 101(2) Requirement for Service 'Under Conditions Other Than Dishonorable,'" https://uploads-ssl .webflow.com/5ddda3d7ad8b1151b5d16cff/5efed0ac6dc9fc718786414b_Petition%20 to%20amend%20regulations%20implementing%2038%20USC%20101(2).pdf, accessed October 7, 2021.

82. US Department of Veterans Affairs, "Update and Clarify Regulatory Bars to Benefits Based on Character of Discharge," *Federal Register*, July 10, 2020, https://www .federalregister.gov/documents/2020/07/10/2020-14559/update-and-clarify-regulatory -bars-to-benefits-based-on-character-of-discharge.

83. Jasper Craven, "On His Way out the Door, Trump Privatizes Another Critical VA Service," *Battle Borne*, November 20, 2020, https://battleborne.substack.com/p/on-his -way-out-the-door-trump-privatizes.

84. Nikki Wentling, "GAO Finds VA Contractors Not Meeting Timeliness, Accuracy Standards on Exams," *Stars and Stripes*, November 13, 2018, https://www.stripes.com /news/veterans/gao-finds-va-contractors-not-meeting-timeliness-accuracy-standards -on-exams-1.556460.

85. Glassdoor, "Reviews: VES," 2020, https://www.glassdoor.com/Reviews/Veterans -Evaluation-Services-Reviews-E480923.htm.

86. Patty Ryan, "VA Contractor Sent Patients to Tampa Doctor as Prosecutors Tried to Send Him to Prison," *Tampa Bay Times*, August 23, 2015, https://www.tampabay .com/news/courts/criminal/va-contractor-sent-patients-to-tampa-doctor-as -prosecutors-tried-to-send/2242416/.

87. Jasper Craven, "The VA Is Socialism in Action. We Must Defend It from Privatization," *The Nation*, March 18, 2019, https://www.thenation.com/article/archive /veterans-administration-socialism-privatization/.

CHAPTER 7: PLAYING THE VETERAN CARD

Epigraph: Lindsay Schnell, "Teamwork Puts Women Veterans in Office," *USA Today*, November 23, 2018, https://www.emilyslist.org/news/entry/tough-talk-tough-women -new-house-members-come-together-to-form-the-badasses; Matt Flegenheimer, "Tammy Duckworth Is Nothing and Everything Like Joe Biden," *New York Times*, August 1, 2020, https://www.nytimes.com/2020/08/01/us/politics/tammy-duckworth -biden-vp.html.

1. Paul Rieckhoff, *Chasing Ghosts: A Soldier's Fight for America from Baghdad to Washington* (London: Penguin Publishing Group, 2006), 309.

2. Leo Shane III, "The Number of Veterans in Congress Will Drop to Lowest Level since at Least World War II," *Military Times*, December 2, 2020, https://www .militarytimes.com/news/pentagon-congress/2020/12/02/the-number-of-veterans-in -congress-will-drop-to-lowest-level-since-at-least-ww-ii/.

3. With Honor, home page, https://withhonor.org/, accessed December 13, 2020.

4. Jennifer Steinhauer, "Veterans Turned Lawmakers Form a Political Band of Like Minds," *New York Times*, April 7, 2019, https://www.nytimes.com/2019/04/06/us /politics/democrats-military-veterans.html.

5. Jennifer Steinhauer, "Female Veterans in Congress, and They Want Reinforcement," *New York Times*, May 10, 2019, https://www.nytimes.com/2019/05/09/us /politics/female-veterans-democrats-elections.html. VoteVets's conservative rival and sometimes ally, the Concerned Veterans of America, spent $6 million on congressional races in 2018, but according to its director, Nate Anderson, doesn't "believe in electing veterans simply because they are veterans. We believe in electing leaders who will advance good policy, and it's great if they happen to be veterans."

6. Carol Giacomo, "New to Congress, Wise to the World," *New York Times*, April 22, 2019, https://www.nytimes.com/2019/04/21/opinion/democratic-veterans-congress.html.

7. For more on the challenges that female veterans face when they seek elected office, see Rebecca Best, Kyleanne Hunter, and Katherine Hendricks Thomas, "Fighting for a Seat at the Table: Women's Military Service and Political Representation," *Journal of Veterans Studies*, 7 (2): 19–33, https://journal-veterans-studies.org/articles/10.21061 /jvs.v7i2.266/galley/298/download/.

8. John Kerry, *Every Day Is Extra* (New York: Simon & Schuster, 2018), 298.

9. Jennifer Steinhauer, "Confronting Ghosts of 2000 in South Carolina," *New York Times*, October 19, 2007, https://www.nytimes.com/2007/10/19/us/politics/19mccain.ht.

10. Dan Nowicki and Bill Muller, "McCain Profile," AZCentral, March 1, 2007, http://archive.azcentral.com/news/election/mccain/articles/2007/03/01/20070301mccainbio-chapter10.html.

11. "John McCain: The Ultimate Public Servant" (editorial), *San Francisco Chronicle*, August 26, 2018, https://www.sfchronicle.com/opinion/editorials/article/Editorial-John-McCain-the-ultimate-public-13183692.php.

12. Ken Rudin, "Long-Time War Hawk, Murtha Is an Angry Dove," NPR, November 18, 2005, https://www.npr.org/templates/story/story.php?storyId=5018733.

13. Jasper Craven, "Democrats Are Ignoring One Key Voting Group: Veterans," *New York Times*, October 10, 2018, https://www.nytimes.com/2018/10/10/magazine/veterans-democrats-midterm-elections.html.

14. Natasha Korecki, "Tammy Duckworth Bursts into VP Contention," *Politico*, July 12, 2020, https://www.politico.com/news/2020/07/12/tammy-duckworth-vp-contention-357234.

15. Kyle Swenson, "Rep. Duncan D. Hunter: Tequila Shots, Golf Outings and Airfare for Pet Alleged in Indictment," *Washington Post*, August 22, 2018, https://www.washingtonpost.com/news/morning-mix/wp/2018/08/22/how-duncan-d-hunter-a-house-conservative-star-imploded-following-campaign-spending-indictment/.

16. Eric Gordon, "Can Republican Rep. Duncan Hunter Keep His Southern California Seat?," *LA Progressive*, August 1, 2019, https://www.laprogressive.com/duncan-hunter/.

17. David Philipps, *Alpha: Eddie Gallagher and the War for the Soul of the Navy SEALS* (New York: Crown Publishing, 2021), 275.

18. For more on the Gallagher case, see Steve Early and Suzanne Gordon, "The Right Is Embracing the Reactionary Brutality of 'Special Operators' like Eddie Gallagher," *Jacobin*, October 22, 2021, https://jacobinmag.com/2021/10/spec-ops-eddie-gallagher-navy-seals-trump-military-celebrities.

19. Jason Kander, "Jason Kander," in *Why I Run: 35 Progressive Candidates Who Are Changing Politics*, ed. Kate Childs Graham (New York: Abrams Image, 2019), 107.

20. Dave Philipps, "Rising Star Pauses to Confront War's Demons," *New York Times*, August 26, 2019, https://www.nytimes.com/2019/08/25/us/jason-kander-ptsd.html.

21. Philipps, "Rising Star."

22. Philipps, "Rising Star."

23. Steve LeBlanc, "Military Vet Moulton Joins 2020 Presidential Race," AP News, April 22, 2019, https://apnews.com/article/bd9279193f814528a4d07eb3dbb96c25.

24. Seth Moulton, "Congressman Seth Moulton Introduces the Faster Care for Veterans Act," January 14, 2016, https://moulton.house.gov/press-releases/congressman-seth-moulton-introduces-the-faster-care-for-veterans-act.

25. Reid Epstein, "How Biden Could Learn from Conor Lamb's Victory in Trump Country," *New York Times*, August 16, 2020, https://www.nytimes.com/2020/08/16/us/politics/joe-biden-conor-lamb-trump.html?searchResultPosition=7.

26. Joe Violante, Steve Robertson, and Dennis Cullinan, "Nancy Pelosi—a Proven Leader for America's Veterans," *The Hill*, November 20, 2018, https://thehill.com/blogs/congress-blog/politics/417626-nancy-pelosi-a-proven-leader-for-americas-veterans.

27. Jennifer Steinhauer, "Two Veterans Groups, Left and Right, Join Forces against the Forever Wars," *New York Times*, March 17, 2019, https://www.nytimes.com/2019/03/16/us/politics/vote-vets-concerned-veterans-america.html.

28. Michael Gold, "An N.Y. Street Is Named for Robert E. Lee, Officials Want That Changed," *New York Times*, June 11, 2020, https://www.nytimes.com/2020/06/11/nyregion/general-lee-avenue-fort-hamilton-brooklyn.html.

29. Medea Benjamin and Nicolas J. S. Davies, "War, Peace, and Presidential Candidates," Code Pink, March 27, 2019, https://www.codepink.org/war_peace_and_presidential_candidates.

30. Catie Edmondson, "House Moves Again to Cut Off Support to Saudi War in Yemen," *New York Times*, July 11, 2019, https://www.nytimes.com/2019/07/11/us/politics/house-democrats-saudi-arabia.html.

31. Andrea Germanos, "More Testing, Not More Bombs," Common Dreams, May 19, 2020, https://www.commondreams.org/news/2020/05/19/more-testing-not-more-bombs-29-house-democrats-demand-cuts-pentagon-budget-amid.

32. Daniel Sjursen, *Ghost Riders of Baghdad: Soldiers, Civilians, and the Myth of the Surge* (Lebanon, NH: University Press of New England, 2015), 200.

33. Danny Sjursen, "Discredited Russian Bounty Story Exposes Media's Role in Status Quo," *Scheerpost*, September 28, 2020, https://scheerpost.com/2020/09/28/discredited-russian-bounty-story-exposes-medias-role-in-status-quo/.

34. Crow reportedly experienced significant backlash for his involvement in this bipartisan initiative, and, in the words of one congressional staffer, "it was a gigantic fuckup."

35. Nan Levinson, "The Vet Conundrum and America's Wars," *TomDispatch*, July 12, 2020, https://tomdispatch.com/nan-levinson-the-vet-conundrum-and-america-s-wars/.

36. Donald Shaw, "Dems Voting against Pentagon Cuts Got 3.4x More Money from the Defense Industry," *Sludge*, July 22, 2020, https://readsludge.com/2020/07/22/dems-voting-against-pentagon-cuts-got-3-4x-more-money-from-the-defense-industry/.

37. Matthew Hoh, "Heaven Protect Us from Men Who Live the Illusion of Danger," *CounterPunch*, February 26, 2020, https://www.counterpunch.org/2020/02/26/heaven-protect-us-from-men-who-live-the-illusion-of-danger-pete-buttigieg-and-the-us-military/.

38. For more on "lateral entry" into the military, see Andrew Tilghman, "The Pentagon's Controversial Plan to Hire Military Leaders off the Street," *Military Times*, June 19, 2016, https://www.militarytimes.com/2016/06/19/the-pentagon-s-controversial-plan-to-hire-military-leaders-off-the-street/. In a recent *New Yorker* profile, Mitch McConnell acknowledged that he joined the Army Reserves early in his career because "it was smart politically." He was discharged after five weeks due to an eye condition—and possibly political pull as well. Dorothy Wickenden, "Mitch McConnell, the Most Dangerous Politician in America," *New Yorker: Politics and More* (podcast), April 16, 2020, https://www.newyorker.com/podcast/political-scene/mitch-mcconnell-the-most-dangerous-politician-in-america.

39. Reid J. Epstein, "Buttigieg's Bet: After Iran Strike, Military Experience Matters Even More," *New York Times*, January 5, 2020, https://www.nytimes.com/2020/01/05/us/politics/pete-buttigieg-military-iran.html.

40. Michael Sandel, "Disdain for the Less Educated Is the Last Acceptable Prejudice," *New York Times*, September 2, 2020, https://www.nytimes.com/2020/09/02/opinion/education-prejudice.html?auth=login-email&login=email.

41. Peter Dreier, "Why Is Socialism Becoming Less Scary?," *Portside*, October 29, 2020, https://portside.org/2020-10-29/why-socialism-becoming-less-scary.

42. Ally Schweitzer, "Progressives Are Ready to Strengthen Labor Unions in Virginia. Moderate Democrats, Not So Much," *DCist.com*, January 21, 2021, https://dcist.com/story/21/01/19/progressives-face-battle-to-scrap-right-to-work-law-virginia/.

43. After his 2018 campaign defeat, Richard Ojeda started a Political Action Committee called No Dem Left Behind to aid other candidates, like himself, running as Democrats in rural, conservative districts. As the 2022 midterm elections approached, his PAC was backing several veterans against right-wing Republican House members. Among them was Marcus Flowers, an African American Army vet seeking the Democratic nomination to run against US Representative Marjorie Taylor Greene in Georgia. For details, see https://www.nodemleftbehind.com.

44. The Intercept, "Glenn Greenwald Interviews Kerri Harris: Can the Insurgency Now Defeat a Centrist U.S. Senator?," YouTube video, September 5, 2018, https://theintercept.com/2018/09/05/kerri-harris-glenn-greenwald-interview/.

45. Catie Edmondson, "G.O.P. Pins House Hopes on Profile That's Lifted Democrats," *New York Times*, May 20, 2020, https://www.nytimes.com/2020/05/19/us/politics/republicans-house-diversity-election.html.

46. Jeremy Peters and Kathleen Gray, "Are Michigan Democrats in Trouble in the Senate Race?," *New York Times*, October 19, 2020, https://www.nytimes.com/2020/10/19/us/politics/michigan-senate-peters-james.html.

47. Annie Karni, "Ronny Jackson, Ex–White House Doctor, Wins Texas House Runoff," *New York Times*, July 14, 2020, https://www.nytimes.com/2020/07/14/us/politics/ronny-jackson-texas.html.

48. Bob Moser, "Mitch McConnell Defends His Turf," *Nation*, September 22, 2020, https://www.thenation.com/article/politics/mitch-mcconnell-amy-mcgrath/.

49. Berry Craig, "Can Amy McGrath Stop Mitch's Laughter?," *LA Progressive*, October 22, 2020, https://www.laprogressive.com/can-amy-mcgrath-stop-mitchs-laughter/?

50. Mary Jennings Hegar, *Shoot like a Girl: One Woman's Dramatic Fight in Afghanistan and on the Home Front* (New York: Berkley, 2017), 74–80.

51. Patrick Svitek, "M. J. Hegar Defeats Royce West in Democratic Runoff for U.S. Senate," *Texas Tribune*, July 14, 2020, https://www.texastribune.org/2020/07/14/mj-hegar-john-cornyn-texas-senate-royce-west/.

52. Jennifer Steinhauer, "Trump's Actions Rattle the Military World," *New York Times*, June 12, 2020, https://www.nytimes.com/2020/06/12/us/politics/trump-polls-military-approval.html.

53. Catie Edmondson, "G.O.P. Senators on the Ropes Come Out Swinging against China," *New York Times*, June 14, 2020, https://www.nytimes.com/2020/06/13/us/politics/faced-with-crisis-and-re-election-senate-republicans-blame-china.html.

54. Katie Glueck, Matt Flegenheimer, and David E. Sanger, "Much Changed World, Same Joe Biden Seeking to Undo What Trump Has Done," *New York Times*, August 18, 2020, https://www.nytimes.com/2020/08/18/us/politics/joe-biden-foreign-policy.html.

CHAPTER 8: VETERANS AND THE 2020 ELECTION
Epigraph: Jennifer Steinhauer, "Trump Cites the v.a. as a Central Achievement. But Troubles Simmer," *New York Times*, August 19, 2020, https://www.nytimes.com/2020/08/19/us/politics/trump-veterans.html.

1. Andrew J. Bacevich, *America's War for the Greater Middle East: A Military History* (New York: Random House, 2016), 368.

2. Neta Crawford, "The Numbers," *The Nation*, September 2, 2021, 18, https://www.thenation.com/article/society/costs-war-deaths/.

3. Susan B. Glasser, "Mike *Pompeo, the Secretary of Trump*," *New Yorker*, August 19, 2019, https://www.newyorker.com/magazine/2019/08/26/mike-pompeo-the-secretary-of-trump.

4. Andrew Bacevich, "A Greatest Generation We Are Not," Common Dreams, May 5, 2020, https://www.commondreams.org/views/2020/05/05/greatest-generation-we-are-not.

5. In 2020, both Kolfage and Bannon were indicted for defrauding donors to this project. Before Donald Trump left office in January 2021, he pardoned Bannon, but not Kolfage. Caitlin M. Kenney, "Feds Say Veteran Brian Kolfage Secretly Took Donor Money Meant for Building Border Wall," *Stars and Stripes*, August 20, 2020, https://www.stripes.com/news/us/feds-say-veteran-brian-kolfage-secretly-took-donor-money-meant-for-building-border-wall-1.642015.

6. "v.a. Secretary Robert Wilkie: This Is Not the 'Scandal-Plagued v.a. of the Obama Administration,'" *Fox across America*, podcast, June 18, 2020, https://radio.foxnews.com/2020/06/18/va-secretary-robert-wilkie-this-is-not-the-scandal-plagued-v-a-of-the-obama-administration/.

7. Daniel. A. Sjursen, *Patriotic Dissent: America in the Age of Endless War* (Berkeley, CA: Heyday, 2020), 31.

8. Steve Hendrix and Joshua Partlow, "How Pete Buttigieg Went from War Protester to 'Packing My Bags for Afghanistan,'"*Washington Post*, July 29, 2019, https://www.washingtonpost.com/politics/2019/07/29/how-pete-buttigieg-went-war-protester-packing-my-bags-afghanistan/?arc404=true.

9. Allan Smith, "Mayor Pete Buttigieg Rips Trump for Possible Pardons of War Criminals," NBC News, May 26, 2019, https://www.nbcnews.com/politics/donald-trump/mayor-pete-buttigieg-rips-trump-possible-pardons-war-criminals-n1010406.

10. Steve Early and Suzanne Gordon, "The Inside Story of Mayor Pete's Wine Cave Caper," *Portside*, December 27, 2019, https://portside.org/2019-12-27/inside-story-mayor-petes-wine-cave-caper.

11. Seth Harp, "Bernie Sanders Leads Trump, All 2020 Candidates in Donations from Active-Duty Troops," *Rolling Stone*, January 31, 2020, https://www.rollingstone.com/politics/politics-news/bernie-sanders-leads-trump-all-2020-candidates-in-donations-from-active-duty-troops-946188/.

12. Steve Beynon, "Wilkie Says Socialism Poses a Serious Risk to the VA," *Stars and Stripes*, March 2, 2020, https://www.stripes.com/news/veterans/wilkie-says-socialism -poses-a-serious-risk-to-the-va-1.621023.

13. Steve Beynon, "Biden Says US Must Maintain Small Force in Middle East, Has No Plans for Major Defense Cuts," *Stars and Stripes*, September 10, 2020, https://www .stripes.com/news/us/biden-says-us-must-maintain-small-force-in-middle-east-has -no-plans-for-major-defense-cuts-1.644631.

14. Joseph R. Biden Jr., "Plan to Keep Our Sacred Obligation to Our Veterans," JoeBiden.com, July 29, 2020, https://joebiden.com/veterans/.

15. Steve Beynon, "Biden's Plan to Boost VA: Increase Wages for Health Care Work-ers to Compete with the Private Sector," *Stars and Stripes*, September 11, 2020, https:// www.stripes.com/news/us/biden-s-plan-to-boost-va-increase-wages-for-health-care -workers-to-compete-with-the-private-sector-1.644747.

16. Leo Shane III, "How Will Trump and Biden Handle Veterans Issues? Here's What They Told Us," *Military Times*, October 14, 2020, https://www.militarytimes.com /news/election-2020/2020/10/14/how-will-trump-and-biden-handle-veterans-issues -heres-what-they-told-us/.

17. Suzanne Gordon and Steve Early, "Will Biden's Surprise VA Pick Halt the Slide toward Privatization?," *American Prospect*, December 18, 2020, https://prospect.org /cabinet-watch/will-bidens-surprise-veterans-affairs-pick-halt-the-slide-toward -privatization/.

18. David Ignatius, "Acting Navy Chief Fired Crozier for 'Panicking'—and before Trump Could Intervene," *Washington Post*, April 6, 2020, https://www.washingtonpost .com/opinions/2020/04/05/acting-navy-chief-fired-crozier-panicking-before-trump -might-intervene/.

19. Eric Schmitt and Thomas Gibbons-Neff, "Navy Inquiry Faults Two Top Officers aboard Roosevelt for Handling of Virus," *New York Times*, June 19, 2020, https://www.nytimes.com/2020/06/19/us/politics/carrier-roosevelt-coronavirus -crozier.html.

20. Julian E. Barnes, "U.S. Military Seeks More Funding for Pacific Region after Pandemic," *New York Times*, April 5, 2020, https://www.nytimes.com/2020/04/05/us /politics/us-china-military-funding-virus.html.

21. Alex Emmons, "Progressives Plan to Push Big Cuts to Defense Spending, Citing Coronavirus Crisis," *The Intercept*, June 24, 2020, https://theintercept.com/2020/06/24 /defense-spending-coronavirus-bernie-sanders/.

22. Jake Johnson, "Time to 'Reinvest in People' and 'Cut Weapons of War': Barbara Lee Unveils Plan to Cut up to $350 Billion from Pentagon," Common Dreams, June 16, 2020, https://www.commondreams.org/news/2020/06/16/time-reinvest-people-and -cut-weapons-war-barbara-lee-unveils-plan-cut-350-billion?cd-.

23. Jake Johnson, "'The Fight Isn't Over,' Say Anti-war Groups as 139 House Demo-crats Vote with GOP to Reject 10% Pentagon Budget Cut," Common Dreams, July 21, 2020, https://www.commondreams.org/news/2020/07/21/fight-isnt-over-say-anti-war -groups-139-house-democrats-vote-gop-reject-10-pentagon.

24. Tammy Duckworth, "Tucker Carlson Doesn't Know What Patriotism Is" (opinion), *New York Times*, July 9, 2020, https://www.nytimes.com/2020/07/09/opinion/tammy-duckworth-tucker-carlson.html.

25. C. Kube and K. Dilanian, "U.S. Commander: Intel Still Hasn't Established Russia Paid Taliban 'Bounties' to Kill U.S. Troops," NBC News, September 14, 2020, https://www.nbcnews.com/politics/national-security/u-s-commander-intel-still-hasn-t-established-russia-paid-n1240020.

26. Eric Lipton et al., "He Could Have Seen What Was Coming: Behind Trump's Failure on the Virus," *New York Times*, April 11, 2020, https://www.nytimes.com/2020/04/11/us/politics/coronavirus-trump-response.html.

27. Eric Lipton, "The 'Red Dawn' Emails: 8 Key Exchanges on the Faltering Response to the Coronavirus," *New York Times*, April 11, 2020, https://www.nytimes.com/2020/04/11/us/politics/coronavirus-red-dawn-emails-trump.html.

28. Tom Engelhardt, "Might the Coronavirus Be a Peacemaker?," Common Dreams, April 14, 2020, https://www.commondreams.org/views/2020/04/14/might-coronavirus-be-peacemaker.

29. Peter Baker, "Trump's New Coronavirus Message: Time to Move on to the Economic Recovery," *New York Times*, May 7, 2020, https://www.nytimes.com/2020/05/06/us/politics/trump-coronavirus-recovery.html.

30. Helene Cooper, "Milley Apologizes for Role in Trump Photo Op: 'I Should Not Have Been There,'" *New York Times*, June 11, 2020, https://www.nytimes.com/2020/06/11/us/politics/trump-milley-military-protests-lafayette-square.html.

31. Thomas Gibbons-Neff and Eric Schmitt, "Pentagon Ordered National Guard Helicopters' Aggressive Response in D.C.," *New York Times*, June 6, 2020, https://www.nytimes.com/2020/06/06/us/politics/protests-trump-helicopters-national-guard.html.

32. Jake Johnson, "'This Isn't a Healthy Democracy': Warnings of Domestic Military Threat as Top US General Walks DC Streets in Combat Fatigues," Common Dreams, June 2, 2020, https://www.commondreams.org/news/2020/06/02/isnt-healthy-democracy-warnings-domestic-military-threat-top-us-general-walks-dc.

33. Cotton's only slightly less restrained opinion piece for the *New York Times* led to major upheaval on the newspaper staff—and later resignation of the editor responsible for running it. Tom Cotton, "Send in the Troops," *New York Times*, June 3, 2020, https://www.nytimes.com/2020/06/03/opinion/tom-cotton-protests-military.html.

34. They included retired admiral Mike Mullen, former Joint Chiefs chairman Martin Dempsey, former NATO commander James Stavridis, and retired four-star Marine general John Allen. In the pages of *Foreign Policy*, Allen warned that "the appearance of U.S. soldiers carrying out the president's intent by descending on American citizens . . . could wreck the high regard Americans have for their military, and much more." David E. Sanger and Helene Cooper, "Trump and the Military: A Mutual Embrace Might Dissolve on America's Streets," *New York Times*, June 4, 2020, https://www.nytimes.com/2020/06/04/us/politics/trump-military-protests.html.

35. Thomas Gibbons-Neff, Eric Schmitt, and Helene Cooper, "Aggressive Tactics by National Guard, Ordered to Appease Trump, Wounded the Military, Too," *New York*

Times, June 10, 2020, https://www.nytimes.com/2020/06/10/us/politics/national-guard -protests.html.

36. Thomas Gibbons-Neff, H. Cooper, Eric Schmitt, and Jennifer Steinhauer, "Former Commanders Fault Trump's Use of Troops against Protesters," *New York Times*, June 2, 2020, https://www.nytimes.com/2020/06/02/us/politics/military-national -guard-trump-protests.html.

37. Common Defense email, "Tell the Pentagon to Stop Giving War Weapons to the Police," June 20, 2020.

38. Mike Baker, "A 'Wall of Vets' Joins the Front Lines of Portland Protests," *New York Times*, July 25, 2020, https://www.nytimes.com/2020/07/25/us/a-wall-of-vets -joins-the-front-lines-of-portland-protests.html.

39. According to an audit released by the Pentagon's top watchdog in 2020, "a significant amount of that equipment was likely unwanted or unneeded by police forces across the country." J. Keller, "Police Departments Don't Really Need Excess Military Gear, Pentagon IG Says," *Task and Purpose*, October 9, 2020, https://taskandpurpose .com/news/military-surplus-equipment-inspector-general-audit/.

40. Jennifer Steinhauer, "Veterans Fortify the Ranks of Militias Aligned with Trump's Views," *New York Times*, September 11, 2020, https://www.nytimes.com/2020 /09/11/us/politics/veterans-trump-protests-militias.html.

41. Del Quentin Wilber, "Prosecutors' Challenge in Capitol Riot Probe: The Oath Keeper Who Didn't Go Inside," *Los Angeles Times*, April 20, 2021, https://www.latimes .com/politics/story/2021-04-20/oath-keepers-leaders-poses-challenge-for-doj -investigation-of-capitol-assault.

42. Jeffrey Goldberg, "James Mattis Denounces President Trump, Describes Him as a Threat to the Constitution," *The Atlantic*, June 4, 2020, http://www.theatlantic.com /politics/archive/2020/06/james-mattis-denounces-trump-protests-militarization /612640/.

43. Ashley Curtin, "Secretary of Defense Opposes Invoking Insurrection Act, a Rebuke to President Trump," Nation of Change, June 3, 2020, https://www.nationofchange .org/2020/06/03/secretary-of-defense-opposes-invoking-insurrection-act-a-rebuke-to -president-trump/.

44. In his published account of these events a year later, *Wall Street Journal* reporter Michael Bender credited both Esper and Milley with being a restraining influence on Trump at a time when other White House advisers were busy drafting a June 1, 2020, proclamation that would have invoked the Insurrection Act as a prelude to deploying ten thousand troops. See Bender, *Frankly, We Did Win This Election: The Inside Story of How Trump Lost* (New York: Twelve, 2021).

45. Eric Schmitt, Thomas Gibbons-Neff, and Peter Baker, "Trump Agrees to Send Home Troops from Washington, Easing Tensions with the Pentagon," *New York Times*, June 5, 2020, https://www.nytimes.com/2020/06/04/us/politics/trump-troops -washington-pentagon.html.

46. Greg Myre, "Trump Orders National Guard to Pull Out of Washington," NPR, June 7, 2021, https://www.npr.org/sections/live-updates-protests-for-racial-justice /2020/06/07/871701963/trump-orders-national-guard-to-pull-out-of-washington.

47. Cooper, "Milley Apologizes."

48. Michael Gold, "An N.Y. Street Is Named for Robert E. Lee. Officials Want That Changed," *New York Times*, June 11, 2020, https://www.nytimes.com/2020/06/11 /nyregion/general-lee-avenue-fort-hamilton-brooklyn.html.

49. Barbara Starr and Ryan Browne, "Trump Launches Unprecedented Attack on Military Leadership He Appointed," CNN, September 8, 2020, https://www.cnn.com /2020/09/07/politics/trump-attack-military-leadership/index.html.

50. Catie Edmondson and Emily Cochrane, "Defying Trump, Lawmakers Move to Strip Military Bases of Confederate Names," *New York Times*, July 20, 2020, https:// www.nytimes.com/2020/07/20/us/politics/congress-trump-confederate-base-names .html.

51. Peter Baker and Helene Cooper, "Trump Rejects Renaming Military Bases Named after Confederate Generals," *New York Times*, June 11, 2020, https://www .nytimes.com/2020/06/10/us/politics/trump-rejects-renaming-military-bases.html.

52. Michael Crowley, "Trump's Campaign Talk of Troop Withdrawals Doesn't Match Military Reality," *New York Times*, October 11, 2020, https://www.nytimes.com /2020/10/11/us/politics/trump-troop-withdrawals-war.html.

53. Jennifer Steinhauer, "Trump's Actions Rattle the Military World: 'I Can't Support the Man,'" *New York Times*, June 12, 2020, https://www.nytimes.com/2020/06/12/us /politics/trump-polls-military-approval.html.

54. Katie Rogers, "Trump Encourages Racist Conspiracy Theory about Kamala Harris," *New York Times*, August 14, 2020, https://www.nytimes.com/2020/08/13/us /politics/trump-kamala-harris.html.

55. A Reuters poll conducted in mid-2020 revealed that 78 percent of Americans surveyed—92 percent Democrats and 67 percent Republicans—believed that "a well-functioning United States Postal Service is important to having a smooth and successful election during the coronavirus pandemic." J. Corbett, "Ahead of Key House Vote, Polling Shows Bipartisan Majority of Americans Want More Funding for USPS," Common Dreams, August 19, 2020, https://www.commondreams.org/news/2020/08 /19/ahead-key-house-vote-polling-shows-bipartisan-majority-americans-want-more -funding?cd-.

56. Lee Moran, "Veterans Group Taunts Donald Trump for 'Finally' Going to War . . . with the Postal Service," *Huffington Post*, August 14, 2020, https://www.huffpost.com/entry /veterans-group-donald-trump-post-office_n_5f3673ccc5b6959911e3105e?guccounter=1.

57. Igor Derysh, "With Trump Donor in Charge, USPS May Shut Locations, Cut Service before Election," *Truthout*, July 31, 2020, https://truthout.org/articles/with -trump-donor-in-charge-usps-may-shut-locations-cut-service-before-election/.

58. Jake Johnson, "Lawmakers Demand Removal of Postmaster General DeJoy," *Truthout*, August 10, 2020, https://truthout.org/articles/lawmakers-demand-removal -of-postmaster-general-dejoy/.

59. Maryam Jameel and Ryan McCarthy, "Insufficient COVID Protections for Postal Workers Pose Threat to Mail-in Voting," *Truthout*, October 27, 2020, https://truthout .org/articles/insufficient-protections-for-postal-workers-pose-threat-to-mail-in -voting/.

60. Conor Friedersdorf, "Trump Adviser: Hillary Clinton 'Should Be Shot in a Firing Squad for Treason,'" *The Atlantic*, August 16, 2016, https://www.theatlantic.com/politics/archive/2016/08/clinton-baldasaro/496199/.

61. Andrew Blake, "Secret Service Says It's Investigating Al Baldasaro, a Trump Adviser, over Clinton Comments," *Washington (DC) Times*, July 21, 2016, https://www.washingtontimes.com/news/2016/jul/21/al-baldasaro-a-trump-adviser-is-under-secret-servi/.

62. Megan Henney, "GOP Candidate Sean Parnell Slams Biden, Democrats over 'Contempt for Middle America,'" Fox News, August 25, 2020, https://www.foxnews.com/politics/sean-parnell-republican-national-convention.

63. Katie Glueck and Sydney Ember, "Biden, Speaking to National Guard Group, Takes Aim at Republican Criticism on Crime," *New York Times*, August 29, 2020, https://www.nytimes.com/2020/08/29/us/politics/biden-trump-crime.html.

64. As *Military Times* reported, 44 percent of the troops surveyed self-identified as political independents. About 40 percent said they were Republican or Libertarian, and only 13 percent said they were Democrats. Thirteen percent of those polled in mid-2020 planned to vote for a third-party candidate, and nearly 9 percent didn't intend to vote at all. Leo Shane III, "Trump's Popularity Slips in Latest Military Times Poll." *Military Times*, August 31, 2020.

65. Monmouth University Polling Institute, "Biden Competitive across State," September 15, 2020, https://www.monmouth.edu/polling-institute/reports/monmouthpoll_fl_091520/.

66. Jeffrey Goldberg, "Trump: Americans Who Died in War Are 'Losers' and 'Suckers,'" *The Atlantic*, September 3, 2020, https://www.theatlantic.com/politics/archive/2020/09/trump-americans-who-died-at-war-are-losers-and-suckers/615997/.

67. Jennifer Steinhauer, "After Report That Trump Disparaged War Dead, Democrats See Chance to Win Over Military Voters," *New York Times*, September 4, 2020, https://www.nytimes.com/2020/09/04/us/politics/trump-military-vote-democrats.html.

68. VoteVets email, "How We Win in November," August 29, 2020.

69. Scott Bourque, "More Than 100 Veterans Sign Letter Condemning Sen. McSally," KJZZ (Phoenix, AZ), June 19, 2020, https://kjzz.org/content/1593645/more-100-veterans-sign-letter-condemning-sen-mcsally.

70. As usual, Trump was incorrect. Hunter Biden did not receive a "dishonorable discharge." After failing a drug test for cocaine, he was given a less severe administrative discharge.

71. "Read the Full Transcript from the First Presidential Debate between Joe Biden and Donald Trump," *USA Today*, October 4, 2020, https://news.yahoo.com/read-full-transcript-first-presidential-171037222.html.

72. "National Exit Polls: How Different Groups Voted," *New York Times*, November 3, 2020, https://www.nytimes.com/interactive/2020/11/03/us/elections/exit-polls-president.html.

73. Jed Kolko and Toni Monkovic, "The Places That Had the Biggest Swings toward and against Trump," *New York Times*, December 7, 2020, https://www.nytimes.com/2020/12/07/upshot/trump-election-vote-shift.html.

74. David Choi, "Trump Campaign Witness Says It's 'Odd' That US Troops Voted for Biden in Large Numbers," *Business Insider*, November 11, 2020, https://www.businessinsider.com/military-veteran-vote-joe-biden-trump-lawsuit-2020-11.

75. Sam Knight, "Silicon Valley Campaign Cash Complicates Democrats' Plan to Break Up Tech Giants," *Truthout*, October 25, 2020, https://truthout.org/articles/silicon-valley-campaign-cash-complicates-democrats-plan-to-break-up-tech-giants/.

76. Joan Walsh and John Nichols, "Joe Biden's Presidency Depends on Georgia," *The Nation*, November 12, 2020, https://www.thenation.com/article/politics/georgia-senate-warnock-ossoff/.

77. Catie Edmondson, "Virus Diagnosis and Secret Texts Upend a Critical Senate Race in a Single Night," *New York Times*, October 3, 2020, https://www.nytimes.com/2020/10/03/us/politics/coronavirus-thom-tillis-cal-cunningham-north-carolina.html.

78. Glen Johnson and Alayna Treene, "Schumer's Regrets," *Axios*, December 1, 2020, https://www.axios.com/schumer-regrets-democrats-senate-chances-1bc586cb-46d1-4aa0-97f1-0274cfed1c00.html.

79. Brian Slodysko, "Skarlatos Congressional Candidate Funds Questioned," Associated Press, October 2, 2021, https://www.opb.org/article/2021/10/02/alek-skarlatos-oregon-campaign-funds-questioned/.

80. Marquise Francis, "Can an Afro-Latina Combat Veteran Make a Run at Congress in 'Trump District' Staten Island?," *Yahoo News*, March 6, 2021, https://www.yahoo.com/now/can-an-afro-latina-combat-veteran-make-a-run-at-congress-in-trump-district-aka-staten-island-200042802.html?guccounter=1.

81. As *Military Times* explains, "Congressional records on veterans serving in elected office before then are incomplete." L. Shane, "The Number of Veterans in Congress Will Drop to Lowest Level since at Least World War II," *Military Times*, December 2, 2020, https://www.militarytimes.com/news/pentagon-congress/2020/12/02/the-number-of-veterans-in-congress-will-drop-to-lowest-level-since-at-least-ww-ii/.

82. Veterans Campaign, "2020 Election Analysis: Veterans Heading to Congress and How Vets Voted," 2020, http://www.veteranscampaign.org/2020-election-analysis.

83. Ally Mutnick, "Republicans Draft Veteran Candidates to Reclaim House Majority," *Politico*, April 9, 2021, https://www.politico.com/news/2021/04/09/republicans-veteran-candidates-house-majority-480646.

84. Michael Scherer and Josh Dawsey, "Would-be Speaker Kevin McCarthy Walks the Trump Tightrope, Pursuing a GOP House," *Washington Post*, October 22, 2021, https://www.washingtonpost.com/politics/2021/10/22/kevin-mccarthy-trump/.

85. Will Weissert, "Veterans Are Prized Recruits as Congressional Candidates," *AP News*, August 22, 2021, https://apnews.com/article/veterans-9cad3c4211a0e15852c44c8d75681254.

CONCLUSION

1. Patricia Kime, "6 Major Veterans Orgs to White House: Fire VA Secretary Wilkie Now," *Military.com*, December 20, 2020, https://www.military.com/daily-news/2020/12/16/6-major-veterans-orgs-white-house-fire-va-secretary-wilkie-now.html.

2. US Department of Veterans Affairs, "Senior VA Officials' Response to a Veteran's Sexual Assault Allegations," Office of Inspector General, December 10, 2020, iv–viii, https://www.va.gov/oig/pubs/VAOIG-20-01766-36.pdf.

3. Nine months after he left office, Wilkie publicly criticized the VSOs for seeking expanded VA benefits and services, "rather than catering to veterans with specific military-related needs." See Leo Shane III, "Vets Should Be Getting Fewer Disability Benefits, More Help in Post-Military Life, Says Former SECVA," *Military Times*, November 9, 2021, https://www.militarytimes.com/military-honor/salute-veterans/2021/11/09/vets-should-be-getting-fewer-disability-benefits-more-help-in-post-military-life-says-former-secva/.

4. Luke Broadwater, "Senator Describes Push to Stop Deportation of Veterans," *New York Times*, July 8, 2021, https://www.nytimes.com/2021/07/07/us/politics/veterans-deported-duckworth.html.

5. Franco Ordoñez and Quil Lawrence, "Biden Selects Denis McDonough as VA Secretary," NPR, December 10, 2020, https://www.npr.org/sections/biden-transition-updates/2020/12/10/944980660/biden-selects-denis-mcdonough-as-va-secretary.

6. Megan Cassella and Alex Thompson, "Biden to Tap Denis McDonough for Veterans Affairs," *Politico*, December 10, 2020, https://www.politico.com/news/2020/12/10/denis-mcdonough-veterans-affairs-secretary-444213.

7. US Department of Veterans Affairs, "VA Pilots Evaluation Model to Determine Potential Exposure to Environmental Hazards While Serving," press release, November 11, 2021, https://www.va.gov/opa/pressrel/pressrelease.cfm?id=5739.

8. VA Office of Public and Intergovernmental Affairs, "VA Prepares to Get Ahead of Surge in Backlogged Cases," press release, October 13, 2021, https://www.va.gov/opa/pressrel/pressrelease.cfm?id=5728.

9. US Senate Committee on Veterans Affairs, "Hearing to Consider Pending Nomination," January 27, 2021, https://www.veterans.senate.gov/hearings/hearing-to-consider-pending-nomination.

10. Liam Rose et al., "Assessment of Changes in U.S. Veterans Health Administration Care Delivery Methods during the COVID-19 Pandemic," JAMA Network, October 14, 2021, https://jamanetwork.com/journals/jamanetworkopen/article-abstract/2784999.

11. Suzanne Gordon, "In an Article on 'Value-Based' Veterans' Care, Vested Interests and Misinformation," Veterans Healthcare Policy Institute, Spring 2021, https://a34b5402-33e3-45c7-a5a2-cbf950e8aff5.filesusr.com/ugd/23193b_36bb9117024d4330ac7 1633086a86a5d.pdf.

12. Nurses Organization of Veterans Affairs, "NOVA Community Care Survey Comments," September 2021, https://cdn.ymaws.com/www.vanurse.org/resource/resmgr/2021_files/advocacy/2021_community_care_survey_r.pdf.

13. Terri Tanielian et al., "Ready or Not? Assessing the Capacity of New York State Health Care Providers to Meet the Needs of Veterans," RAND Corporation, 2018, https://www.rand.org/pubs/research_reports/RR2298.html.

14. AVAPL, "AVAPL Community Care Survey," September 2021, https://avapl.org/advocacy/pubs/Community%20Care%20Survey%20Final%206-26-21.pdf.

15. Phillip Longman and Suzanne Gordon, "Longman-Gordon Report—VA Health-care: A System Worth Saving," American Legion, 2018, 6–10, https://www.legion.org/publications/238801/longman-gordon-report-va-healthcare-system-worth-saving.

16. US Department of Health and Human Services, "Report to Congress on the Nation's Substance Abuse and Mental Health Workforce Issues," SAMHSA, January 24, 2013, https://store.samhsa.gov/shin/content/PEP13-RTC-BHWORK/PEP13-RTC-BHWORK.pdf.

17. Clifford Marks, "America's Looming Primary Care Crisis," New Yorker, July 25, 2020, https://www.newyorker.com/science/medical-dispatch/americas-looming-primary-care-crisis; Reed Abelson, "Doctors without Patients: 'Our Waiting Rooms Are like Ghost Towns,'" New York Times, May 5, 2020, https://www.nytimes.com/2020/05/05/health/coronavirus-primary-care-doctor.html.

18. Cecil G. Sheps Center for Health Care Services Research, "176 Rural Hospital Closures: January 2005–Present (134 since 2010)," University of North Carolina, https://www.shepscenter.unc.edu/programs-projects/rural-health/rural-hospital-closures/, accessed November 30, 2020.

19. Hoag Levins, "Already in Fiscal Crisis, Rural Hospitals Face COVID-19," Leonard Davis Institute of Health Economics, University of Pennsylvania, June 2020, https://ldi.upenn.edu/news/already-fiscal-crisis-rural-hospitals-face-covid-19.

20. CISION PR Newswire, "One in Four U.S. Rural Hospitals at High Financial Risk of Closing as Patients Leave Communities for Care," April 8, 2020, https://www.prnewswire.com/news-releases/one-in-four-us-rural-hospitals-at-high-financial-risk-of-closing-as-patients-leave-communities-for-care-301037081.html.

21. Chris Pomorski, "Death of a Hospital," New Yorker, June 7, 2021, https://www.newyorker.com/magazine/2021/06/07/the-death-of-hahnemann-hospital.

22. David Himmelstein and Steffie Woolhandler, "The 'Public Option' on Health Care Is a Poison Pill," The Nation, October 2, 2019, https://www.thenation.com/article/archive/insurance-health-care-medicare/.

23. See September 2021 online petition, "Stop Direct Contracting Entities from Taking Over Traditional Medicare," circulated by Physicians for a National Health Program at https://pnhp.salsalabs.org/DCEpetitionSeptember2021/index.html.

24. Mark Miller, "Medicare's Private Option Is Gaining Popularity and Critics," New York Times, February 21, 2020, https://www.nytimes.com/2020/02/21/business/medicare-advantage-retirement.html.

25. Lisa Rein, "Trump Alumni Launch Group to Push His VA Policies—and Blunt Biden's," Washington Post, August 19, 2021, https://www.washingtonpost.com/politics/veterans-trump-biden/2021/08/18/fa39b5f2-ff68-11eb-ba7e-2cf966e88e93_story.html.

26. Walt Buteau, "Lawsuit Claims 'Another Scandal Is Brewing' with VA Patient Wait Times," News Channel 8, July 20, 2021, https://www.wfla.com/8-on-your-side/lawsuit-claims-another-scandal-is-brewing-with-va-patient-wait-times/.

27. Jill Castellano, "The Mission Act Is Supposed to Help US Veterans Get Health Care Outside the VA. For Some, It's Not Working," USA Today, November 1, 2021, https://www.usatoday.com/in-depth/news/investigations/2021/11/01/mission-act-aid-veterans-healthcare-va-isnt-letting-it/8561618002/.

28. Jill Castellano, "Are You a Veteran Who Needs Medical Help Outside the va? Start Here," Inewsource, November 1, 2021, https://inewsource.org/2021/11/01/mission -act-appeals-guide/.

29. Congressional Budget Office, "The Veteran's Community Care Program: Background and Early Effects," October 2021, 10, https://www.cbo.gov/system/files/2021-10 /57257-VCCP.pdf.

30. David C. Chan, David Card, and Lowell Taylor, "Is There a va Advantage? Evidence from Dually Eligible Veterans," National Bureau of Economic Research, November 2020, http://conference.nber.org/conf_papers/f145428.pdf.

31. Suzanne Gordon and Russell Lemle, "New Study Settles the Privatization Debate: va Produces Better Outcomes at Lower Cost," Veterans Healthcare Policy Institute Blog, March 23, 2021, https://www.veteranspolicy.org/post/new-stanford -study-settles-the-privatization-debate-va-produces-better-outcomes-at-lower -cost.

32. L. Bilmes, "Long-Term Costs of United States Care for Vets," Costs of War Project, August 18, 2021, https://watson.brown.edu/costsofwar/files/cow/imce/papers /2021/Costs%20of%20War_Bilmes_Long-Term%20Costs%20of%20Care%20for %20Vets_Aug%202021.pdf.

33. Kayla Williams, "Coronavirus Pandemic Illustrates the Need to Maintain a Strong va," The Hill, March 18, 2020, https://www.navso.org/news/coronavirus -pandemic-illustrates-need-maintain-strong-va.

34. Commission on Care, "Final Report," June 30, 2016, 201–3, https://www.stripes .com/polopoly_fs/1.417785.1467828140!/menu/standard/file/Commission-on-Care _Final-Report_063016_FOR-WEB.pdf.

35. October 12, 2021, letter to va Secretary Denis McDonough from Senators Bernie Sanders and Richard Blumenthal. Copy in possession of the authors.

36. C. Flanders, "Amid Hospital Crunch, va to Offer Mental Health Beds to Nonveterans," Seven Days, November 4, 2021, https://www.sevendaysvt.com/OffMessage /archives/2021/10/27/amid-hospital-crunch-va-to-offer-mental-health-beds-to -nonveterans.

37. Govinfo, "HR3590 (IH)—GI Bill of Health," https://www.govinfo.gov/app/details /BILLS-104hr3950ih, accessed February 2, 2021.

38. Ann Devroy and Bill McAllister, "Derwinski Quits Bush's Cabinet," Washington Post, September 27, 1992, https://www.washingtonpost.com/archive/politics/1992/09 /27/derwinski-quits-bushs-cabinet/c5153015-c6a1-48d9-bd51-881562f53cde/.

39. Carl Forsling, "Unpacking the Veteran Entitlement Spectrum," Task and Purpose, October 6, 2014, https://taskandpurpose.com/community/unpacking-veteran -entitlement-spectrum/.

40. C. J. Chivers, "At War: The Military's Unpreparedness for Covid-19," New York Times, April 10, 2020, https://nims360.blogspot.com/2020/04/at-war-militarys -unpreparedness-for.html.

41. Michelle Miller-Adams, "We Need Tuition-Free College. For Adults," New York Times, May 14, 2020, https://www.nytimes.com/2020/05/14/opinion/free-college-adults -covid.html.

42. Will Fischer, "A Veteran's Case for Canceling Student Debt and Making Higher Education Tuition-Free," Nation of Change, February 11, 2020, https://www .nationofchange.org/2020/02/11/a-veterans-case-for-canceling-student-debt-and -making-higher-education-tuition-free/.

43. Les Leopold, *The Man Who Hated Work and Loved Labor: The Life and Times of Tony Mazzocchi* (White River Junction, VT: Chelsea Green, 2007), 483.

44. Thomas Kaplan and Katie Glueck, "Biden, Courting Liberals, Backs Tuition-Free College for Many Students," *New York Times*, March 15, 2020, https://www .nytimes.com/2020/03/15/us/politics/biden-backs-free-college.html.

45. Shane Goldmacher and Sydney Ember, "Biden, Seeking Democratic Unity, Reaches Left toward Sanders's Ideas," *New York Times*, April 9, 2020, https://www .nytimes.com/2020/04/09/us/politics/biden-sanders-medicare-student-debt.html.

46. Jenny Gross, "Can Biden's $109 Billion Plan for Free Community College Work?," *New York Times*, July 7, 2021, https://www.nytimes.com/2021/07/10/business /dealbook/does-free-college-work.html.

47. Rory Fanning, "A Truly Antiwar Agenda Must Include Free College and Medicare for All," *Truthout*, January 15, 2020, https://truthout.org/articles/a-truly-antiwar -agenda-must-include-free-college-and-medicare-for-all/.

48. Jack Brewster, "Biden Won't Support Progressive Student-Loan Forgiveness Plan, He Says," *Forbes*, May 21, 2021, https://www.forbes.com/sites/jackbrewster /2021/05/21/biden-wont-support-progressive-student-loan-forgiveness-plan-he -says/.

49. SVA president Carrie Wofford as quoted by Stacy Cowley, "Veterans Hurt by For-Profits Get Victory," *New York Times*, March 12, 2021, https://www.nytimes.com /2021/03/11/business/veterans-for-profit-schools-gi-bill.html.

50. National Nurses United, "Medicare for All," https://www.nationalnursesunited.org /medicare-for-all, accessed October 7, 2021.

51. Pete Lucier, Kyleanne Hunter, and Joe Plenzler, "We're Combat Veterans. We Support the Students Demanding Gun Control," *Washington Post*, February 20, 2018, https://www.washingtonpost.com/news/checkpoint/wp/2018/02/20/were-combat -veterans-we-support-the-students-demanding-gun-reform/.

52. Martin Kuz, "Can Veterans Lead the Way on Preventing Suicide?," *Christian Science Monitor*, December 31, 2019, https://www.csmonitor.com/USA/Military/2019/1231 /Can-veterans-lead-the-way-on-preventing-suicide.

53. "VA Secretary Vows to Empower Federal Workforce, Encourage Union Organizing," *AFGE Insider*, April 26, 2021, https://www.afge.org/article/va-secretary-vows-to -empower-federal-workforce-encourage-union-organizing/.

54. Hamilton Nolan, "Enormous VA Union Contract Moves towards Uncertain Conclusion under New Biden Administration," *In These Times*, February 5, 2021, https://inthesetimes.com/article/va-union-contract-biden-veterans-affairs.

55. AFGE, "New Data: White Employees Twice as Likely to Be Promoted Than Black Employees at the Veterans Affairs Department," press release, October 15, 2020, https://www.afge.org/publication/new-data-white-employees-twice-as-likely-to-be -promoted-than-black-employees-at-the-veterans-affairs-department.

56. Jim Tankersley and Emily Cochrane, "Hurdle for Biden as Stimulus Bill Drops State Aid," *New York Times*, December 18, 2020, https://www.nytimes.com/2020/12/17/business/stimulus-state-local-aid.html.

57. Mark Brenner, "Will the Stimulus Stop States from Slashing More Jobs?," *Labor Notes*, April 2021, https://labornotes.org/2021/03/will-stimulus-stop-states-slashing-more-jobs.

58. Jake Johnson, "DeJoy Is the Real Life Grinch: Postmaster General's Pre-election Sabotage Fuels Christmas Delivery Delays," Common Dreams, December 22, 2020, https://www.commondreams.org/news/2020/12/22/dejoy-real-life-grinch-postmaster-generals-pre-election-sabotage-fuels-christmas?cd-.

59. Keith Combs, "One Way to Honor Vets? Protect the Postal Service," *Postal Reporter*, November 6, 2019, http://www.postal-reporter.com/blog/one-way-to-honor-vets-protect-the-postal-service/.

60. As quoted by Hailey Fuchs, "Bipartisan Bill Aims to Rescue Postal Service," *New York Times*, May 20, 2021, https://www.nytimes.com/2021/05/19/us/politics/postal-service-reform-legislation.html.

61. "A Plan for a Better Post Office. Finally," editorial, *New York Times*, May 29, 2021, https://www.nytimes.com/2021/05/28/opinion/post-office-postal-service.html.

62. David Dayen, "Postal Banking Test in the Bronx Yields No Customers," *American Prospect*, November 9, 2021, https://prospect.org/economy/postal-banking-test-in-the-bronx-yields-no-customers/.

63. Brittany DeBarros, letter to About Face supporters, October 15, 2020, authors' private collection.

64. Max Boot, "COVID Is Killing Off Traditional Notions of National Defense," *Washington Post*, March 31, 2020, https://www.washingtonpost.com/opinions/2020/03/31/covid-19-is-killing-off-our-traditional-notions-national-defense/?arc404=true.

65. Jake Johnson, "Ilhan Omar Rips Congress for Approving $740.5 Billion Pentagon Budget while Skimping on Covid Relief," Common Dreams, December 9, 2020, https://www.salon.com/2020/12/12/ilhan-omar-rips-congress-for-approving-7405-billion-pentagon-budget-while-skimping-on-covid-relief_partner/.

66. Nguyen Phan Que Mai, "Neglected Victims of Agent Orange," *New York Times*, May 2, 2021, https://www.nytimes.com/2021/04/30/opinion/sunday/agent-orange-vietnam-war-anniversary.html. In May 2021, US Representative Barbara Lee (D-CA) introduced legislation seeking financial compensation for Vietnamese victims of Agent Orange exposure and their children, in addition to the $125 million that the United States has spent over the last thirty years. See Marjorie Cohn, "Barbara Lee Introduces Bill to Help Vietnamese Victims of Agent Orange," *Truthout*, June 3, 2021, https://truthout.org/articles/barbara-lee-introduces-bill-to-help-vietnamese-victims-of-agent-orange/?eType=EmailBlastContent&eId=9f37b01e-91bf-4f34-b93e-8c9c8d59d233.

67. Catie Edmondson, "Senate Sends Military Bill to Trump's Desk, Spurning His Veto Threat," *New York Times*, December 11, 2020, https://www.nytimes.com/2020/12/11/us/politics/senate-military-bill-trump-veto-threat.html.

68. Danny Sjursen, "A Certain Kind of Diversity: Secretary of Defense Lloyd Austin," *LA Progressive*, December 11, 2020, https://www.laprogressive.com/secretary-of-defense-lloyd-austin/.

69. "Gen. Lloyd Austin's Full Opening Statement in Senate Confirmation Hearing," video, *PBS NewsHour*, January 19, 2021, https://www.pbs.org/newshour/politics/watch -gen-lloyd-austins-full-opening-statement-in-senate-confirmation-hearing.

70. Jennifer Steinhauer, "Diversity Push Inside Military Spurs Backlash," *New York Times*, June 6, 2021, https://www.nytimes.com/2021/06/10/us/politics/military -diversity.html. As Steinhauer reported, Cotton objected to what he claimed was man- datory training on "police brutality, white privilege, and systemic racism," while his House colleague, Crenshaw, created a whistleblower page on his website so equally of- fended active-duty troops could register complaints about "woke-ness" in the military.

71. Rory Fanning, "July 4 Glorifies the US Military—a Force with White Supremacy at its Core," *Truthout*, July 4, 2021, https://truthout.org/articles/july-4-glorifies-the-u-s -military-a-force-with-white-supremacy-at-its-core/.

72. Andrea Mazzarino, "Changing the Way the Military Handles Sexual Assault," *TomDispatch*, May 24, 2021, https://tomdispatch.com/changing-the-way-the-military -handles-sexual-assault/.

73. Alexander Stockton and Lucy King, "There's a Sexual Assault Crisis in the Mili- tary. Congress Can Stop It," *New York Times*, June 2, 2021, https://www.nytimes.com /2021/06/01/opinion/sexual-assault-military-ernst-gillibrand.html?campaign.

74. Zoe Carpenter, "Chain of Command," *The Nation*, August 9–16, 2021, https:// www.thenation.com/article/society/military-sexual-harassment-gillibrand/.

75. David Dayen, "Gillebrand Slams 'Four Men' for Watering Down Military Sexual Assault Reform," *The American Prospect*, December 8, 2021, https://prospect.org/politics /gillibrand-slams-four-men-for-watering-down-military-sexual-assault-reform/.

76. As quoted by Jennifer Steinhauer, "U.S. 'Forever War' Veterans Back Biden on Withdrawal," *New York Times*, July 7, 2021.

77. Trump's full remarks can be found at https://www.rev.com/blog/transcripts/donald -trump-perry-georgia-rally-speech-transcript-september-25. Even though he did not appear in uniform, Lance Corporal Hunter Clark soon found himself under investigation by the Marines for possible improper participation in "partisan political" activities. See https://goodwordnews.com/sailor-investigated-for-speaking-at-trump-rally-in-georgia/.

78. William Rivers Pitt, "Biden Breaks Campaign Promise, Approves Arms Sale to Saudi Arabia," *Truthout*, April 15, 2021, https://truthout.org/articles/biden-breaks -campaign-promise-approves-arms-sale-to-saudi-arabia/.

79. Stephen Semler, "The Flow of Military Equipment to Police through Q1 of 2021," *Speaking Security Newsletter*, April 2, 2021, https://stephensemler.substack.com/p/the -flow-of-military-equipment-to.

80. Stephen Semler, "House Committee Approves $25 Billion Increase to Mili- tary Budget," *Speaking Security Newsletter*, September 1, 2021, https://stephensemler .substack.com/p/house-committee-approves-25bn-increase. As Semler reports, when House progressives proposed, for the second year in a row, a 10 percent cut in overall military spending, that amendment received fewer votes than the similar legislative effort in 2020 described in chapter 8.

81. Sharon Zhang, "Bernie Sanders Announces He's Voting No on $778 Billion Defense Bill," *Truthout*, November 17, 2021, https://truthout.org/articles/sanders -announces-hes-voting-no-on-778-billion-defense-bill/.

82. Jake Johnson, "'A $753,000,000,000 Defense Budget Is a Failure': Biden Pentagon Request Rebuked," *Common Dreams*, May 28, 2021, https://www.commondreams.org/news/2021/05/28/753000000000-defense-budget-failure-biden-pentagon-request-rebuked. As reported by the *New York Times*, in mid-2021, the Biden administration did signal to Congress that it was open to "tightening the much stretched 2001 law that serves as the domestic legal basis for open ended 'forever wars' against terrorists around the word." See Charlie Savage, "Biden Administration Is Open to Tightening Law Authorizing War on Terror," *New York Times*, August 4, 2021, https://www.nytimes.com/2021/08/03/us/politics/biden-war-powers.html.

83. Quincy Institute for Responsible Statecraft, homepage, https://quincyinst.org, accessed January 5, 2021.

84. Andrew Bacevich, "So It Goes," *Nation of Change*, June 28, 2021, https://www.nationofchange.org/2021/06/28/so-it-goes/.

85. Eisenhower Media Network, proposal, September 11, 2020, personal communication.

86. Catherine Lutz and Andrea Mazzarino, eds., *War and Health: The Medical Consequences of the Wars in Iraq and Afghanistan* (New York: New York University Press, 2019).

87. Costs of War, Watson Institute for International and Public Affairs, Brown University, homepage, https://watson.brown.edu/costsofwar/, accessed January 5, 2021.

88. Letter to Speaker Nancy Pelosi, November 16, 2020, https://winwithoutwar.org/wp-content/uploads/2020/11/2020.11.16_Castro-HFAC-Organizational-Endorsement-Letter.pdf.

89. Catie Edmondson and Luke Broadwater, "5 Veterans Leave Positions to Advise Arizona Senator, Citing Obstacles to Progress," *New York Times*, October 22, 2021, https://www.nytimes.com/2021/10/21/us/politics/sinema-veterans-resign.html.

90. Max Greenwood, "Ruben Gallego Is Left's Favorite to Take on Sinema," *The Hill*, October 7, 2021, https://thehill.com/homenews/campaign/575675-democrats-eye-gallego-amid-growing-frustration-with-sinema.

91. Jennifer Steinhauer, "In Battle at Capitol, Veterans Fought on Opposite Sides," *New York Times*, February 8, 2021, https://www.nytimes.com/2021/02/08/us/politics/capitol-riot-trump-veterans-cops.html.

92. Luke Broadwater and Nicholas Fandos, "Police at the Capitol Recount the Horror of January 6," *New York Times*, July 27, 2021. https://www.nytimes.com/2021/07/27/us/jan-6-inquiry.html?

93. VA Undersecretary for Health Dr. Richard Stone, as quoted by Howard Altman, "Mobile Vet Centers Deployed at Capitol to Provide Mental Health Resources for Siege Survivors, Responders," *Military Times*, February 3, 2021, https://www.militarytimes.com/news/pentagon-congress/2021/02/02/mobile-vet-centers-deployed-at-capitol-to-provide-mental-health-resources-for-seige-survivors-responders/.

SELECTED BIBLIOGRAPHY

Ackerman, Elliot. *Places and Names: On War, Revolution, and Returning.* New York: Penguin Press, 2019.

Ackerman, Spencer. *Reign of Terror: How the 9/11 Era Destabilized America and Produced Trump.* New York: Viking, 2021.

Adler, Amy B., Carl Andrew Castro, and Thomas W. Britt, eds. *Military Life: The Psychology of Serving in Peace and Combat.* Westport, CT: Praeger Security International, 2006.

Alimahomed-Wilson, Jake, and Ellen Reese, eds. *The Cost of Free Shipping: Amazon in the Global Economy.* London: Pluto, 2020.

Allen, Thomas, and Paul Dickson. *The Bonus Army: An American Epic.* London: Walker Books, 2004.

Bacevich, Andrew J. *The Age of Illusions: How America Squandered Its Cold War Victory.* New York: Metropolitan Books, 2020.

Bacevich, Andrew J. *Breach of Trust: How Americans Failed Their Soldiers and Their Country.* New York: Metropolitan Books, 2013.

Bacevich, Andrew J. *Washington Rules: America's Path to Permanent War.* New York: Metropolitan Books, 2010.

Bannerman, Stacy. *Homefront 911: How Families of Veterans Are Wounded by Our Wars.* New York: Arcade, 2015.

Bateson, John. *The Last and Greatest Battle: Finding the Will, Commitment, and Strategy to End Military Suicides.* Oxford: Oxford University Press, 2015.

Bauman, Robert H., and Dina Rasor. *Shattered Minds: How the Pentagon Fails Our Troops with Faulty Helmets.* Lincoln, NE: Potomac Books, 2019.

Belew, Kathleen. *Bring the War Home: The White Power Movement and Paramilitary America.* Cambridge, MA: Harvard University Press, 2018.

Bellesiles, Michael. *A People's History of the U.S. Military: Ordinary Soldiers Reflect on Their Experience of War, from the American Revolution to Afghanistan.* New York: New Press, 2012.

Bennett, Michael J. *When Dreams Came True: The GI Bill and the Making of Modern America*. Washington, DC: Brassey's, 1996.

Bergen, Peter. *Trump and His Generals: The Cost of Chaos*. New York: Penguin Press, 2019.

Best, Mat. *Thank You for My Service*. New York: Bantam Books, 2020.

Bhagwati, Anuradha. *Unbecoming: A Memoir of Disobedience*. New York: Atria Books, 2019.

Bilmes, Linda J., and Joseph Stiglitz. *The Three Trillion Dollar War: The True Cost of the Iraq Conflict*. New York: W. W. Norton, 2008.

Bonior, David E. *Whip: Leading the Progressive Battle during the Rise of the Right*. Westport, CT: City Point Press, 2018.

Bonior, David E., Steven Champlin, and Timothy Kolly. *The Vietnam Veteran: A History of Neglect*. New York: Praeger, 1984.

Boudreau, Tyler E. *Packing Inferno: The Unmaking of a Marine*. Port Townsend, WA: Feral House, 2008.

Boulton, Mark. *Failing Our Veterans: The G.I. Bill and the Vietnam Generation*. New York: New York University Press, 2014.

Butalla, S. Fabian, ed. *We Are Not Invisible*. Ashland, OR: Hellgate Press, 2019.

Carnevale, David, and Camilla Stivers. *Knowledge and Power in Public Bureaucracies: From Pyramid to Circle*. New York: Routledge, 2020.

Carver, Ron, David Cortright, and Barbara Doherty, eds. *Waging Peace in Vietnam: US Soldiers and Veterans Who Opposed the War*. New York: New Village Press, 2019.

Castro, Carl Andrew, and Sanela Dursun, eds. *Military Veteran Reintegration: Approach, Management, and Assessment of Military Veterans Transitioning to Civilian Life*. London: Academic Press, 2019.

Chivers, C. J. *The Fighters: Americans in Combat*. New York: Simon & Schuster, 2018.

Cockburn, Andrew. *The Spoils of War: Power, Profit and the American War Machine*. New York: Verso, 2021.

Cohen, Donald, and Allen Mikaelian. *Privatization of Everything: How the Plunder of Public Goods Transformed America and How We Can Fight Back*. New York: New Press, 2021.

Cortright, David. *Soldiers in Revolt: GI Resistance during the Vietnam War*. Chicago: Haymarket Books, 1975.

Darda, Joseph. *How White Men Won the Culture Wars: A History of Veteran America*. Berkeley: University of California Press, 2021.

Denton-Borhaug, Kelly. *And Then Your Soul Is Gone: Moral Injury and U.S. War-Culture*. Sheffield, UK: Equinox Publishing, 2021.

Duckworth, Tammy. *Every Day Is a Gift: A Memoir*. New York: Grand Central, 2021.

Engelhardt, Tom. *A Nation Unmade by War*. Chicago: Haymarket Books, 2018.

Fanning, Rory. *Worth Fighting For: An Army Ranger's Journey out of the Military and across America*. Chicago: Haymarket Books, 2014.

Finkel, David. *Thank You for Your Service*. New York: Macmillan, 2013.

Finley, Erin P. *Fields of Combat: Understanding PTSD among Veterans of Iraq and Afghanistan*. Ithaca, NY: Cornell University Press, 2011.

Fountain, Ben. *Billy Lynn's Long Halftime Walk*. New York: HarperCollins, 2012.

Gade, Daniel and Daniel Huang. *Wounding Warriors: How Bad Policy Is Making Veterans Sicker and Poorer.* Washington: Ballast Books, 2021.

Gallagher, Eddie, and Andrea Gallagher. *The Man in the Arena: From Fighting ISIS to Fighting for My Freedom.* Washington: Ballast Books, 2021.

Germano, Kate, and Kelly Kennedy. *Fight Like a Girl: The Truth behind How Female Marines Are Trained.* Amherst: Prometheus Books, 2018.

Gibson, Chris. *Rally Point: Five Tasks to Unite the Country and Revitalize the American Dream.* New York: Hachette, 2017.

Glantz, Aaron. *The War Comes Home: Washington's Battle against America's Veterans.* Berkeley: University of California Press, 2009.

Gordon, Suzanne. *The Battle for Veterans' Healthcare: Dispatches from the Frontlines of Policy Making and Patient Care.* Ithaca, NY: Cornell University Press, 2017.

Gordon, Suzanne. *Wounds of War: How the VA Delivers Health, Healing, and Hope to the Nation's Veterans.* Ithaca, NY: Cornell University Press, 2018.

Graham, Kate Childs, ed. *Why I Run: 35 Progressive Candidates Who Are Changing Politics.* New York: Abrams Image, 2019.

Grossman, Dave. *On Killing: The Psychological Cost of Learning to Kill in War and Society.* New York: Little, Brown, 1995.

Guelzo, Allen C. *Abraham Lincoln: Redeemer President.* Grand Rapids: Wm. B. Eerdmans, 1999.

Harding, Scott, and Seth Kershner. *Counter-recruitment and the Campaign to Demilitarize Public Schools.* New York: Palgrave Macmillan, 2015.

Hatch, James, and Christian D'Andrea. *Touching the Dragon: And Other Techniques for Surviving Life's Wars.* New York: Knopf, 2018.

Hendricks Thomas, Kate, and Kyleanne Hunter, eds. *Invisible Veterans: What Happens When Military Women Become Civilians Again.* Santa Barbara: Praeger, 2019.

Hickman, Joseph. *The Burn Pits: The Poisoning of America's Soldiers.* New York: Skyhorse, 2016.

Holmstedt, Kirsten. *Band of Sisters: American Women at War in Iraq.* Mechanicsburg, PA: Stackpole Books, 2007.

Jamail, Dahr. *The Will to Resist: Soldiers Who Refuse to Fight in Iraq and Afghanistan.* Chicago: Haymarket Books, 2009.

Jones, Ann. *They Were Soldiers: How the Wounded Return from America's Wars—the Untold Story.* Chicago: Haymarket Books, 2013.

Jones, Richard Seelye. *A History of the American Legion.* Indianapolis: Bobbs-Merrill, 1946.

Junger, Sebastian. *Tribe: On Homecoming and Belonging.* New York: Hachette, 2016.

Kander, Jason. *Outside the Wire: Ten Lessons I've Learned in Everyday Courage.* New York: Hachette, 2018.

Kennard, Matt. *Irregular Army: How the U.S. Military Recruited Neo-Nazis, Gang Members, and Criminals to Fight the War on Terror.* New York: Verso, 2015.

Kennedy, Kelly. *They Fought for Each Other: The Triumph and Tragedy of the Hardest Hit Unit in Iraq.* New York: MacMillan, 2011.

Kerry, John. *Every Day Is Extra.* New York: Simon & Schuster, 2018.

Ketwig, John. *Vietnam Reconsidered: The War, the Times, and Why They Matter*. Chicago: Independent Publishers Group, 2018.

Kieran, David. *Signature Wounds: The Untold Story of the Military's Mental Health Crisis*. New York: New York University Press, 2019.

Klay, Phil. *Redeployment*. New York: Penguin Press, 2014.

Klein, Robert. *Wounded Men, Broken Promises: How the Veterans Administration Betrays Yesterday's Heroes*. New York: Macmillan, 1981.

Kovic, Ron. *Born on the Fourth of July*. 1976. Reprint, New York: Akashic Books, 2016.

Lembcke, Jerry. PTSD: *Diagnosis and Identity in Post-empire America*. Lanham, MD: Lexington Books, 2013.

Lembcke, Jerry. *The Spitting Image: Myth, Memory, and the Legacy of Vietnam*. New York: New York University Press, 1998.

Leopold, Les. *The Man Who Hated Work and Loved Labor: The Life and Times of Tony Mazzocchi*. White River Junction, VT: Chelsea Green, 2007.

Levinson, Nan. *War Is Not a Game: The New Antiwar Soldiers and the Movement They Built*. New Brunswick, NJ: Rutgers University Press, 2016.

Lewis, Michael. *The Fifth Risk*. New York: W. W. Norton, 2018.

Lewis, Michael. *The Premonition*. New York: W. W. Norton, 2021.

Lombardi, Chris. *I Ain't Marching Anymore: Dissenters, Deserters, and Objectors to America's Wars*. New York: New Press, 2020.

Lutz, Catherine, and Andrea Mazzarino, eds. *War and Health: The Medical Consequences of the Wars in Iraq and Afghanistan*. New York: New York University Press, 2019.

MacGillis, Alec. *Fulfillment: Winning and Losing in One-Click America*. New York: Farrar, Straus and Giroux, 2021.

MacLeish, Kenneth T. *Making War at Fort Hood: Life and Uncertainty in a Military Community*. Princeton, NJ: Princeton University Press, 2013.

Maurer, James. *It Can Be Done: The Autobiography of James Hudson Maurer*. New York: Rand School Press, 1938.

Meagher, Robert Emmet, and Douglas A. Pryer, eds. *War and Moral Injury: A Reader*. Eugene, OR: Cascade Books, 2018.

Messner, Michael. *Guys like Me: Five Wars, Five Veterans for Peace*. New Brunswick, NJ: Rutgers University Press, 2019.

Messner, Michael. *Unconventional Combat: Intersectional Action in the Veterans' Peace Movement*. New York: Oxford University Press, 2021.

Mettler, Suzanne. *Soldiers to Citizens: The G.I. Bill and the Making of the Greatest Generation*. Oxford: Oxford University Press, 2005.

Michaels, Jon D. *Constitutional Coup: Privatization's Threat to the American Republic*. Cambridge, MA: Harvard University Press, 2017.

Miller, Thomas, ed. *The Praeger Handbook of Veterans' Health: History, Challenges, Issues, and Developments*. Santa Barbara: Praeger, 2012.

Mittelstadt, Jennifer. *The Rise of the Military Welfare State*. Cambridge, MA: Harvard University Press, 2015.

Moore, Ellen. *Grateful Nation: Student Veterans and the Rise of the Military-Friendly Campus*. Durham, NC: Duke University Press, 2019.

Nicosia, Gerald. *Home to War: A History of the Vietnam Veterans' Movement.* New York: Carroll & Graf, 2001.

Philipps, David. *Alpha.* New York: Crown Publishing, 2021.

Plate, Andrea. *Madness: In the Trenches of America's Troubled Department of Veterans Affairs.* Tarrytown, NY: Marshall Cavendish, 2019.

Roach, Mary. *Grunt: The Curious Science of Humans at War.* New York: W. W. Norton, 2016.

Roberts, Lawrence. *Mayday 1971: A White House at War, a Revolt in the Streets, and the Untold History of America's Biggest Mass Arrest.* New York: Houghton Mifflin Harcourt, 2020.

Roncoroni, Jason, and Shauna Springer. *Beyond the Military: A Leader's Handbook for Warrior Reintegration.* San Bernadino: Lioncrest, 2019.

Roth-Douquet, Kathy, and Frank Schaeffer. *AWOL: The Unexcused Absence of America's Upper Classes from Military Service—and How It Hurts Our Country.* New York: HarperCollins, 2006.

Rumer, Thomas. *The American Legion: An Official History, 1919–1989.* New York: M. Evans and Company, 1990.

Schake, Kori, and Jim Mattis, eds. *Warriors and Citizens: American Views of Our Military.* Stanford, CA: Hoover Institution Press, 2016.

Severo, Richard, and Lewis Milford. *The Wages of War: When America's Soldiers Came Home—from Valley Forge to Vietnam.* New York: Simon & Schuster, 1989.

Shay, Jonathan. *Odysseus in America: Combat Trauma and the Trials of Homecoming.* New York: Scribner's, 2002.

Sherman, Nancy. *Afterwar: Healing the Moral Wounds of Our Soldiers.* New York: Oxford University Press, 2015.

Shulkin, David J. *It Shouldn't Be This Hard to Serve Your Country: Our Broken Government and the Plight of Veterans.* New York: Public Affairs, 2019.

Shulkin, David J., Shereef Elnahal, Ellen Maddock, and Megan Shaheen, eds. *Best Care Everywhere.* Washington, DC: US Department of Veterans Affairs, 2017.

Sjursen, Daniel. *Ghost Riders of Baghdad: Soldiers, Civilians, and the Myth of the Surge.* Lebanon, NH: University Press of New England, 2015.

Sjursen, Daniel A. *Patriotic Dissent: America in the Age of Endless War.* Berkeley, CA: Heyday, 2020.

Sjursen, Daniel. *A True History of the United States: Indigenous Genocide, Racialized Slavery, Hyper-capitalism, Militarist Imperialism, and Other Overlooked Aspects of American Exceptionalism.* Lebanon, NH: Steerforth, 2021.

Starr, Paul. *The Discarded Army: Veterans after Vietnam.* New York: Charter House, 1973.

Vine, David. *Base Nation: How U.S. Military Bases Abroad Harm America and the World.* New York: Skyhorse, 2017.

Waller, Willard Walter. *The Veteran Comes Back.* San Francisco: Dryden Press, 1944.

White, Greg Cope. *The Pink Marine: One Boy's Journey through Bootcamp to Manhood.* Los Angeles: About Face Books, 2016.

Williams, Kayla. *Love My Rifle More Than You: Young and Female in the U.S. Army.* New York: W. W. Norton, 2005.

Williams, Kayla. *Plenty of Time When We Get Home.* New York: W. W. Norton, 2014.

Wilson, S. Brian. *Don't Thank Me for My Service: My Viet Nam Awakening to the Long History of US Lies.* Atlanta: Clarity, 2018.

Wright, Ann, and Susan Dixon. *Dissent: Voices of Conscience.* Asheville, NC: Koa Books, 2008.

INDEX

Consumer Financial Protection Bureau (CFPB), 91, 92
Consumer Watchdog (organization), 104
Cook, Samuel R., 35–37
Cooper, Bradley, 87
Cooper, Chris, 193
Cooper, Shawn, 90
Cope White, Greg, 29
Cornyn, John, 197, 218–19
coronavirus pandemic, 82–84; CARES Act on, 102–3; during election of 2020, 205–7; essential workers during, 235–36; jobs eliminated during, 240; mental healthcare during, 226; military spending during, 188; Postal Service during, 213–15; VA during, 167–70; VA employees during, 171; VHA during, 19
Cortright, David, 3
Cosgrove, Toby, 129
Costs of War Project (organization), 51–52, 206, 231–32, 248
Cotting, Dave I., 30
Cotton, Tom, 146, 208, 215, 220, 298n33
Court, Jamie, 104
COVID-19 pandemic. See coronavirus pandemic
Cox, J. David, 170
Cox, Paul, 47, 171
Crenshaw, Dan, 220, 246
Crow, Jason: on Afghanistan troop levels, 188, 219, 245–46; during January 6 insurrection, 250; on military spending, 189
Crozier, Brett, 205
Cruise, Tom, 18
Cunningham, Cal, 197, 219

Dallas (Texas), 67
David, Christopher, 209–10
Davis, Ronald, 68
Dayen, David, 103
deaths: caused by hazing, 32; noncombat, 50
DeBarros, Brittany Ramos, 148–51, 220, 243
debts: COVID stimulus funds and, 103; of service members, 34–36; student loan debt, 89, 237
DeFazio, Peter, 188, 195, 206, 214, 219–20
Defense, Department of (DOD): budget of, 17, 187–90, 205–6; direct commission officer

program of, 190–91; equipment sold to local police by, 246; extremism task force in, 244–45; names of Confederates used for bases by, 211–12
defense industry: as employer of veterans, 63–64; political contributions by, 190
Defense Logistics Agency, 246
DeJoy, Louis, 214, 242
Del Gaudio, Andrew, 42
Democratic Party: presidential primary race of 2020 in, 191, 201; veterans as candidates for, 180–82; veterans as congressmembers in, 177–78
Dennehy, Brian, 88
Derwinski, Edward J., 234
DeVos, Betsy, 89–92
Direct Contracting Entities, 227
Disabled American Veterans (DAV), 112; on VA care, 163; Vietnam-era veterans in, 120; on Vietnam Veterans Act, 119
discharges: categories of, 21; review procedures for, 174
Disney Corp., 137
divorce, 46
D'Olier, Franklin, 114
Donald J. Trump Foundation, 97
Dong, Roger, 109
draft (conscription), 4; replaced by all-volunteer military, 6
Duckworth, Tammy, 176; born in Thailand, 212–13; in election of 2006, 181; during January 6 insurrection, 250; on MISSION Act, 165; in Senate, 223; on Trump, 206–8; on war in Syria, 189
Duke Energy (firm), 147
Durbin, Dick, 181
DynCorp, 69

Eastwood, Clint, 195
Eaton, Paul, 211
Edstrom, Erik, 10, 30, 31, 85
Edwards, Chet, 123
Eisch, Brian, 44
Eisenhower, Dwight D., 115
Eisenhower Media Network (EMN), 247–48
Eitel, Robert, 91
election of 2016, 11–12, 199

Trump administration, 92, 274n25; Asset and Infrastructure Review under, 229–30; compensation and pension (c&p) exams under, 175; Iraq and Afghanistan Wars during, 207–8; MISSION Act under, 164–67; nontraditional treatments funded by, 99; private-sector mental health contractors and, 93–96; suicide initiative of, 99; VA under, 143, 157–62; voter supersession by, 213–15

Trump University, 90

Truusa, Tiia-Triin, 32

Trynosky, Stephen, 132

Underwood, Lauren, 173

unemployment: among Vietnam-era veterans, 118; during COVID-19 pandemic, 83

unions: at Amazon, 102; during Biden administration, 239–40; meetings at veterans' service organizations' halls, 278n8; of VA staff, 170–72; Veterans Organizing Institute and, 138–39, 249; VoteVets supported by, 147

United Confederate Veterans, 112

Urban, David, 63

USAA (firm), 103

US Chamber of Commerce, 105

US Chamber of Commerce Foundation, 99

VA Accountability and Whistleblower Protection Act (2017), 159–60

VA Choice Act (2014), 128–30

VA Commission on Care, 129–30

Van Dam, Andrew, 266n11, 278n9

Verardo, Mike, 97

Verardo, Sarah, 97–99

veterans: definition of, 21; elected to House and Senate in 2020, 220; suicides among, 51; women as, 3–4, 46–47

Veterans Affairs, US Department of (VA): American Legion and, 111; Asset and Infrastructure Review Commission in, 229–30; during Biden administration, 223–28, 239–40; budget and functions of, 18–19; during coronavirus pandemic, 167–70; discharge review procedures of, 174; expanding services of, 232–34; Faster Care for Veterans Act on, 185; Hannon Act

on, 172–74; healthcare coverage from, 4–5; after January 6 insurrection, 250; medical marijuana prescribed by, 122; MISSION Act on, 164–67; motto of, 222; outsourcing of services of, 130–31, 230–32; post-9/11 veterans' service organizations' criticisms of, 154; price of prescription drugs negotiated by, 106; private-sector mental health contractors for, 93–96; regulatory powers of, 92; Rieckhoff on, 142, 143; scandal in, 126–28; services to women by, 143–44; as target of veterans' anger, 80–81; during Trump administration, 12, 157–62; Trump on, 217; unions for staff of, 170–72; VA Choice Act on, 128–29; VA Commission on Care on, 129–30; vendors to, 132–33; veterans' service organizations on care given by, 162–63; Vietnam-era veterans and, 119–20; voucherization of, 123. *See also* Veterans Health Administration

Veterans and Military Families Council, 181

Veterans Benefits Administration (VBA), 18, 124–25, 224

Veterans' Cannabis Coalition (VCC), 122

Veterans Choice Program, 128, 143

Veterans Community Care and Access Act (2017), 131

Veterans Community Care Program, 230

Veterans Community Project, 184

Veterans Evaluation Services (VES; firm), 175

Veterans 4 America First Institute (organization), 228

Veterans for Peace (VFP), 74, 118, 141; DeBarros on, 150; on Raytheon, 248; VA employees supported by, 171–72

Veterans for Responsible Leadership (VFRL), 13–14

Veterans for Trump (organization), 215–16

Veterans Health Administration (VHA): during Biden administration, 224; congressional criticisms of, 17; coordinated care model of, 231; during coronavirus pandemic, 167; expanding services of, 232–34; during government shutdown, 58; MISSION Act on, 164–67, 228; outsourcing by, 160–61; privatization of, 156–57; research sponsored by, 19; skills of staff of, 16; spending on compensation and pensions by, 22; veterans eligible for care by, 19–20, 256n49; veterans employed by, 64. *See also* fourth mission of VHA

Veterans of Foreign Wars (VFW): on Bonus Marchers, 115; during Cold War, 116; creation and history of, 112, 113; decline in membership of, 121; on expanding VA care, 234; PAC created by, 120; on private-sector treatments for PTSD, 94; on VA care, 162; on Vietnam Veterans Act, 119; during Vietnam War, 117

Veterans Organizing Institute (VOI), 138–39, 249

veterans' service organizations (VSOS), 24; Biden and, 223; Big Six, 112–14; Cold War veterans in, 116–18; Concerned Veterans for America, 123–25; decline in memberships of, 120–22; on expanding VA care, 234, 235; federal charters for, 278n9; on Hannon Act, 174; Iraq and Afghanistan Veterans of America, 139–45; legislative lobbying by, 104–7; post-9/11, 136–37; Student Veterans of America, 134–36; on VA care, 162–63; on Vietnam Veterans Act, 119; VoteVets, 146–48; on withdrawal from Afghanistan, 245; women in, 151–54

Vets for Black Lives (organization), 248

Vets for the People (organization), 151, 154

Vets Forward (organization), 217

Vet Voice Foundation (VVF), 146

Vietnam-era veterans, 118–20; American Legion and, 110–11; care for, 18; feelings of, 74–75; other-than-honorable discharges for, 53; stereotypes of, 59

Vietnam Veterans Act (proposed), 119

Vietnam Veterans Against the War (VVAW), 3; creation and history of, 116–18

Vietnam Veterans of America (VVA), 112, 113, 119–20; creation of, 116

Vietnam War: draft during, 5–6; movement against, 3, 116–17

Villanueva, Jeremy, 135

Vine, David, 60

violence: "intimate partner violence," 78–80; mass shooters, 78–80; by police, 67; sexual assaults, 48–50

VoteVets (organization), 146–48; Buttigieg supported by, 202; DeBarros on, 150–51; in

election of 2018, 178; in election of 2020, 216–17; get-out-the-vote campaign of, 212; on saving Postal Service, 214; on use of military against demonstrators, 208

VoteVets Action Fund, 146–48

VoteVets Political Action (organization), 146

Walmart (firm), 99–100

Walsh, Joe, 181

Ward-Smith, Linda, 169

Warren, Elizabeth, 139

water pollution, 38–39

Webb, Cameron, 195

Weidman, Rick, 27, 29; Agent Orange exposure of, 37–38; on Steven Cohen, 95; on Faster Care for Veterans Act, 185

Weinstein, Adam, 103

Wellman, Fred, 216, 218

Wells Fargo (firm), 137

West, Royce, 197

West Point, US Military Academy at, 31; careers of graduates of, 61; Trump's commencement address at, 212

Wheeler, Dan, 131

White, Dennis, 7, 193

white supremacist groups, 82

Whitmer, Gretchen, 236

Wilkie, Robert: AFGE and, 170; during coronavirus pandemic, 167, 170; Inspector General's report on, 222–23; MISSION Act administered under, 164–67; nontraditional treatments funded by, 99; on Sanders, 202; on Trump, 200; as VA secretary, 12, 58–59, 98, 160, 200; veterans' service organizations and, 303n3

Wilkins, Roy, 115

Willenz, June, 116

Williams, Brian, 141

Williams, Kayla: as Army linguist, 10, 51; on Big Six veterans' service organizations, 136; as Center for Women Veterans director, 143; on expanding population eligible for benefits, 235; expanding VA services proposed by, 232; on new veterans' service organizations, 137; on VA services for women, 144

Wilson, Brian, 117

With Honor Fund (Super PAC), 100, 177, 221